# Research Involving Participants with Cognitive Disability and Differences

# Research Involving Participants with Cognitive Disability and Differences

## *Ethics, Autonomy, Inclusion, and Innovation*

*Edited by*

M. ARIEL CASCIO AND ERIC RACINE

OXFORD
UNIVERSITY PRESS

**OXFORD**
UNIVERSITY PRESS

Great Clarendon Street, Oxford, OX2 6DP,
United Kingdom

Oxford University Press is a department of the University of Oxford. It furthers the University's objective of excellence in research, scholarship, and education by publishing worldwide. Oxford is a registered trade mark of Oxford University Press in the UK and in certain other countries



First Edition published in 2019

Impression: 1



Published in the United States of America by Oxford University Press
198 Madison Avenue, New York, NY 10016, United States of America

British Library Cataloguing in Publication Data

Data available

Library of Congress Control Number: 2019938557

ISBN 978–0–19–882434–3

Printed and bound by
CPI Group (UK) Ltd, Croydon, CR0 4YY

# Preface

This volume emerged from our interest in research involving participants who might be considered (especially by research ethics committees or institutional review boards) to be vulnerable by virtue of some sort of "cognitive impairment," a notion in need of deconstruction. In our experience, both the notion of vulnerability and the notion of cognitive impairment have often been left poorly defined (Racine and Bracken-Roche, 2019), even if they guide many practices. Our own research experience has included a number of studies involving vulnerabilities linked to cognitive impairment in research involving participants with autism, cerebral palsy, and mental health conditions. While we are concerned with protecting participants in situations of vulnerability (to undue influence, to coercion, to unnecessary discomfort), we, like others, are also worried that potential participants might be vulnerable to unjusitied exclusion. We knew that several researchers around the globe have been and are still successfully including people with cognitive impairments, cognitive disability, or cognitive difference in research, and that many people concerned (including researchers, potential participants, and broader communities) are passionate about research inclusion. We hope that this volume helps fill gaps caused by the limited insight in research ethics and methods guidebooks that address ethics, autonomy, and inclusion for these participants.

We would like to acknowledge many people who made this work possible. Thank you to Charlotte Holloway at Oxford University Press, for managing the publication side of this process, answering questions, and keeping us on task. Thank you also to current and former members of the Pragmatic Health Ethics Research Unit at the Institut de recherches cliniques de Montréal, who provided feedback on this volume from its earliest stages. We especially thank Wren Boehlen, Gabrielle Doré, Sara Ferwati, Justine Fortin, Corinne Lajoie, Jelena Poleksic, and Stephanie Simpson for their assistance with the editorial process at various stages.

Finally we would like to thank the writers for the excellent chapters and commentaries they have contributed and for their continued engagement in this work and this topic.

## Reference

Racine, E. and Bracken-Roche, D. (2019). "Enriching the Concept of Vulnerability in Research Ethics: An Integrative and Functional Account." *Bioethics* 33/1: 19–34.

# Contents

# Contributors

**John Aspler**, Pragmatic Health Ethics Research Unit, Institut de recherches cliniques de Montréal, Canada, and Integrated Program in Neuroscience, McGill University, Canada

**Deborah R. Barnbaum**, Department of Philosophy, Kent State University, USA

**Pamela Block**, Department of Anthropology, University of Western Ontario, Canada

**Allison Bloom**, Department of Sociology and Anthropology, Moravian College, USA

**Leonardo Carbonieri Campoy**, Department of Social Sciences, Pontifícia Universidade Católica—Paraná, Brazil

**Franco A. Carnevale**, Ingram School of Nursing, McGill University, Canada

**M. Ariel Cascio**, Pragmatic Heath Ethics Research Unit, Institut de recherches cliniques de Montréal, Neurology & Neurosurgery, McGill University, Canada, and College of Medicine, Central Michigan University, USA

**Hajer Chalghoumi**, School of Psychology, University of Ottawa, Canada

**Virginie Cobigo**, School of Psychology, University of Ottawa, Canada, CHEO Research Institute, Canada, and Centre for Research on Educational and Community Services, University of Ottawa, Canada

**Caitlin Courchesne**, Faculty of Medicine, The University of British Columbia, Canada

**Vanessa Cox**, School of Health and Rehabilitation Sciences, Western University, Canada

**Pamela Cushing**, Disability Studies, Kings University College, Western University, Canada

**Laura B. Dunn**, Department of Psychiatry and Behavioral Sciences, Stanford University, USA

**Donald Fogelberg**, School of Medicine, University of Washington, USA

**Paul J. Ford**, NeuroEthics Program, Cleveland Clinic, USA

**Casey Fulford**, School of Psychology, University of Ottawa, Canada

**Mariam Hanna**, School of Psychology, Carleton University, Canada

**Paul E. Holtzheimer**, National Center for PTSD, Executive Division, White River Junction VA Medical Center, USA

**Britteny M. Howell**, Division of Population Health Sciences and National Resource Center for Alaska Native Elders, University of Alaska Anchorage, USA

**Judy Illes**, Canada Research Chair in Neuroethics, The University of British Columbia, Canada

**Eva Kahana**, Department of Sociology, Case Western Reserve University, USA

**Elizabeth Anne Kinsella**, School of Occupational Therapy, Western University, Canada

**Eran Klein**, Department of Neurology, Oregon Health and Science University, USA and Department of Philosophy, University of Washington, USA

**Anne Kohler**, Department of Sociology and Anthropology, Colgate University, USA

**Benjamin Majewski**, Independent Scholar, USA

**Saira A. Mehmood**, Department of Sociology and Anthropology, Spelman College, USA

**Marjorie Montreuil**, Pragmatic Health Ethics Research Unit, Institut de recherches cliniques de Montréal (IRCM), Canada, and Ingram School of Nursing, McGill University, Canada

**Treena Orchard**, School of Health Studies, Western University, Canada

**Melissa Park**, School of Physical and Occupational Therapy, Faculty of Medicine, McGill University, Canada

**Stephanie Patterson**, School of Health Technology and Management, Stony Brook University, USA

**Natasha Plourde**, School of Psychology, University of Ottawa, Canada

**Lynne A. Potvin**, School of Psychology, University of Ottawa, Canada

**Eric Racine**, Pragmatic Health Ethics Research Unit, Institut de recherches cliniques de Montréal, Department of Medicine and Department of Social and Preventive Medicine, Université de Montréal and Departments of Neurology and Neurosurgery andMedicine, and Biomedical Ethics Unit, McGill University, Canada

**Kenneth A. Richman**, Center for Health Humanities, School of Arts and Sciences, MCPHS University, USA

**Mackenzie Salt**, Department of Linguistics and Languages and McMaster Autism Research Team, McMaster University, Canada

**Lauren R. Sankary**, NeuroEthics Program, Cleveland Clinic, USA

**Christine Schneider**, Department of Sociology, Case Western Reserve University, USA

**Karrie A. Shogren**, Department of Special Education and Kansas University Center on Developmental Disabilities, University of Kansas, USA

**Whitney D. Taylor**, School of Psychology, University of Ottawa, Canada

**Gail Teachman**, School of Occupational Therapy, Faculty of Health Sciences, Western University, Canada

**Jack Trammell**, Chair of Sociology, Criminal Justice, and Human Services Department, Mount Saint Mary's University, USA

**Megan S. Wright**, Penn State Law and Departments of Humanities and Public Health Sciences, Penn State College of Medicine, USA

# Introduction

Traditionally, research ethics aims to protect research participants from undue risk and ensure that they are informed about the implications of their research participation. The pursuit of these all-important goals is complicated for participants who think, learn, or interact differently as a result of cognitive differences, impairments, or disabilities. Indeed, the history of research ethics illustrates how participants with various cognitive impairments (e.g., mild cognitive impairment) or cognitive styles/differences (e.g., autism), or a combination of both, have been taken advantage of and abused, exposed to unjustified risks, and misinformed. This is perhaps most notable in the 1950s–1960s hepatitis study conducted at the Willowbrook State School for people with intellectual and developmental disabilities in Staten Island, NY, USA. Resident children were deliberately infected with hepatitis as part of research into immunity (Carlson, 2013; Rothman, 1991; see also Chapter 4). There are also everyday concerns about unethical conduct in research revealed in these chapters, such as adults with autism reporting being coerced into research as children (Chapter 7) and the implication that researchers might specifically study children too young to assent simply in order to rely only on proxy consent, rather than getting consent or assent from participants directly (Chapter 4). Accordingly, the goals of protection and information embedded in research ethics are quintessential for participants who have cognitive impairments or are cognitively different. This has often been expressed through the idea that these research participants are vulnerable, an idea we come back to later. That being said, the protective stance taken by traditional research ethics has been a source of potential overprotection and exclusion (Fisher, 2003; Martino and Schormans, 2018). Accordingly, research ethics can sometimes become disabling to participants because it is premised on strong equations between cognitive impairment/difference with a need for stringent protection and blanket assumptions about lack of decision-making capacity, which perpetuate exclusionary attitudes and practices. The chapters in this volume address the titular themes of ethics, autonomy, inclusion, and innovation with respect to research involving participants considered to have "impaired cognition" (as an experience, of long or short duration) or "cognitive impairments" (as part of a diagnosis), thus putting into question common ways that research ethics deals with participation affected by cognitive impairment, or with cognitively different participants. Some chapters provide overarching views on the topic, situated within legal and academic approaches to ethics; some report challenges faced by researchers, while others report success stories of inclusion and engagement.

We have deliberately chosen to include in the title of this volume both the terms cognitive disability and cognitive difference, to stress the plurality of experiences and perspectives to capture groups of participants often clustered together but who have wide-ranging conditions, support needs, and abilities. By these terms we mean people who may be considered vulnerable (by researchers, research ethics committees, or other gatekeepers) by virtue of something to do with the mind, brain, or nervous system. This collection of "cognitive disability and cognitive difference" encompasses a range of people who face common research ethics issues, but sometimes radically different personal and social experiences. We therefore spend some time in this introduction unpacking these experiences and the language of impairment, disability, and difference.

Our initial working title for this volume focused on "impaired cognition," with the idea that it is the cognition that is impaired and not the person, and being intentionally open to both temporary and permanent different ways of being in the world and situations that might change a person's habitual way of thinking, learning, or interacting (or making decisions). The language of impairment motivated this volume, as it mirrors the language often used by research ethics committees in identifying vulnerable populations. However, a focus on impairments also has downsides as identified by the disability rights movement. Many (though not all) disability rights activists and scholars make a distinction between impairment and disability in which impairment is an individual limitation of function (physical, mental, or otherwise), whereas disability is the social condition of lost or limited opportunities due to physical, social, or other barriers (Oliver, 2017). A focus on impairment is generally associated with the biomedical model of disability, which locates the cause of any limitations within the individual. A focus on disability is generally associated with the social model, which locates this cause in social context. Not all impairments imply disability. An impairment can be more or less disabling based on how a society accommodates diversity. In this volume, we assert that research ethics can be enabling or disabling toward people with cognitive impairments. We therefore shift the focus in our title from impairment to disability.

However, the term cognitive disability also provides some limitations. The concept of disability is not simply a social framing of the biomedicalized notion of impairment. People can also identify as disabled or as people with disabilities. The term "cognitive disability" has been used in the ethics literature to include "conditions like autism, dementia, Alzheimer's," as well as intellectual disability (Kittay and Carlson, 2010). However, this volume also includes situations that people might not label as disability. We do include a number of chapters on autism (as do Kittay and Carlson, 2010), which many autistic people assert is a difference and not a disability although there are also many autistic people who do identify with the disability rights movement. We also address the notion of cognition, capacity, or cognitive differences in situations of mental illness, as people living under the label of mental illness also face assumptions about cognition and decision-making (Bracken-Roche et al., 2016). Kittay and Carlson do not include mental illness in their volume on ethics and cognitive disability, but the anthropological treatment of cognitive impairment and "the ethics of possibility" (Ginsburg and Rapp, 2018) does draw from the anthropology of mental illness (McKearney and Zoanni, 2018) and recognizes work on, for example, schizophrenia, as within the same lineage as work on intellectual disability (Ginsburg and Rapp, 2018). While our intention is not to claim that intellectual disability, mental illness, autism, dementia, and so on can be equated to each other, our intention is to highlight the similar experiences of marginalization, exclusion, and erasure people living with these experiences and labels face—especially in research—as a result of experiences or assumptions about cognition. For this reason, we have included in our title also "cognitive difference," to encompass cognitive experiences not considered disabilities. The chapters in this volume address a range of experiences assembled under the label or presumption of cognitive impairment.

Just as "cognitive disability" cannot be a catch-all, neither can "cognitive difference," which risks being euphemistic by erasing impairment. Our volume does include chapters about participants with disabilities related to many different kinds of impairments, including dysfunctions or conditions that are acquired during development, subsequent to injury, or during aging. Memory impairments caused by dementia provide just one example of how a cognitive change can be experienced as a disabling impairment leading to frustration and challenges, not just as a difference. Many people would not describe their experience primarily as a difference in being and thinking. We therefore choose to use plural terminology to reflect the range of experiences faced by individuals who may have similar cognitive conditions but whose experiences may be radically different. A person with mild cognitive impairment may actually experience deep suffering due to a fragile ability to remember and learn. It would be an inappropriate euphemism to describe this person's condition as cognitive difference and risk erasing the harm people experience because of such conditions. This is in line with disability rights concerns, advocating that scholars not deny impairment generally (Oliver, 2017; Shakespeare, 1999), and not rely on euphemism specifically (Brown, 2013; crippledscholar, 2017).

However, describing someone who has different cognitive processing abilities for visual-spatial information because of their cerebral palsy (CP) acquired at birth as cognitively impaired or disabled may be profoundly disrespectful and further stigma and stereotypes against people who are cognitively different. These differences may be disabling in some contexts, if people are not supported or if there are no accommodations made, but people with CP may be rightly offended by being labeled as cognitively impaired (see, e.g., Larivière-Bastien et al., 2011). Similarly, while some autistic people identify as disabled and see neurodiversity as a disability rights movement, others may take umbrage at being labeled with cognitive disability, experiencing autism as diversity but not disability (see, e.g., Ripamonti, 2016). People living with mental illness may draw from many different models, ranging from a neurodiversity approach seeing mental illness as a different way of thinking to a social constructivist model to an illness model separating the experience of mental illness from the person entirely (Estroff, 1993; Graby, 2015).

Accordingly, we recognize that impairment and difference are on a spectrum, and may overlap and interact, notably over time. It may be that the same condition is experienced radically differently (as an impairment or as a difference) by different people or by the same person in different situations. Both terms are needed to describe what people experience and the realities that they live and want to project. We understand that for some scholars all cognitive impairments should be equated with cognitive difference, although we do not wish to impose this view on those individuals who experience cognitive impairment as a challenging and frustrating condition. However, we clearly disagree that all cognitive differences should be boiled down to cognitive impairment.

The contributors in this volume address a range of experiences: intellectual and development disability broadly (Chapters 3, 4, 6, 10, and 11); autism (Chapters 5, 7, and 8), fetal alcohol spectrum disorder (Chapter 15), Down syndrome (Chapter 17), and neurological conditions of childhood specifically (Chapter 12); psychiatric diagnosis/mental illness (Chapters 1, 12–14); and neurodegenerative diseases associated with aging (Chapters 1 and 9). Wright also raises the question of disorders of consciousness and addiction (Chapter 2). These chapters also showcase a range of fields and disciplines (anthropology, sociology, neuroethics, child studies, health and rehabilitation sciences, philosophy, and law).

Research participants with cognitive disability and difference may be considered a vulnerable population, but, at the same time, should also be empowered to participate in research. However, cognitive disability and difference may pose challenges to ethical research, particularly with respect to the research ethics principle of autonomy. National guidelines such as the US Belmont Report and international guidelines such as the Declaration of Helsinki link the principle of autonomy to key obligations, perhaps most notably informed consent, although there are several others. Exercising autonomy in the research process may be difficult for people with cognitive disability and difference for a variety of reasons, often linked to notions of decision-making capacity but including also communication styles, and experiences of exploitation in broader social contexts beyond the research setting. However, several alternative or modified strategies, for example when obtaining informed consent, have been used by researchers. The chapters in this volume explore these strategies, drawing on both empirical and normative research to offer suggestions for research design, research ethics, and best practices that empower people with cognitive disability and difference to participate in clinical and social/behavioral research while respecting and managing potential vulnerabilities to coercion or undue influence. For research participants with cognitive disability and difference, participating in relevant research follows the Disability Rights Movement's call "Nothing About Us Without Us" (Brown, 2012; Charlton, 2000) and is a vital component of the bioethical principle of justice. Accordingly, this book provides a guide for researchers working with populations experiencing impaired cognition, with a particular focus on informed consent and decision-making in the context of clinical and non-clinical research.

This volume is organized into four sections: (1) Conceptual Frameworks; (2) Challenges; (3) Successes; and (4) Commentaries. The remainder of this introduction provides a section-by-section overview and presents some general comments to readers.

## Section 1: Conceptual Frameworks

This section sets the stage for future sections by exploring the conceptual, ethical, and normative foundations for a discussion of autonomy and research ethics pertinent to people with cognitive disability and difference.

Lauren Sankary and Paul Ford (Chapter 1) draw on their work in implanted neural device trials to provide an overview of various options for consent to research for participants who may not be able to give traditional informed consent. These options include double consent, proxy consent (with participant assent), advanced consent, and process consent. The chapter therefore provides a useful overview of options for consent useful for researchers working with diverse participants in any type of study.

Megan Wright (Chapter 2) analyzes legal and policy guidelines with respect to proxy consent, asking who is authorized to provide consent on behalf of a participant who is not legally able to provide their own consent. She also explores innovations in guardianship reform and supported decision making. Both Chapters 1 and 2 are situated within US law and policy, such as the Common Rule, but their ideas have broad applicability.

Continuing the theme of proxy consent, Howell and Shogren (Chapter 3) provide an overview of empirical research on research ethics for participants and potential participants with intellectual disability, focusing particularly on differing perspectives between people with intellectual disability, their parents and guardians, and research ethics committee members. They argue for strategies to increase self-determination and facilitate meaningful inclusion in research, which is in line with the priorities of many people with intellectual disability.

Deborah Barnbaum's chapter (Chapter 4) delves more directly into the question of consent in the absence of a proxy. Focusing on individuals with mild or moderate cognitive impairment who may be able to consent to research participation but are not often given the chance, Barnbaum addresses directly the question of capacity and autonomy—what capacities are needed to make autonomous decisions about consent, and what conceptual errors might limit those capacities? Barnbaum argues that participants without cognitive disabilities are not, in fact, always autonomous, and participants with cognitive disabilities may not be so impaired when it comes to consent. Kenneth Richman (Chapter 5) similarly addresses directly the characteristics of participants whose capacities are sometimes doubted, specifically those diagnosed with autism. He surveys common characteristics of autism that may impact autonomy and consent to research and provides suggestions for a more autism-friendly research process. Both Chapters 4 and 5 focus on empowerment for individual research participants and are best positioned as being discussions of cognitive differences.

With this groundwork laid, the next two sections provide concrete examples of empirical research involving participants with various cognitive differences facing actual or presumed impairments in cognition.

## Section 2: Challenges

This section reflects on cases where researchers faced challenges achieving their goals of inclusion or the research stopped short of such initial goals.

Stephanie Patterson and Pamela Block (Chapter 6) focus on administrative barriers to research at the national level in the US. They describe efforts to change the language of the US Common Rule away from "mentally disabled persons" to "individuals with impaired decision-making ability." This chapter challenges the assumption that people with disabilities are inherently vulnerable or homogenous with respect to impairment and capacity to consent. It draws on the experiences of the researchers and their colleagues in attempting to conduct research involving participants or co-researchers labeled as cognitively disabled.

Mackenzie Salt (Chapter 7) writes about the ethical issues he encountered planning and executing a study involving participants who, like Salt, are adults on the autism spectrum. He focuses particularly on conversations with the multiple research ethics boards involved in approving this study, and their assumptions about consent capacity and autism.

Leonardo Campoy's study (Chapter 8) also addresses autism, though from a very different angle. An anthropologist, Campoy writes about the ethical tensions he experienced during fieldwork regarding his own role in conversations between children with autism, parents, and doctors. He posits that ethnographers can serve as anthropological therapists, translating between these different actors' worlds and perspectives. This chapter considers research ethics not only with respect to the role of the researcher, but also by explaining the complex relationship between research and care.

Christine Schneider and Eva Kahana (Chapter 9) write about challenges encountered recruiting participants from a US Veterans Affairs Medical Center for a study on the experience of forgetting. Schneider and Kahana's participants can be understood as "doubly vulnerable" by virtue of both veteran status and mild cognitive impairment. The authors identify several barriers at administrative, interpersonal, and personal levels and propose some solutions to increase recruitment.

Vanessa Cox and colleagues (Chapter 10) write about the engaging intersection of research with a vulnerable population and research on a sensitive topic in their qualitative study of the socio-sexual relationships of adults with mild intellectual disability. They focus largely on challenges with gatekeepers—parents, staff, and others who might be involved as intermediaries in the interactions between researchers and research participants. The researchers write about how they kept participants actively involved in negotiating their participation, and in how dependence on others impacts both research participation and participants' socio-sexual lives.

Finally, Jack Trammell (Chapter 11) writes about research on college programs for students with intellectual disability. While the number and visibility of such programs has increased, research has been limited, particularly in the extent to which studies include the perspectives of the students themselves. This chapter presents a case study of one such program, reviews research on these programs, and provides suggestions for better including the voices of students with intellectual and developmental disability in future studies.

## Section 3: Successes

This section responds to challenges raised in Section 2 by documenting success stories across a range of studies.

Marjorie Montreuil, Gail Teachman, and Franco Carnevale (Chapter 12) focus specifically on the experiences of children with cognitive disabilities and differences, specifically communication differences and mental health diagnoses. The authors detail examples of research projects that strive to center the perspectives of children, whose perspectives are often excluded from research—doubly so when they are doubly vulnerable by virtue of a neurodevelopmental or mental health condition and of being children or youth. The innovative works described in this chapter challenge that exclusion.

Eran Klein (Chapter 13) demonstrates the value of consulting with potential research participants to understand ethical issues, in an important form of empirical research on human research ethics. His social research study asks participants in the clinical research study about their perspectives on the consent process, identifying concerns and raising suggestions to improve practice.

Saira Mehmood (Chapter 14) describes ethnographic research with participants with chronic mental illness, who might experience variations in capacity to consent over the course of a study. Mehmood highlights the value of ethnographic research not just as a methodological tool, but as an ethical tool allowing the researcher to gain insight into capacity in a context where it might shift daily.

John Aspler (Chapter 15) details several strategies for successfully including people with fetal alcohol spectrum disorders (FASD) in focus groups as part of a study on FASD and media content. He also addresses the benefits and difficulties of engaging with stakeholders about research design, and the tensions between different innovations as solutions may raise new ethical questions themselves.

Virginie Cobigo and colleagues (Chapter 16) respond in a sense to chapters in Section 2 on the challenges of working with research ethics committees on protocols involving participants with intellectual and developmental disabilities. They share their conversations with research ethics committees across a range of projects, including examples of documents they have used.

Anne Kohler's chapter (Chapter 17) similarly engages with research ethics, most notably creating an accessible research ethics training module with her research assistant, who has Down syndrome. Kohler's chapter also uses the lens of feminist care ethics in detailing other methodological innovations for a qualitative study on the experiences of adolescents and adults with Down syndrome.

## Section 4: Commentaries

In this spirit of broadening the conversation and the tradition of journals such as *Current Anthropology* and the *American Journal of Bioethics*, and of related volumes such as Fein and Rios's (2018) *Autism in Translation*, we have chosen to include in this volume commentaries, which reflect upon the major themes presented in this volume, providing new perspectives for readers. Some commentaries address only one chapter and others address multiple. While they are best read in context with these other chapters, they may also stand alone to offer new perspectives.

Commentaries by chapter contributors themselves (Deborah Barnbaum, Megan Wright, Leonardo Campoy, and Jack Trammell) draw connections between chapters. Anne Kohler and Benjamin Majewski's commentary expands upon Anne Kohler's chapter by providing reflections between lead researcher Kohler and her research assistant Majewski on the role of people with Down syndrome as collaborators in research. Other commentaries present new perspectives, sharing additional data or research experiences about the topic (Laura Dunn and Paul Holtzheimer (Chapter 18), Allison Bloom (Chapter 23)), or considering the applicability of the chapter's concerns to other participant groups (Caitlin Courchesne and Judy Illes (Chapter 19)). Finally, we editors have each written commentaries that address all of the volume's chapters together (Eric Racine (Chapter 29), Ariel Cascio (Chapter 30)).

There are a few specific cross-cutting themes we want to draw the reader's attention to. Readers particularly interested in the role of research ethics committees should read the chapters by Mackenzie Salt (Chapter 7), Britteny Howell and Karrie Shogren (Chapter 3), Christine Schneider and Eva Kahana (Chapter 9), and Virginie Cobigo and colleagues (Chapter 16). Readers interested in the role of third parties in consent or as quasi-participants are directed to the chapters by Virginie Cobigo and colleagues (Chapter 16); Vanessa Cox and colleagues (Chapter 10); Anne Kohler (Chapter 17); John Aspler (Chapter 15); Marjorie Montreuil (Chapter 12); Britteny Howell and Karrie Shogren (Chapter 3); and Kenneth Richman (Chapter 5). Many of these chapters detail how to manage the involvement of others, a valuable topic that has been raised as a tension in studies involving support persons for participants with such needs (Llewellyn, 2009). Readers interested in the role of people who might be labeled with cognitive differences as researchers (not just research participants) might be particularly interested in the chapter by Mackenzie Salt (Chapter 7), a researcher on the autism spectrum; the commentary by Anne Kohler and Benjamin Majewski (Chapter 26), the latter of whom reflects on his role as a research assistant with Down syndrome in a study on experiences of people with this syndrome; and the chapter by Stephanie Patterson and Pamela Block (Chapter 6), which describes a study with a co-researcher with traumatic brain injury. Readers interested in the experiences of children should read the chapter by Marjorie Montreuil and colleagues (Chapter 12), as well as the commentary by Caitlin Courchesne and Judy Illes (Chapter 19).

Taken together, this volume seeks to fill a gap in the literature on research ethics by bringing explicit attention to ongoing and innovative work on research involving participants with cognitive disabilities or differences. It should therefore be useful to researchers, students, and trainees who are planning and conducting such studies because it provides an example of how researchers have addressed ethical challenges and a resource for thinking through new issues. Potential research participants and those close to them might also want to read this book, as it provides an inside look into researchers' work and thought processes. This inside look could be interesting to someone who is approached by a researcher and asked to take part, or to give permission for the researcher to ask their family member, student, client, or patient if they want to participate. Overall, we assert that research ethics pervades the everyday experiences of researchers, participants, and other concerned parties, and that a focus on research ethics not only protects participants from harms and discomfort, but also empowers representation and inclusion.

## References

Bracken-Roche, D., Bell, E., and Racine, E. (2016). "The 'Vulnerability' of Psychiatric Research Participants Why This Research Ethics Concept Needs to Be Revisited." *The Canadian Journal of Psychiatry*, 61: 335–339.

Brown, L. X. Z. (2012). "Include Us in the Conversation: What 'Nothing About Us Without Us' Means," https://www.autistichoya.com/2012/03/include-us-in-conversation-what-nothing.html (accessed November 5, 2018).

Brown, L. X. Z. (2013). "How 'Differently Abled' Marginalizes Disabled People," https://www.autistichoya.com/2013/08/differently-abled.html (accessed March 12, 2019).

Carlson, L. (2013). "Research Ethics and Intellectual Disability: Broadening the Debates." *Yale Journal of Biology & Medicine*, 86: 303–314.

Charlton, J. I. (2000). *Nothing about Us Without Us: Disability Oppression and Empowerment*. Berkeley, CA: University of California Press.

crippledscholar (2017). "Euphemisms for Disability are Infantalizing," https://crippledscholar.com/2017/11/12/euphemisms-for-disability-are-infantalizing/ (accessed March 12, 2019).

Estroff, S. (1993). "Identity, Disability, and Schizophrenia: The Problem of Chronicity," in Lindenbaum, S. and Lock, M. (eds.) *Knowledge, Power and Practice: The Anthropology of Medicine and Everyday Life*. Berkeley, CA: University of California Press, pp. 247–287.

Fein, E. and Rios, C. (2018). *Autism in Translation: An Intercultural Conversation on Autism Spectrum Conditions*. London: Palgrave Macmillan.

Fisher, C.B. (2003). "Goodness-of-Fit Ethic for Informed Consent to Research Involving Adults with Mental Retardation and Developmental Disabilities." *Mental Retardation and Developmental Disabilities Research Reviews*, 9: 27–31.

Ginsburg, F. and Rapp, R. (2018). "Cognitive Disability: Towards an Ethics of Possibility." *The Cambridge Journal of Anthropology*, 36: 113–119.

Graby, S. (2015). "Neurodiversity: Bridging the Gap Between the Disabled People's Movement and the Mental Health System Survivors' Movement," in Spandler, H., Anderson, J., and Sapey, B. (eds.) *Madness, Distress and the Politics of Disablement*. Bristol: Policy Press, pp. 231–244.

Kittay, E.F. and Carlson, L. (2010). *Cognitive Disability and Its Challenge to Moral Philosophy*. Hoboken, NJ: Wiley.

Larivière-Bastien, D., Majnemer, A., Shevell, M., and Racine, E. (2011). "Perspectives of Adolescents and Young Adults with Cerebral Palsy on the Ethical and Social Challenges Encountered in Healthcare Services." *Narrative Inquiry on Bioethics: A Journal of Qualitative Research*, 1: 43–54.

Llewellyn, P. (2009). "Supporting People with Intellectual Disabilities to Take Part in Focus Groups: Reflections on a Research Project. *Disability & Society*, 24: 845–856

Martino, A.S. and Schormans, A. F. (2018). "When Good Intentions Backfire: University Research Ethics Review and the Intimate Lives of People Labeled with Intellectual Disabilities." *Forum Qualitative Sozialforschung* 19/3.

McKearney, P. and Zoanni, T. (2018). "Introduction: For an Anthropology of Cognitive Disability." *The Cambridge Journal of Anthropology*, 36: 1–22.

Oliver, M. (2017). "Defining Impairment and Disability." *Disability and Equality Law*, 3.

Ripamonti, L. (2016). "Disability, Diversity, and Autism: Philosophical Perspectives on Health." *The New Bioethics*, 22: 56–70.

Rothman, D.J. (1991). *Strangers at the Bedside: A History of How Law and Bioethics Transformed Medical Decision Making*. New York: Basic Books.

Shakespeare, T. (1999). "'Losing the Plot'? Medical and Activist Discourses of Contemporary Genetics and Disability." *Sociology of Health & Illness*, 21: 669–688.

# SECTION 1
# CONCEPTUAL FRAMEWORKS

# 1

# Ongoing Consent in Situations of Cognitive Vulnerability

## Special Considerations in Implanted Neural Device Trials

*Lauren R. Sankary and Paul J. Ford*

### Introduction: The ethical imperative to research conditions of those who are cognitively vulnerable

Advances in clinical research into neurological and mental health disorders often depend upon the participation of cognitively vulnerable patient populations. This includes research participants whose cognitive abilities may fluctuate over the course of research participation, either due to neurodegenerative disease processes, exacerbation of mental health disorders, or research interventions affecting central nervous system function. When fluctuations in cognition affect capacity to make decisions regarding research participation, special ethical considerations complicate the process of obtaining ongoing consent from research participants. Ethical and regulatory safeguards must balance the ongoing interests and responsibilities of various stakeholders, including research participants, caregivers, and other legally authorized representatives, researchers, sponsors, and research oversight boards.

Ongoing consent is framed by the expectations set out in the initial informed consent process of any clinical trial. While specific regulatory and ethical safeguards address the initial informed consent process, few guidelines specifically address the periodic re-evaluation of capacity or the process of obtaining *ongoing* consent to continued participation in research. Under the Belmont Report, the ethical principle of respect for persons requires that research practices recognize the autonomy of capacitated research participants and protect those with diminished autonomy. Protections for incapacitated individuals range from introducing safeguards to the informed consent process to altogether excluding entire classes of individuals from research participation. The Belmont Report maintains that these protections should be titrated to the risk of harm and the likelihood of benefit research participation entails. According to the Belmont Report, "The judgment that any individual lacks autonomy should be periodically re-evaluated and will vary in different situations." This acknowledges that capacity may fluctuate over time and should be re-evaluated over the course of research participation and as circumstances change.

The notion of promoting respect for persons and protecting those with diminished autonomy through informed consent to research participation is affirmed in US regulations for the protection of human subjects (including the Department of Health and Human Services "Common Rule" policies in 45 CFR 46 and the Food and Drug Association (FDA) human subject protection regulations in 21 CFR 50). Both the Common Rule and FDA regulation recognize the importance of the circumstances under which consent may be obtained: "An investigator shall seek such consent only under circumstances that provide the prospective subject or the representative sufficient opportunity to consider whether or not to participate and that minimize the possibility of coercion or undue influence" (21 CFR 50 Protection of Human Subjects Subpart B Sec. 50.20). Circumstances that do not lead to coercion during the initial consent process may become coercive over the course of research participation. Informed consent requires assuring participants maintain the right to withdraw from research and ongoing voluntariness of participation. Regulations 45 CFR 46.116 (a)(8) and 21 CFR 50.25 (a)(8) require that research subjects be informed they "may discontinue participation at any time without penalty or loss of benefits to which the subject is otherwise entitled." Protecting the right to withdraw from research requires a careful assessment of what benefits of research participation may function as a penalty to research participants if lost upon withdrawal and therefore serve to coerce continued participation.

Similar guidelines are expressed in international codes of ethics. For instance, in the 2013 version of the Declaration of Helsinki, Article 28 (World Medical Association, 2013) specifically outlines that subjects who cannot consent for themselves should not be involved in risky research with no likelihood of benefit unless the research fulfills three criteria: minimal risk and burden, inability to conduct the research with capacitated subjects, and the aim of promoting health in subjects' respective patient populations. These guidelines continue to show an uneasy tension between over- and under-protection of research subjects who do not have full capacity to decide for themselves.

Addressing the concern of unjust exclusion of potential research participants necessitates the development of consent practices that maximize the ability of individuals with cognitive limitations to participate meaningfully in decisions regarding participation in clinical research. In addition, proper authorization to participate and good protection of participant's interests must be assured. The unnecessary exclusion of individuals with cognitive impairments from participation in research deprives these individuals of the potential for direct benefit in some trials and the opportunity to contribute to generalizable knowledge that may help future patients. Further, this exclusion of potential research participants may delay or entirely obstruct research progress and the development of effective clinical treatments by limiting the feasibility of recruiting and enrolling needed participants and discouraging investigators and sponsors from conducting or funding this research. This argument is strengthened when considering ongoing consent, particularly when research risks have already been assumed and the remainder of research that is needed to get proper results is of low risk. Ultimately, excluding subjects from study enrollment or continued participation may exacerbate disparities in the allocation of public resources, increasing the burden of neurological and mental health disorders on patients and families. In this chapter, we discuss best ethical practices in clinical research for a context-specific approach to maximize the ability of those with cognitive impairments and those likely to become cognitively impaired to contribute to decisions regarding continued participation in clinical research.

## Vulnerability of clinical research participants whose cognition fluctuates

The perceived vulnerability of individuals with fluctuating or impaired cognition may present a barrier to enrollment in research. During the process of obtaining and maintaining informed consent to participation in clinical research, vulnerability is negatively associated with voluntariness and appreciation of the implications of participation in research (Ford, 2009). Discourse around vulnerability in human subjects research has misguidedly conceived of vulnerability as a static quality of classes of potential research participants, including children, pregnant women, and individuals with cognitive impairments (Bell et al., 2014). This conception of vulnerability overlooks relational and situational dimensions of vulnerability, often leading to the unjust and unnecessary exclusion of potential research participants. Importantly, these relational and situational dimensions are frequently the aspects of vulnerability that are most subject to intervention through research design, conduct, and regulation. Characterizing relational aspects of vulnerability is essential to the identification of best practices in obtaining informed consent to participation in research.

In Kenneth Kipnis' taxonomy of vulnerability in research (2001), he identifies six kinds of vulnerability that describe circumstances affecting the efficacy of an individual's consent to participate in research. The first form of vulnerability described in Kipnis' bioethical taxonomy is cognitive vulnerability, referring to circumstances that limit a potential research participant's "capacity to deliberate about and decide whether to participate in the study" (Kipnis, 2001). This aligns closely with the criteria used for evaluations of capacity to make decisions regarding medical care (Appelbaum and Grisso, 1988). Circumstances suggesting cognitive vulnerability include delays in and disorders affecting cognitive development, dementia, and certain mental health disorders. Cognitively vulnerable research participants may also be subject to the other kinds of vulnerability under Kipnis' taxonomy, including juridic vulnerability (subordination to formal authority), deferential vulnerability (the tendency to be influenced or pressured by others), medical vulnerability (presence of a health condition for which no existing clinical therapies provide satisfactory remedies), and allocational or infrastructural vulnerability (potential exploitation of those who lack access to social and economic resources) (Kipnis, 2001). Vulnerability may be exacerbated by therapeutic misconception, or a lack of appreciation for the overarching purpose of research to produce generalizable knowledge, regardless of the potential for research participants to experience direct clinical benefit (Kipnis, 2001; Henderson et al., 2007). Therapeutic misconception may lead to the overestimation of the clinical benefits of an investigational intervention and under-appreciation of intervention-related risks (Lidz et al., 2004; Henderson et al., 2007).

Kipnis' taxonomy points to circumstances researchers should be attentive to in seeking voluntary and informed consent to research participation. Instead of excluding potential research participants on the basis of binary capacity determinations or categorical assignments to vulnerable subpopulations, researchers should carefully assess cognitive, relational, and situational factors that may limit the voluntariness of informed consent and identify which of those factors can be mitigated. Cognitive limitations can be mitigated by including caregivers and loved ones in informed consent discussions, modifying communication of study-related information, and providing additional time for deliberation. Relational aspects of vulnerability can be mitigated by integrating independent research participant advocates and consent monitors into the consent process. To minimize potential exploitation related to disparities in access to health-related goods, risks and benefits of participation must be examined in relation to a participant's access to important social and economic resources.

## Existing models for obtaining consent to research participation

Several approaches to research consent have been proposed for those with cognitive vulnerabilities to attempt to account for later changes in capacity. These include double consent, proxy consent with participant assent, advance consent, and process consent. Each of these models establishes relationship-based protections for ongoing consent as new decision points arise over the course of participation in research.

Under the practice of obtaining double consent to research participation, researchers obtain surrogate or proxy consent in addition to the consent of a capacitated research participant when cognition is expected to decline during research participation (High, 1993; Sachs et al., 1994). Double consent may become a practical necessity since participants often depend on caregivers who serve as proxies to support the planning, transportation, and motivation research participation may require (Jongsma and van de Vathorst, 2015). However, double consent may be considered disrespectful of the autonomy of fully capacitated research participants and a barrier to enrollment for potential participants who lack the resources or family support to involve a surrogate or proxy in the informed consent process.

When individuals lack capacity to provide consent for their own participation in research, consent may be obtained under a similar model of proxy consent with participant assent. Assent signifies affirmation of a participant's initial and ongoing willingness to participate in research, while dissent signifies refusal to participate regardless of proxy consent (Slaughter et al., 2007). A participant's assent or dissent may be communicated through direct verbal expressions, body language suggesting comfort or distress, or behavioral indications of cooperation or lack of cooperation (Slaughter et al., 2007). While obtaining assent may promote the continued involvement of persons with cognitive impairments in informed consent conversations, proxy consent practices have been criticized for their susceptibility to exclusionary consent practices, such as only contacting persons with cognitive impairments after consent has been obtained from a proxy (Dewing, 2002; Slaughter et al., 2007). Practices that ignore the importance of assent reduce the moral status of individuals with cognitive impairments (Dewing, 2002) and overlook vital ways in which participants can meaningfully engage in the informed consent process.

Advance consent refers to the use of research advance directives for capacitated individuals to indicate preference about future participation in research. Research advance directives may provide useful guidance to proxies and members of the research team regarding an incapacitated individual's previously held views toward participation in research. The use of research advance directives may promote the inclusion of individuals with cognitive impairments in research in a manner that is consistent with the participant's long-term values. However, this model is criticized for privileging the precedent or former autonomy of previously capacitated individuals over the present interests of persons with dementia or other neurodegenerative disorders (Dewing, 2002). Further, advance directives fail to appreciate many situational and relational aspects that may be important factors in decisions regarding research participation. The utility of advance directives is limited to the circumstances they anticipate and the stability of the preferences and values they reflect (Jongsma and van de Vathorst, 2015). While they may serve as a useful supplement to other consent practices, research advance directives have not been widely adopted (Jongsma and van de Vathorst, 2015; Muthappan et al., 2005).

Process consent describes an "inclusionary" and person-centered approach to obtaining initial and ongoing consent to research participation among individuals without legal capacity to provide informed consent (Dewing, 2007). Inspired by Carol Gilligan's feminist ethics of care, this model rejects competency-based approaches to obtaining consent that overlook situational and relational aspects of capacity that may be present beyond the legal threshold of capacity. Process consent seeks to involve individuals with cognitive impairments as active participants and collaborators in research (Dewing, 2007). This process respects each individual in their full integration in a network of social supports which are extensions and aspects of the individual. Including partners from the participant's social network is not a matter of obtaining "dual consent"; rather, it is a natural reflection of the way most people make decisions in relationship to others. In this way, a participant who lacks a specific component of capacity could reasonably rely on a trusted friend to supply that aspect and together they would be considered to be capacitated as a unit for purposes of providing consent to research participation.

Under the process consent model, researchers establish a basis for initial consent and ongoing consent monitoring through a process of observation and information gathering. Researchers collect cues about a potential participant's well-being, triggers, or indications of disruptions to their well-being, and observe how the person provides consent to participate in activities or procedures in their day-to-day life (Dewing, 2007). During the initial consent process, participants are informed about the study in which they are being asked to participate using communication methods tailored to their cognitive abilities through adaptations to written information and use of pictorial information and props, as needed (Dewing, 2007). Researchers then look for "evidence of assent or non-objection" rather than merely relying on the absence of verbal or non-verbal indications of dissent (Dewing, 2007). In monitoring for ongoing consent, researchers look for any evidence that a participant's feelings about research participation have changed. Any behavioral, verbal, or non-verbal sign that a participant no longer wishes to participate in research prompts a full re-visitation of consent (Dewing, 2007). Finally, researchers provide feedback relevant to the participant's well-being to caregivers, as appropriate, to support participants as they transition back to day-to-day life upon exiting from the research setting (Dewing, 2007).

Dewing's process consent model provides an approach to move beyond a binary, competency-based approach and to maximize the ability of individuals with cognitive impairments to participate in decisions regarding research participation. While her recommendations may not apply to the individual circumstances and cognitive abilities of every potential research participant, they describe best practices for tailoring the informed consent process to the vulnerabilities and strengths of individuals with cognitive impairments as they are situated in social and environmental contexts. In considering a broader range of cognitive impairments, best practices involve a blend of aspects of each of the models described earlier. Researchers should encourage potential participants and their proxies to anticipate situations that may affect decisions about continued enrollment in research after initial consent has been provided.

## Ongoing consent

Beyond obtaining initial consent as participants enroll in clinical research, researchers must ensure ongoing consent to research participation remains voluntary and informed. When there is reason to expect cognition to decline or fluctuate meaningfully over the course of research participation, researchers should develop a plan to re-evaluate ongoing capacity for continued consent to research participation. Reassessments of capacity should not merely test for a participant's recitation of the contents of an informed consent checklist. Open-ended questions should be used to evaluate a participant's understanding of the nature of their participation in research in contrast to standard clinical care, understanding of salient risks and potential benefits of study participation, appreciation for how these trade-offs may affect his/her life, and reasons for continued participation. These requirements mirror those for initial consent.

Research protocols should identify procedures for the re-evaluation of capacity to provide ongoing consent to address circumstances in which a participant's behavior raises suspicion of a meaningful decline in capacity and define intervals at which a specific disease process are reasonably expected to cause meaningful decline in capacity. Developing a timeline for the reassessment of capacity entails anticipating circumstances that call into question the presumption of ongoing capacity, such as the presence of a neurological or mental health disorder or foreseeable side effects of an intervention that affects central nervous system function. Points of re-evaluation should be tailored to expectations regarding rate of cognitive decline, other aspects of disease progression, or changes in medical management that may affect cognition. In interventional studies, capacity should be re-evaluated as participants are exposed to initial and ongoing intervention-related risks. In the example of brain device trials (discussed in greater detail in the section "Special considerations in implanted neural device trials: An example"), capacity should be evaluated during initial consent to participate in research and reassessed immediately prior to research interventions, including the surgical implantation and removal of a device.

Capacity should again be reassessed in response to substantial changes in the research protocol that require participants to re-consent to or otherwise acknowledge updates to procedures or other aspects of clinical trial participation. Researchers should also define procedures for the re-evaluation of capacity in response to unforeseen circumstances, such as unexpected adverse events. Finally, the process by which participants exit or withdraw from a clinical trial may prompt reassessment of capacity, especially if this process poses additional risks to participants' health or well-being. The below example of a device-related research trial highlights this challenge.

Practical considerations for how to best respect ongoing consent hinge on the nature of a study. Studies that are primarily observational pose different ongoing risks than primarily interventional clinical trials; however, many protocols blend observational and interventional features or phases. For example, biobanks and other biorepositories collect biosamples and health data obtained from blood draws, lumbar punctures, or other interventions, sometimes undertaken primarily for clinical rather than research purposes. These biosamples and data are processed and then stored for future scientific investigation, most of which can be understood as observational and presenting no additional risks to study participants beyond ongoing risks to confidentiality. However, a primarily interventional study of an implanted brain device, such as responsive neurostimulation for epilepsy, may involve a significant period of observation after the device has been implanted. Data collected through closed-loop neurostimulation devices are often stored by researchers for further analysis, and may be shared with other researchers. It is important to disclose the nature and timing of these risks during the informed consent process and reaffirm ongoing consent as participants encounter these risks over the course of a clinical trial. Another consideration is the continuum of capacity to consent for participation in research is always judged along axis of risk and complexity of what is being asked. It is reasonable to expect that even if a subject were to lose capacity to consent to a complicated surgery, they may continue to have capacity to consent to the collection and storage of simple questionnaire data.

## Revoking consent

The revocation of consent to research participation can happen in several different circumstances for patients whose capacity to consent diminishes during a protocol. The most common circumstances are when a participant asks to discontinue involvement, when a legally authorized representative asks for withdrawal, or when the research team believes that additional consent is needed but no mechanism exists to attain it.

Even when participants are deemed to lack capacity to make independent decisions regarding research participation, they should continue to be included in research-related decisions, including decisions regarding study withdrawal. Assent and agreement continue to be important concepts across the spectrum of changes in cognition. Individuals who lack full capacity to consent frequently retain the ability to express preferences, goals, values, and concerns that can inform a proxy and the research team or be interpreted as indications of assent or dissent. Despite a general consensus that any indication of distress should cause a participant to be removed from the study, some argue signs of dissent should instead prompt further evaluation before a subject's participation is terminated, particularly in studies involving a very high benefit to risk ratio (Slaughter, 2007).

Protections need to be in place to limit the extent to which proxies can retroactively withdraw consent that had been provided by research participants while they retained capacity. It is important to respect the wishes of previously capacitated individuals, especially when research-related risks have already been undertaken and continued participation does not expose participants to unforeseen risks. When participants have provided first-person consent to participation in research, the burden falls on a proxy who wishes to act in a way that is inconsistent with these express directives to justify withdrawing consent to ongoing circumstances. While unforeseen circumstances, such as an unexpected deterioration in the participant's health condition, may justify an inconsistent decision about ongoing enrollment, this decision needs to be reconciled with evidence of the participant's long-term values.

## Special considerations in implanted neural device trials: An example

A specific example of a class of research, clinical trials of implanted neural devices, is useful to demonstrate how these considerations impact the process of obtaining ongoing consent to research participation. In clinical trials of implanted neural devices, ethical safeguards become particularly important for research involving cognitively vulnerable patient populations. This includes patients with existing cognitive deficits or in the early stages of a progressive neurodegenerative disease. Participation in implanted neural device trials is frequently only available to patients who have exhausted established therapies. These circumstances suggest that medical vulnerability may exacerbate cognitive vulnerabilities in the patient populations targeted for recruitment in these clinical trials. Since potential participants may be invited to participate in implanted device research by their treating clinicians and encouraged to participate by family members on whom they are functionally dependent, these individuals may also experience significant deferential vulnerability. Significant costs associated with implanted brain device therapies, including surgical, device-related, and follow-up care costs, may result in allocational and infrastructural vulnerabilities. Since relatively few surgical centers possess the expertise and resources to support clinical research in implanted brain devices, potential participants usually have few clinical trial options to choose between when enrolling in research or obtaining post-trial follow-up care.

Once a participant has decided to enroll in an implanted neural device trial, this research presents challenges for establishing ongoing consent. Potential side effects associated with surgical implantation and ongoing stimulation may impact cognitive and affective aspects of decision-making, potentially limiting decision-making capacity over the course of research participation (Ford, 2007). Beyond the risks of surgical implantation, neural devices expose participants to ongoing hardware-related risks, including infection, skin erosion, or lead migration (Doshi, 2011). Further, the need for hardware-related follow-up care, including battery replacement or stimulation reprogramming, introduces additional complexity to the ongoing consent process. Finally, as participants exit clinical trials, they encounter additional risks and complex decisions related to the surgical removal (explant) of investigational devices. Since explant of neural devices such as deep brain stimulators may present greater risks for surgical complications such as intracerebral hemorrhage than the initial implantation of these devices (Liu, 2012), explant-related risks may not be adequately foreseen upon enrollment in clinical trials. Each of these considerations may introduce unanticipated risks to safety and well-being. Even if a participant does not feel coerced into enrolling in a clinical trial, they may feel coerced into continued participation or may be unduly influenced by their inability to access device-related care outside of the context of a clinical trial. In clinical trials of neurostimulation devices, both explanting the device and leaving the device implanted pose ongoing risks to safety and well-being.

Another source of potential undue influence relates to whether a participant will become financially responsible for costs related to device programming or removal if he or she withdraws from a clinical or declines to participate in an optional follow-up phase (Ford, 2007). These circumstances may coerce continued participation and constitute a penalty or loss of benefits prohibited under 21 CFR 50.25 (a)(8). However, there are limits to the resources available to researchers to account for participants making choices that go against a protocol. If a researcher has budgeted for surgical explant of the device, but the subject refuses and insists on indefinite follow-up care, this could create an unreasonable burden on the researcher stemming directly from the participant's choice to go against an agreed-upon protocol. Participant choices have costs associated with them and careful consideration needs to be undertaken to understand which costs are coercive and which are simply the natural consequences of a participant breaking the agreement. Of course, when a participant who no longer has full capacity refuses to have a surgery performed, substantial weight is placed on not violating his or her inalienable right to bodily integrity.

In light of the distribution of research-related risks over the course of participation in a clinical trial, it is important to engage potential participants in an informed consent process that anticipates exit considerations at the time of initial enrollment and to provide opportunities to re-evaluate consent as additional risks are undertaken. In these clinical trials, researchers can enhance the initial consent using techniques from the consent models previously mentioned. While obtaining dual consent might not be necessary in most clinical trials, researchers might want to encourage participants to involve family in the informed consent process to promote respect for a participant's decision enroll in the trial and to identify an individual to represent the participant's preferences if he or she loses capacity. Undertaking a dual consent process allows the proxy decision-maker to hear exactly why the participant is entering the trial. This can be referenced later when the proxy may need to make decisions about ongoing participation after a participant's capacity has diminished. Although requiring a capacitated participant to have another person also give consent could be experienced as disrespectful to an individual's autonomy and has the potential to exclude those who lack a person in their lives that fill this role, it can be justified in implanted device trials when there is an anticipated future decision point, such as device explant, that will require robust consent for participants who likely will not have full capacity at a later date.

Researchers should encourage participants and their proxies to contemplate decisions that will need to be made later in the course of study participation, including choices about device removal and exit from the clinical trial. Finally, elements of process consent can be employed to obtain ongoing consent from participants with temporarily or progressively diminished capacity. In revisiting consent in light of concerns about a participant's ongoing capacity, researchers should modify their approach to conveying and assessing understanding of study-related information. Regardless of formal determinations of capacity, these practices promote the ability of participants to express preferences and values that inform ethically robust decisions regarding ongoing participation in research.

## Conclusion

This chapter expands upon existing models for obtaining informed consent from cognitively vulnerable research participants to describe best practices for obtaining ongoing consent to continued participation in clinical research. In seeking to minimize coercion and maximize the ability of individuals with cognitive vulnerabilities to participate in initial and ongoing consent discussions, it is important to avoid considering cognitive vulnerability in isolation. Drawing on relationship-based approaches to obtaining informed consent, these recommendations can be used to support researchers in recognizing and addressing aspects of vulnerability that can affect the ability of individuals with cognitive impairments to participate in research-related decisions. Using the example of clinical research in implanted neural devices to explore clinical and practical considerations for ongoing consent, the ethical analysis outlined above supports the development of research practices that maximize the ability of cognitively vulnerable research participants to contribute to decisions regarding ongoing research participation.

## References

Appelbaum, P. S. and Grisso, T. (1988). "Assessing Patients' Capacities to Consent to Treatment." *New England Journal of Medicine*, 319: 1635–1638.

Bell, E., Racine, E., Chiasson, P., Dufourcq-Brana, M., Dunn, L.B., Fins, J.J., Ford, P.J., Glannon, W., Lipsman, N., Macdonald, M.E., and Mathews, D.J. (2014). "Beyond Consent in Research: Revisiting Vulnerability in Deep Brain Stimulation for Psychiatric Disorders." *Cambridge Quarterly of Healthcare Ethics*, 23/3: 361–368.

Dewing, J. (2002). "From Ritual to Relationship: A Person-centred Approach to Consent in Qualitative Research With Older People Who Have a Dementia." *Dementia*, 1/2: 157–171.

Dewing, J. (2007). "Participatory Research: A Method for Process Consent With Persons Who Have Dementia." *Dementia*, 6/1: 11–25.

Doshi, P.K. (2011). "Long-term Surgical and Hardware-related Complications of Deep Brain Stimulation." *Stereotactic and Functional Neurosurgery*, 89/2: 89–95.

Ford, P.J. (2007). "Neurosurgical Implants: Clinical Protocol Considerations." *Cambridge Quarterly of Healthcare Ethics*, 16/3: 308–311.

Ford, P.J. (2009). "Vulnerable Brains: Research Ethics and Neurosurgical Patients." *Journal of Law, Medicine and Ethics*, 37/1: 73–82.

Henderson, G.E., Churchill, L.R., Davis, A.M., Easter, M.M., Grady, C., Joffe, S., Kass, N., King, N.M., Lidz, C.W., Miller, F.G., and Nelson, D.K. (2007). "Clinical Trials and Medical Care: Defining the Therapeutic Misconception." *PLoS Medicine*, 4/11: e324.

High, D.M. (1993). "Advancing Research with Alzheimer Disease Subjects: Investigators' Perceptions and Ethical Issues." *Alzheimer Disease and Associated Disorders*, 7/3: 165–178.

Jongsma, K. and van de Vathorst, S. (2015). "Advance Directives in Dementia Research: The Opinions and Arguments of Clinical Researchers—An Empirical Study." *Research Ethics*, 11/1: 4–14.

Kipnis, K. (2001). "Vulnerability in Research Subjects: A Bioethical Taxonomy." *Ethical and Policy Issues in Research Involving Human Participants*, 2: G3.

Lidz, C.W., Appelbaum, P.S., Grisso, T., and Renaud, M. (2004). "Therapeutic Misconception and the Appreciation of Risks in Clinical Trials." *Social Science & Medicine*, 58/9: 1689–1697.

Liu, J.K., Soliman, H., Machado, A., Deogaonkar, M., and Rezai, A.R. (2012). "Intracranial Hemorrhage After Removal of Deep Brain Stimulation Electrodes." *Journal of Neurosurgery*, 116/3: 525–528.

Muthappan, P., Forster, H., and Wendler, D. (2005). "Research Advance Directives: Protection or Obstacle?" *American Journal of Psychiatry*, 162/12: 2389–2391.

Sachs, G.A., Stocking, C.B., Stern, R., Cox, D.M., Hougham, G., and Sachs, R.S. (1994). "Ethical Aspects of Dementia Research: Informed Consent and Proxy Consent." *Clinical Research*, 42/3: 403–412.

Slaughter, S., Cole, D., Jennings, E., and Reimer, M.A. (2007). "Consent and Assent to Participate in Research From People With Dementia." *Nursing Ethics*, 14/1: 27–40.

World Medical Association (2013). "World Medical Association Declaration of Helsinki. Ethical Principles for Medical Research Involving Human Subjects." *JAMA*, 310/20: 2191.

# 2

# Who Decides? Legal Changes to Facilitate Inclusion of Participants with Impaired Cognition in Research

*Megan S. Wright*

## Introduction

The research enterprise relies on human volunteers. While many of these volunteers are able to provide voluntary, informed consent to participate in research, a requirement under established bioethical principles and existing human research subjects regulation, other prospective participants may have impaired consent capacity.[1] These individuals may thus be excluded from research.

Excluding potential research participants with cognitive impairments is not an optimal solution for many research questions, however. Conducting research with participants with impaired cognition will sometimes be necessary for clinical trials testing an intervention that targets a disorder causing the impaired cognition. For example, the efficacy of deep brain stimulation to treat disorders of consciousness may need to be assessed with persons who are unable to consent or even assent. Persons with impaired cognition may also be invited to participate in behavioral science research that seeks to understand the workings of an (impaired) brain. This is the case for psychological studies about schizophrenia, which necessarily include participants who may have fluctuating capacity due to mental illness. Additionally, participants with impaired cognition may be engaged with social science research about the lived experiences of persons with such conditions. This occurs when, for instance, sociologists ask persons with dementia or who are addicted to psychoactive substances about their lived experiences. There may be no other way to know about their experiences without asking them.

Beyond the scientific rationale for including persons with impaired cognition in research, there are ethical reasons to do so. The Belmont Report, one of the foundational documents in the ethics of human subjects research, emphasizes the principle of justice by raising the question "Who ought to receive the benefits of research and bear

[1] In this chapter, terms such as "impaired cognition" and "impaired consent capacity" are used interchangeably. "Human subject" and "research participant" are also used interchangeably because regulations governing research use the word "subject." Additionally, the term "incompetent" is used as a legal term of art to refer to someone who has been adjudicated as incapable of making some decisions for themselves, and decision-making authority has been legally transferred to a guardian.

its burdens?" (National Commission, 1979). In order to prevent injustice in the context of research participation, "the selection of research subjects needs to be scrutinized in order to determine whether some classes ... are being systematically selected simply because of their easy availability, their compromised position, or their manipulability, rather than for reasons directly related to the problem being studied" (National Commission, 1979). However, the Declaration of Helsinki, which provides ethical guidance for physicians involved in medical research with human subjects, states that underrepresented groups should have access to medical research (World Medical Association, 2013, p. 13), a position that is also consistent with international human rights law (United Nations, 1948, 27.1).[2] Policies excluding persons with impaired cognition from research participation as a bright-line rule are thus counter to the principle of justice.

Other ethical principles may weigh against including persons with impaired cognition in a study, however. Respect for persons, another primary principle in The Belmont Report, means respecting autonomy through obtaining voluntary, informed consent, or protecting people with "diminished autonomy" (e.g., because of illness or disability) even to the point of excluding them from research participation (National Commission, 1979). The report notes that for persons with limited comprehension, "respect requires giving them the opportunity to choose to the extent they are able, whether or not to participate in the research" and "also requires seeking the permission of other parties in order to protect the subjects from harm" (National Commission, 1979). The report also advises that "third parties" be able to withdraw the research participant with cognitive impairments if the third party determines continued research participation is not in the participant's best interests.

The Belmont Report also highlights the principle of beneficence in human subjects research, which has implications for research with participants with cognitive impairments. Beneficence necessitates "making efforts to secure [research participants'] well-being" by trying to "maximize possible benefits," including benefits to society, while "minimiz[ing] possible harms" (National Commission, 1979). In attempting to accomplish these aims, it is important to determine whether some groups need special considerations. Multiple codes of ethics have cautioned that when conducting research with persons in "vulnerable" groups, including persons with cognitive impairments, it is necessary to justify why these prospective participants are being recruited, and if conducting research with members of a vulnerable group is not necessary, other volunteers should be sought (World Medical Association, 2013, p. 20; National Commission,

[2] The Universal Declaration of Human Rights (UDHR) (United Nations, 1948) asserts on behalf of the international community, "Everyone has the right freely ... to share in scientific advancement and its benefits" (27.1). Sharing in the burdens and benefits of science is not possible if persons with cognitive impairments are, as a matter of law, policy, or practice, excluded as a class from research participation. Furthermore, the Convention on the Rights of Persons with Disabilities requires signatories "[t]o undertake or promote research and development of, and to promote the availability and use of new technologies, including information and communications technologies, mobility aids, devices and assistive technologies, suitable for persons with disabilities" (United Nations, 2006, 4.1.g). This requirement will in some cases necessitate participation from persons with disabilities that impair cognition.

1979). Furthermore, the Declaration of Helsinki asserts that members of vulnerable groups should directly benefit from their research participation (World Medical Association, 2013, p. 20); that the research should only have minimal risk and burden (World Medical Association, 2013, p. 28); that there should be additional protections (World Medical Association, 2013, p. 19); and that even with the consent of a legally authorized representative, participants' assent sought and dissent respected (World Medical Association, 2013, p. 29).

While scientific justification and ethical analysis informs considerations about whether and how best to involve persons with impaired cognition in research, law and policy regulate the boundaries of permissible research with this population. This chapter explores the legal and regulatory landscape of research with participants with impaired cognition in the United States, focusing on the question of who is authorized to make the decision for a person with a cognitive impairment to participate in research. The chapter concludes by suggesting how the law should be reformed to clearly identify the appropriate legal decision-maker in a manner that facilitates just, respectful, and beneficent research with participants with impaired cognition.

## Legal regulation of research involving participants with impaired cognition

There is a substantial amount of existing law and policy governing research with human subjects, but much less explicit guidance about involving participants with impaired cognition in research. Indeed, one of the most important questions about research with participants with cognitive impairments does not have a clear answer: who can decide to participate? This section seeks to answer this question by reference to US federal law, and select examples of state laws, institutional policies, and professional guidelines that have implications for research with participants with impaired consent capacity.[3]

### Common Rule

The major source of law governing human subjects research in the United States is known as the Common Rule (45 CFR § 46) because the regulations were adopted by multiple federal agencies that oversee human subjects research (Bierer et al., 2017). The Common Rule is based on principles outlined in The Belmont Report, namely respect for persons, beneficence, and justice (National Commission, 1979). The

[3] Other important issues, such as the process of informed consent for participants with impaired cognition and additional research protections, will not be covered in this chapter. This is because the specifics of these issues differ by study population, research question and design, and particular risk–benefit profiles.

Common Rule was revised recently, began taking effect in summer 2018, and is fully in effect as of January 2019 (Federal Register, 2017; Office for Human Research Protections, 2018a).

The initial version of the Common Rule referenced "mentally disabled persons," noting that they need special consideration because they are "vulnerable to coercion or undue influence" (45 CFR § 46.111(a)(3)).[4] The Common Rule required "additional safeguards ... included in the study to protect the rights and welfare" of participants with impaired cognition (45 CFR § 46.111(b)). The term "mentally disabled" has been criticized, however, and the revised Common Rule uses the phrase "individuals with impaired decision-making ability" (Federal Register, 2017, p. 7204).

While the Common Rule requires that human subjects give voluntary, informed consent to participate in research (45 CFR § 46.116), this may not be possible for some persons with impaired cognition. The Common Rule thus permitted a legally authorized representative to provide consent on behalf of the subject (45 CFR §§ 46.102, 116), but never clearly defined who is a legally authorized representative. The Office for Human Research Protection (2009, 2018b) advises that this is a state and local law determination, but acknowledges that many jurisdictions never specify through statute or common law who is a legally authorized representative for research purposes. The Executive Summary of the revised Common Rule states, "The long-standing interpretation by OHRP [Office for Human Research Protection] has been that such laws relating to surrogate consent in the clinical context can be used for purposes of the Common Rule" (Federal Register, 2017, p. 7170). But for states that have no surrogate healthcare decision-making law, the legally authorized representative is determined by local Institutional Review Board (IRB) policy (Federal Register, 2017). The Office for Human Research Protection (2018b) suggests consulting a lawyer if an IRB has questions about who qualifies as a legally authorized representative.

Because lack of clarity about who can be a legally authorized representative may result in the inappropriate inclusion or exclusion of persons with impaired decision-making, the revised Common Rule changed the definition of legally authorized representative to include "an individual recognized by institutional policy as acceptable for providing consent in the nonresearch context to the subject's participation in the procedures involved in the research" (Federal Register, 2017, p. 7171). These changes also were meant to ensure that research with participants who need a legally authorized representative to provide consent could take place in all jurisdictions, consistent with the principles of justice and beneficence. While clinical trials involving medical procedures now should be easier to conduct with persons with impaired cognition, institutions may not have surrogate decision-making policies that apply to social and behavioral science research.

[4] Being a member of a vulnerable group does not necessarily mean that an individual is vulnerable, however (Beauchamp and Childress, 2013, pp. 267–8). As scholars have noted, "for many groups a label covering all members of the group serves to overprotect, stereotype, and even disqualify members capable of making their own decisions" (Beauchamp and Childress, 2013, p. 267).

## State laws

While federal regulations govern much of the human subjects research enterprise, the regulations are silent or vague on many relevant issues. State law interprets and fills gaps in the Common Rule, and also regulates research not covered by the Common Rule. This section will briefly note state laws that matter for conducting research with participants with impaired cognition, focusing on laws that define a legally authorized representative, including guardianship laws.

### Legally authorized representative

The most extensive research on who is a legally authorized representative for research purposes comes from Saks and colleagues' efforts to determine whether proxies can consent to research for persons with decisional impairments. They found that most states do not have law on proxy consent to research participation, but some authorize proxy consent if there is a research advance directive or a durable power of attorney (Saks et al., 2008; see also Office for Human Research Protections, 2009).

Given the absence of direct regulation, inferences from state laws on surrogate healthcare decision-making provide guidance (Saks et al., 2008). Some state laws permit surrogates to make any type of healthcare decisions; other states require use of substituted judgment (i.e., deciding as the incapacitated person would decide); and still other states restrict or prohibit some types of decisions (e.g., reproductive or psychiatric treatment decisions) (Saks et al., 2008). Applying state healthcare decision-making laws to the research context, it seems as though some states would permit proxy consent to research, while others would prohibit it (Saks et al., 2008). There is not a lot of case law litigating the issue of proxy consent, however (Saks et al., 2008), which results in an uncertainty that may discourage investigators from involving research participants who cannot consent or expose investigators to liability for unlawfully including such participants (Office for Human Research Protections, 2009).

A minority of states have detailed laws regulating human subjects research, however. For example, California law governing research not covered by the Common Rule permits proxy consent for medical research if the research is related to patients' incapacity or other serious medical conditions; proxies use the substituted judgment standard of decision-making, or, if not possible, the best interests standard; and the participant does not dissent or resist (California Health and Safety Code, 2004; § 24178).

Some states provide only guidance for conducting research with participants with cognitive impairments. The New York State Task Force on Life and Law (2014), for example, published a report about research with subjects with impaired consent capacity. The report argues that surrogates should be permitted to consent to research participation, based on analogous surrogate consent for health care (Koch, 2014). This recommendation holds even for greater than minimal risk studies with no direct benefit as long as there are additional safeguards, such as demonstrating the research is of "vital importance"; having a consent monitor; relying upon a research advance directive; or submitting to a special panel review of the case (Koch, 2014). While this report is not law, it may create new norms of research conduct if investigators comply with, or IRBs create policies based on, its recommendations.

## Guardianship

Some persons with impaired cognition may be under guardianship. Guardianship is meant to protect the interests of incompetent persons, and some degree of decision-making authority (oftentimes all) is transferred to a judicially appointed guardian. Persons under guardianship may thus not have the authority to decide to participate in research, and the person who would be authorized to consent would be their guardian.

As a recent study has demonstrated, while most states' guardianship laws do not specify guardians' powers with respect to enrolling their ward in research, a significant minority of states do regulate guardians' decisions in this domain, and these states tend to restrict guardians' authority to consent to experimental research or treatment (Wright et al., 2017). For example, Nevada's statute reads "... a guardian shall not consent to ... [t]he participation of a ward in any biomedical or behavioral experiment" (Nevada Revised Statutes, 2007, § 159.0805(1)(c)). A guardian may petition the court to enroll their ward, and the court may authorize participation if there will be direct benefit to the ward; that is, the studied intervention will "assist the ward to develop or regain the ward's abilities" (§ 159.0805(2)-(3)(a)(b)).

For states that do not explicitly regulate research participation by statute, guardians may belong to an organization that has a policy against making this type of decision, or guardians may not be diligent about protecting their wards from inappropriate inclusion in research (Dittrich, 2017). Guardianship status may thus affect access to research.

## Institutional policy and professional guidelines

Without significant state and federal law about research involving participants with impaired cognition, institutional policies and codes of professional ethics have been created to provide guidance (Office for Human Research Protections, 2009), creating law-like rules. The National Institutes of Health (NIH), for example, has a policy on research with participants with "questionable" consent capacity. The NIH recognized that a significant amount of clinical research concerns conditions that may cause cognitive impairment, and that if persons with such impairments cannot participate in these trials, effective treatments and "diagnostic, predictive, and preventative strategies" may not be developed (NIH, 2009). The NIH thus supports involving participants with impaired cognition in research, but with safeguards (NIH, 2009). The safeguards related to who can decide to participate include consent monitors; capacity assessments at multiple time points; modifications to the consent process to increase understanding; obtaining consent from a legally authorized representative who uses substituted judgment or best interests standard of decision-making with a higher evidentiary standard for riskier research; and relying on a research advance directive (NIH, 2009).

Professional codes of conduct also regulate research with participants with impaired cognition. For example, the American Medical Association (AMA) directs physician-researchers to determine whether prospective research participants have decision-making capacity (AMA, 2016, 7.1.2). For participants without capacity, the AMA states that consent of the legally authorized representative will suffice using a reasonable person standard (i.e., "informed and prudent adults would reasonably be expected to volunteer themselves") and if direct benefit is possible (AMA, 2016, 7.1.2(h), (j)). The AMA further advises physicians conducting research that assent also should be obtained from the research participant and dissent respected (AMA, 2016, 7.1.2). Neither the NIH nor the AMA define who a legally authorized representative is, however.

## Legal reform

There remains problematic uncertainty and lack of uniformity in law and policy about who can consent to research participation for participants with impaired cognition (Office for Human Research Protections, 2009). Uncertainty may deter researchers from conducting research involving such participants, which halts scientific progress and may disadvantage people with impaired consent capacity who could benefit from access to research; uncertainty may also lead to unlawful or unethical inclusion of research participants with consent impairments (Office for Human Research Protections, 2009). Lack of regulatory uniformity also results in similarly situated persons being treated differently, some permitted to participate in research and some not, a determination based solely on the rules of the jurisdiction in which they reside, which violates some conceptualizations of justice. Furthermore, lack of uniformity may make it difficult to conduct multi-site research (Office for Human Research Protections, 2009). Legal reform is thus desirable.

Law should clear the path for involving persons with impaired cognition in respectful, beneficent, and just research. This requires clarity about who can appropriately and legally decide whether a person with impaired cognition can participate in a study. This section will discuss and analyze legal tools to identify the decision-maker, including the use of research advance directives, clear statutory definitions about who can be a legally authorized representative, changes to guardianship law, and application of supported decision-making models.

### Research advance directives

A research advance directive operates like other advance directives: it provides written instructions to follow should a person be unable to make their own decisions, or it appoints an agent to make decisions in these circumstances (i.e., power of attorney). The focus of instructions and the locus of decision-making in research advance directives is about research participation. The NIH was a leader in using research advance directives, dating since the late 1980s, and this was possible, in part, because Maryland law permitted healthcare agents to enroll patients in research (Dukoff and Sunderland, 1997).

Research advance directives are beneficial because they clearly identify the legal decision-maker for research consent—either the person prior to their loss of capacity or their agent—and they respect precedent autonomy, but this legal tool is not the most promising avenue of reform for several reasons. First, completion of a research advance directive is not possible for persons with cognitive impairments who have never been legally competent. Second, given that the vast majority of Americans do not complete any type of advance directive (Yadav et al., 2017), it is likely that even fewer would be motivated to complete a research advance directive. Indeed, one study found that only 11% of persons given the opportunity to complete a research advance directive did so (Muthappan et al., 2005). Third, as with any written advance directive, there may be problems with the level of specificity about consent in the document, and it may not be possible to anticipate what kind of research opportunity will be available and what one's preferences will be when recruited for the research (Pierce, 2010).

If institutions opt to promote the use of research advance directives for persons with impaired cognition, they may advise principals to select an agent rather than write instructions. This allows the agent to decide both on the basis of their principal's former values, such as altruism or concern for family members who may be affected by a disorder that causes impaired cognition (Pierce, 2010; Saks et al., 2008), and their current experiential interests, which may be resistant toward participating in a particular study.

## Legally authorized representative clarity

Consulting a legally authorized representative about research participation will be necessary sometimes, like in cases where a prospective participant is unconscious and there is no research advance directive. The law should thus be clear about who can be a legally authorized representative for research consent purposes (Office for Human Research Protections, 2009). Under the Common Rule, deference is given to states and institutions to define "legally authorized representative," but for efficiency and justice reasons, it is preferable to have definitional uniformity.

There is public support for surrogate (i.e., family) consent to dementia research (Kim et al., 2009), support that likely exists for other disorders that cause cognitive impairment. Based on this support, states should authorize by statute a legally authorized representative hierarchy of appointed agents and family members (Saks et al., 2008). Should there be no available family, then perhaps a specially appointed committee (Pierce, 2010) that also includes patient advocates could function as a legally authorized representative for consent purposes.

## Guardianship reform

Saks et al. (2008) recommend that families serve as proxies for research consent rather than involving courts because families know the incapacitated person's preferences, and the protective function of a court is already in place with IRB review. Furthermore, guardianship proceedings are often inefficient and may act as a deterrent to conducting research with persons with decision-making impairments. But not all incapacitated persons have family to protect their interests, and may thus require a guardian.

As noted previously, some states prohibit persons under guardianship from participating in research. While these laws are meant to protect a vulnerable group, these laws may disadvantage some persons who could benefit from participating in research. The harm from exclusion from research may outweigh the benefit of protection in this case, and so this legal safeguard needs to be reconsidered. Wisconsin's nuanced guardianship law permits guardians to consent to research participation for their ward "if the research might help the ward; or if the research might not help the ward but might help others, and the research involves no more than minimal risk of harm to the ward" (Wisconsin Statutes and Annotations, 2016, § 54.25(2)(d)2.b). The exception to this authority is if there is "clear and convincing" evidence the ward would not want to participate in the research, but the presumption is that the ward would want to participate. Even without the prospect of direct benefit and with greater than minimal risks, guardians can enroll their wards in research using the substituted judgment standard and IRB oversight (§ 54.25(2)(d)2.c).

Modeling guardianship laws on Wisconsin's is a promising step toward more inclusive research, but this law remains imperfect. Outside the context of studies with direct benefit, the law only accounts for people who had prior legal competence and known former preferences, which excludes from research some persons with cognitive impairments, such as people with developmental disabilities like Down syndrome who may never have been considered legally competent. Wisconsin's law also does not account for the present preferences or dissent of the person with cognitive impairment. It is thus necessary to examine other legal reforms.

## Supported decision-making

An alternative to guardianship that emerged from advocacy efforts by the development disabilities community is supported decision making. Under this paradigm, a person with a disability that impairs cognition retains legal decision-making authority, but enters into a contract with "supporters" who agree to help the person with the disability make decisions.

Texas adopted supported decision-making "to recognize a less restrictive substitute for guardianship for adults with disabilities who need assistance with decisions regarding daily living" (Texas Estates Code, 2015, § 1357.003). Under Texas law, a person with a disability voluntarily chooses people to assist them in gathering information relevant to making decisions about, for example, healthcare, property management, and living arrangements (§ 1357.056). The supporters, who are fiduciaries, can also provide help with understanding information and communicating decisions to others (§§ 1357.052, 1357.056). The person with a disability is able to specify whether their supporters have access to confidential health and educational information (§ 1357.056), and they can also terminate the agreement (§ 1357.053).[5] Other states have begun adopting supported decision-making into law (Delaware Code Annotated § 9401-9410; Wisconsin Statutes Annotated § 52.01-52.32; District of Columbia Code Annotated § 7-2131-2134).

This model of decision-making emphasizes and promotes agency and self-determination, and is consistent with the values many experts argue should be promoted in the process of deciding to participate in research, regardless of whether a prospective participant has cognitive impairments (Office for Human Research Protections, 2009). Supported decision-making is also relational, which is how people generally tend to make decisions, in consultation and collaboration with others (Wright, 2018). This paradigm works for people who were formerly legally competent, as is the case for many people who develop dementia later in life (Wright, in press). Importantly, however, it also works for people who have never been legally competent, either because of a developmental disability that requires high levels of support or a cognitive impairment acquired while still a minor. As long as a person with a cognitive impairment is conscious and has the ability to make decisions with assistance, then they can make a decision for themselves about whether to participate in a study for which they are recruited. The informed consent process may differ for people using supported decision-making, however, as they may need additional time to consult with their supporters about the risks and benefits of the research. Building in waiting periods for persons with cognitive impairments is already considered a best research practice, however (NIH, 2009).

## Conclusion

While some jurisdictions and institutions permit research involving participants with impaired cognition, this research is often unregulated or prohibited, and there is also uncertainty about who can decide whether a person with impaired consent capacity will participate in research. This chapter has suggested legal reforms to clearly identify who can and should decide whether a person with consent incapacity will participate in research, in order to promote respectful, beneficent, and just inclusion of participants

[5] Texas's supported decision-making law is consistent with and responsive to the Convention on the Rights of Persons with Disabilities (United Nations, 2006), the guiding principles of which include "individual autonomy including the freedom to make one's own choices, and independence of persons" (3a-c). Article 12 of the Convention (United Nations, 2006) requires signatories to "recognize that persons with disabilities enjoy legal capacity on an equal basis with others in all aspects of life" (12.2) and to "take appropriate measures to provide access by persons with disabilities to the support they may require in exercising their legal capacity" (12.3). These measures must "respect the rights, will and preferences of the person" (United Nations, 2006, 12.4).

with impaired cognition in the research enterprise. These reforms include recommending appointment of an agent in a research advance directive, specifying who a legally authorized representative is in statutes, and permitting guardians to consent to research on behalf of their wards. The preferred legal tool is widespread adoption of supported decision-making, so that persons with cognitive impairments can decide for themselves whether to participate in a study. More research is needed about how best to maximize the intended benefits of supported decision making, however, given that to date there is little evidence about its effects (Kohn et al., 2013).

## References


American Medical Association (AMA) (2016). "Opinions on Research & Innovation," in *Code of Medical Ethics*. Chicago, IL: AMA.

Beauchamp, T.L. and Childress, J.F. (2013). *Principles of Biomedical Ethics*, 7th ed. New York: OUP.

Bierer, B.E., Barnes, M., and Fernandez Lynch, H. (2017). "Revised 'Common Rule' Shapes Protections for Research Participants." *Health Affairs*, 36/5: 784–788.

California Health and Safety Code, § 24178 Human Experimentation (2004). 45 C.F.R. § 46, Common Rule.

Delaware Code Annotated, § 9401-9410, Supported Decision-Making Act (2016).

District of Columbia Code Annotated, § 7-2131-2134 (2018).

Dittrich, L. (2017). *Patient H.M.: A Story of Memory, Madness, and Family Secrets*. New York: Random House.

Dukoff, R. and Sunderland, T. (1997). "Durable Power of Attorney and Informed Consent with Alzheimer's Disease Patients: A Clinical Study." *American Journal of Psychiatry*, 154/8: 1070–1075.

Federal Register (2017). *Rules and Regulations*, 82/12: 7149–7274.

Kim, S.Y.H., Kim, K.M., Langa, K.M., Karlawish, J.H.T., Knopman, D.S., and Appelbaum, P.S. (2009). "Surrogate Consent for Dementia Research: A National Survey of Older Americans." *Neurology*, 72/2: 149–155.

Koch, V.G. (2014). "A Policy in Flux: New York State's Evolving Approach to Human Subjects Research Involving Individuals Who Lack Consent Capacity." *Journal of Law, Medicine, and Ethics*, 42/3: 383–388.

Kohn, N.A., Blumenthal, J.A., and Campbell, A.T. (2013). "Supported Decision-Making: A Viable Alternative to Guardianship?" *Penn State Law Review*, 117/4: 1111–1157.

Muthappan, P., Forster, H., and Wendler, D. (2005). "Research Advance Directives: Protection or Obstacle." *American Journal of Psychiatry*, 161/12: 2389–2391.

National Commission for the Protection of Human Subjects of Biomedical and Behavioral Research [National Commission]. (1979). *The Belmont Report: Ethical Principles and Guidelines for the Protection of Human Subjects of Research*. Baltimore, MD: National Commission.

National Institutes of Health (NIH) (2009). "Research Involving Individuals with Questionable Capacity to Consent: Points to Consider," https://grants.nih.gov/grants/policy/questionablecapacity.htm (accessed February 26, 2019).

New York State Task Force on Life and the Law (2014). "Report and Recommendations for Research with Human Subjects Who Lack Consent Capacity," https://www.health.ny.gov/regulations/task_force/docs/report_human_subjects_research.pdf (accessed February 26, 2019).

Nevada Revised Statutes, § 159.0805, Guardianships (2007).

Office for Human Research Protections (2009). "Attachment: Recommendations Regarding Research Involving Individuals With Impaired Decision-Making," https://www.hhs.gov/ohrp/sachrp-committee/recommendations/2009-july-15-letter-attachment/#f1 (accessed February 26, 2019).

Office for Human Research Protections (2018a.) "Revised Common Rule Implementation Timeline," https://www.hhs.gov/ohrp/sites/default/files/Webinar-supplements-July-2018.pdf (accessed February 26, 2019).

Office for Human Research Protections (2018b). "Informed Consent FAQs," https://www.hhs.gov/ohrp/regulations-and-policy/guidance/faq/informed-consent/index.html (accessed February 26, 2019).

Pierce, R. (2010). "A Changing Landscape for Advance Directives in Dementia Research." *Social Science & Medicine*, 70: 623–630.

Saks, E.R., Dunn, L.B., Wimer, J., Gonzalez, M., and Kim, S. (2008). "Proxy Consent to Research: The Legal Landscape." *Yale Journal of Health Policy, Law, and Ethics*, 8/1: 37–92.

Texas Estates Code, § 1357, Supported Decision-Making Agreement Act (2015).

United Nations (1948). *Universal Declaration of Human Rights*. Paris: United Nations.

United Nations (2006). *Convention on the Rights of Persons with Disabilities*. New York: United Nations.

Wisconsin Statutes and Annotations, § 54.25, Duties and Powers of the Guardian of the Person (2016).

Wisconsin Statutes and Annotations, § 52.01-52.32, Supported Decision-Making Agreements (2018).

World Medical Association (WMA) (2013). *Declaration of Helsinki—Ethical Principles for Medical Research Involving Human Subjects*. Helsinki: WMA.

Wright, M.S. (in press). "Dementia, Autonomy, and Supported Healthcare Decision Making." *Maryland Law Review*, 79.

Wright, M.S. (2018). "End of Life and Autonomy: The Case for Relational Nudges in End-of-Life Decision-Making Law and Policy." *Maryland Law Review*, 77/4: 1062-1141.

Wright, M.S., Ulrich, M., and Fins, J.J. (2017). "Guardianship and Clinical Research Participation: The Case of Wards with Disorders of Consciousness." *Kennedy Institute of Ethics Journal*, 27/1: 43–70.

Yadav, K.N., Gabler, N.B., Cooney, E., Kent, S., Kim, J., Herbst, N., Mante, A., Halpern, S.D., and Courtright, K.R. (2017). "Approximately One in Three US Adults Completes Any Type of Advance Directive for End-of-Life Care." *Health Affairs*, 36/7: 1244–1251.

# 3

# Differing Understandings of Informed Consent Held by Research Institutions, People with Intellectual Disability, and Guardians

## Implications for Inclusive, Ethical Research

*Britteny M. Howell and Karrie A. Shogren*

### Introduction

Approximately 1–3% of the world's population experiences an intellectual disability (ID) (Maulik et al., 2011). Despite social and medical gains over the past several decades, people with ID are significantly more likely to experience poorer health and quality of life outcomes than people without (Beadle-Brown et al., 2016; Krahn et al., 2015). Research participation can play an important role in reducing such persistent disparities; however, people with ID remain under-represented in research for a variety of reasons, including the assumption that they are unable to provide informed consent for participation (Brooker et al., 2015). In this chapter, we address differing understandings of informed consent that may be held by research institutions, people with ID, and guardians of people with ID. We also address alternative strategies for increasing participation of people with ID in research, which is necessary for inclusive practice and to increase access to evidence-based practices and quality-of-life outcomes.

Assumptions about the ability to consent and participate in research are often shaped by the understanding of disability adopted by stakeholders. Historically, disability has been understood from a deficits-based perspective, a focus on what people with ID *cannot* do in the process of providing informed consent using standard mechanisms established by research institutions. However, contemporary understandings of disability, rooted in social-ecological models, recognize that disability results from an interaction between personal capabilities and environmental demands; when there is mismatch, a need for support is created (Thompson et al., 2009). By understanding this need for support, alternative participatory strategies can be devised congruent with the needs of people with ID that enable them to engage in the informed consent and research process, respecting the right to self-determination, as well as meeting the demands of research institutions.

Related to conceptualizations of disability, another barrier to increasing research participation of people with ID is that research institutions, people with ID, and guardians of people with ID often disagree on the acceptable levels of risk for research (Slaughter et al., 2007; Swaine et al., 2011). Since approximately half of all people in the United States with ID and developmental disabilities have legal guardians (National Core Indicators, 2016), researchers are frequently required to obtain informed consent from guardians (also called "proxies"). Even when people with ID are not in guardianship arrangements, issues related to providing accessible information that enables informed consent requires consideration. Informed consent is a process that is required by research institutions and/or federal regulations of many nations which aims at ensuring research participants, or their proxies, understand and agree to all aspects and risks of their participation.

In the United States, people with ID have been designated a vulnerable population in the context of research participation, along with other groups, including children, prisoners, and pregnant women. A vulnerable population is defined as one in which the subjects are likely to be susceptible to coercion or undue influence and requires the consideration of additional research safeguards (Office for Human Research Protections, 2009, Subpart A, Section 46.111). The US Office of Human Research Protections (OHRP) provides extensive guidance on involving children and prisoners in research, but none specific to people with ID (US Office for Human Researh Protections, 2018), leaving much of the burden of determining the most useful supports to engage people with ID in the consent process to institutions and individual researchers.

Owing to the high rate of guardianship in the United States mentioned earlier, many adults with ID cannot legally consent to research participation. Generally, when a vulnerable subject, like a child, cannot provide informed consent, researchers must obtain consent from the legal guardian and *assent* from the research subject. However, OHRP defines assent only as "a child's affirmative agreement to participate in research," and does not address how or when adults with ID might provide assent or consent (OHRP, 2009, Subpart D, Section 46.402). Indeed, when adults with ID have a legal guardian, the decisions of the guardians can often supersede the wishes of the individual with ID to participate in research or not.

When an individual does not have a guardianship arrangement, they can consent to participation, but research information must be provided in an understandable way. If consent protocols are not accessible to adults with ID, then obtaining *informed* consent may not be possible and research participation may be restricted. Federal regulation allows research institutions to determine whether or not consent/assent is required for research proposals via individual Institutional Review Boards (IRBs), which results in variation in informed consent/assent procedures both within and between institutions (Grady, 2015). Researchers working with the ID population are often compelled to obtain informed consent from parents and guardians whenever possible in order to comply with IRBs, even when not legally necessary.

Some researchers contend that these informed consent-by-proxy and assent procedures reduce individuals' personhood and self-determination in the research process (Dewing, 2002; Iacono and Murray 2003) and are not consistent with social-ecological models of disability and support needs. Therefore, differing understandings of research risks and informed consent among institutions, individuals, and their guardians result in significant research barriers. This chapter focuses on describing considerations for research institutions, people with ID, and their guardians (when necessary) to understanding and removing such barriers.

## Research institutions

US research institutions have IRBs that provide ethical review and oversight of studies involving human subjects. These boards are made up of community members and researchers, usually from a variety of fields. Since IRBs were created in response to past research abuses, board members tend to hold protective views regarding the need to ensure informed consent in research, often utilizing deficit-based models that assume that people with ID cannot understand research risks and give consent/assent. Best practices dictate the capacity to consent/assent be made on an individual basis; however, IRBs often request set procedures, protocols, and even lengthy assessments be utilized for determining capacity *before* research begins (Iacono, 2006). This introduces challenges to individualizing consent/assent practices based on the support needs of people with ID because the processes and information each participant will need to consent/assent cannot be known before research participation begins. Since IRBs rarely have people with ID or disability advocates on their boards, the people making decisions about capacity to consent are often those without any direct expertise (Klitzman, 2012). This process perpetuates the lack of emphasis on the unique needs of people with ID to participate fully in consent/assent procedures, limiting participation in broader, population-based research studies. When studies directly target people with ID, the lack of individualization of procedures continues to introduce challenges to participation (Iacono and Murray, 2003). Utilizing a "better-safe-than-sorry" model of research ethics may have resulted in a degree of paternalism that has reduced involvement of people with ID in research, rather than promoting their rights and inclusion in research (McDonald and Patka, 2012).

McDonald and colleagues (2016a; 2017) conducted focus groups with IRB members, individuals with ID, their guardians, and others, and found that IRB members consistently underestimated how often people with ID would consent to research and which recruitment strategies they found most appropriate. The authors also report that people with ID believed their exclusion from research to be far more harmful than did IRB members. IRB members were least likely to think that proxy consent procedures were harmful, and were more likely to rate potential psychosocial risks as more harmful than individuals with ID. These are important differences in the way IRB members view research risks and appropriate consent/assent procedures, which likely affects research participation for people with ID.

To promote self-determination and respectful participation in research, policies and practices should not rely solely on the viewpoints of research institutions, but instead should meaningfully incorporate the views of adults with ID and integrate current understanding of disability and support needs. Ideally, people with ID would be included in IRBs, and IRB members would receive training and education on vulnerable populations, guardianship, and accessibility. When IRBs more accurately represent the communities they serve, they may be better able to explore ways to encourage research participation, both in targeted research projects on ID and inclusive, population-based research (Hammel et al., 2016; T. Iacono and Carling-Jenkins, 2012).

## Guardians and other supporters

A guardian is a court-appointed individual with legal authority to care for the personal and property interests of another person, called the ward. A guardian is appointed when a ward is deemed unable to make or communicate safe or sound decisions or has become susceptible to fraud or undue influence (National Guardianship Association, 2018). Social-ecological understandings of disability raise questions about the appropriateness of some guardianship arrangements and propose supports-based alternatives (Glen, 2015). Guardians are often family members or friends of the ward, but there are also paid guardians who support many wards. A guardian or other family member may be asked to consent to research on behalf of an individual with ID not only in the case of legal guardianship, but also when research information and informed consent paperwork is not accessible to the individual with ID. Likewise, IRBs may require proxy consent from family members or staff supports when there is uncertainty about an individual's ability to understand the informed consent document.

When presented with information about studies, researchers have found that guardians may be less likely to consent than the person with ID. Lennox et al. (2005) report a degree of suspicion among guardians regarding participation of their ward in research. They also report that identifying and locating guardians, who often do not have a daily role in decision-making, to obtain informed consent contributed to low recruitment of people with ID in their research. Swaine et al. (2011) found that legal guardians were significantly less likely to consent to research participation (61% willing to participate) than their wards (83%) and people with ID who did not have guardians (86%). These divergent perspectives suggest a need to consider how to balance understandings of risks and benefits across the various stakeholders, including people with disabilities, legal guardians, and researchers. Some argue that guardians may be too restrictive, while others argue that guardians may fear their wards to not understand risk. In either scenario, there must be a discussion of the values, preferences, and needs of people with ID in research participation decisions as each individual person, with or without a disability, will have a unique approach to considering risks and benefits. This is why individualization in the consent/assent process is important (Millar, 2007).

The discrepancies in perspectives may also emerge from past research abuses in the field of ID that increase guardian suspicion of research in general (Iacono, 2006). Family guardians commonly hold the belief that their wards are too trusting, that they will "sign the form if someone was telling [them] to," despite not understanding to what they were agreeing (McDonald et al., 2015). It can be difficult for some parents to recognize when their children with disabilities have become adults, and to adjust their views and expectations from protecting their children to empowering them (Hammel et al., 2008; Kramer, 2018).

Guardians may also be reluctant to consent to research if they are unable to perceive a direct benefit (Hammel et al., 2008; Kramer, 2018). Information about research participation, benefits, and risks may not always be tailored to guardians who need to weigh risks and benefits for their ward. These divergent opinions suggest major barriers to communication about participation in research. Even under guardianship arrangements, there should still be a focus on supporting participation in decision-making and promoting self-determination. It is important that all parties are cognizant of risks and benefits. As the person with ID is ultimately the participant, they should be involved in the decision-making process and fully informed in providing consent/assent.

## People with intellectual disability

For people with ID to participate in consent/assent processes related to research, information needs to be made accessible and relevant using the communication styles they prefer. The amount of information disclosed, the processes followed, and level of individual understanding of consent/assent for research projects vary greatly (Grady, 2015), and research with the ID population is no exception (McDonald and Kidney, 2012). Researchers commonly note that the length, complexity, and required legal language of informed consent may make the paperwork difficult for individuals with and without ID to understand (Cook and Inglis, 2012). However, McDonald et al. (2013) have conducted research into the views of individuals with ID, which indicates that many people do understand that consenting to research is a way to participate meaningfully in activities that potentially benefit themselves or others.

McDonald et al. (2013; 2017) provide interview and focus group data to suggest that many people with ID do not want to be left out of research opportunities that have the ability to increase the community's understanding of the lives of people with disabilities. Indeed, individuals with ID perceive more benefits to their research participation than IRB members or guardians, such as feeling like they are helping others, learning new things, meeting people, doing something new, and ensuring the community learns more about people with disabilities (McDonald et al., 2016b). Such benefits of research participation correspond to the key features of community inclusion that are important for people with ID, ensuring their lives have meaning, choice, and responsibility (Dean et al., 2016).

The work of McDonald et al. (2015) shows that people with ID are more likely to consent/assent to research than IRB members or guardians. It also suggests that people with ID would not indiscriminately agree to participate in *all* research. People with ID can often articulate in which studies they would decline participation, such as medication trials that involve greater risk and uncertainty, or research into very private matters. Contrary to what many guardians assume regarding trust, people with ID indicate *not* being overly trusting of strangers or unfamiliar places because of past experiences. This research suggests more focus is needed on how to create accessible research information and consent/assent procedures for truly ethical practice that focuses on supported participation.

## Obtaining consent/assent from individuals with ID

There is no consensus among researchers outlining best practices to obtaining informed consent/assent from a person with ID to participate in research (Swaine et al., 2011). A variety of techniques have been tried with small samples for acceptability and feasibility, including teach-back methods in which the researcher verifies understanding by having the individual repeat back the study risks and procedures (Tamariz et al., 2013). These approaches have not been systematically integrated into protocols for research participation by adults with ID nor do they always address individualized support needs. Several studies have been conducted by administering assessment instruments to test people for their capacity to consent; however, these consent procedures demand far more of people with ID than for other research participants (Iacono, 2006) and have been criticized for fostering paternalism (Fisher, 2003). Fisher (2003) argues that such strict consent processes focus on the individual's impairments and are so disempowering that these procedures themselves can impair the ability of people with ID to make informed decisions. Further, these methods have not been developed in partnership with people with ID, and as such limit the identification of effective ways to promote consent, assent, and participation from the perspectives of those affected. Some have argued that without including these perspectives of people with ID, it is not possible to enable inclusive research practices that increase understanding and self-determination (McDonald and Raymaker, 2013; Rosner 2015).

Research shows a need for capacity-building and adapted consent/assent procedures rather than the lengthy legalese of the informed consent document (Foe and Larson, 2016; Sigstad, 2014). People with ID may best respond to tailored consent/assent practices that utilize their individual strength and support needs, where consent/assent procedures may look quite different from one participant to the next (Cameron and Murphy, 2007; Ferguson and Murphy 2014). Research institutions and their governing bodies must determine ways to address these needs in current practices. Tailored approaches fit well within recommended best practices for supporting people based on their individual support needs in other life domains (Shogren, 2013a; Shogren et al., 2015); however, current paradigms for understanding disability and support needs have not yet influenced the research participation and consent/assent process. These and other studies suggests that researchers should move away from thinking about people with ID as having an impairment of consent capacity and move towards understanding of support needs of people with ID for meaningful consent and developing responsive, emergent processes that engage the person (Fisher, 2003; McDonald and

Kidney, 2012). The need for supports in decision-making and consent/assent should not be seen as a reason to limit participation, but instead used to devise the best individual support strategies to enable participation and self-determination.

Participatory approaches have the power to enhance participation of people with ID in research and enable informed consent/assent. The principles of participatory research emphasize valuing all types of knowledge and individual strengths to engage in an empowering form of inclusive research focused on productive relationships between researchers and community members that should include the consent/assent process. For example, involving individuals with ID as participant researchers in all steps of a research study was effective at increasing engagement in the study and moving beyond just using simplified language, visual aids, or teach-back methods (Cook and Inglis, 2012). Researchers advocate for more participatory action research approaches for people with ID on the grounds that such methods enable the pursuit of research agendas that better reflect the priorities of people with ID, facilitate knowledge translation, and ensure greater informed and engaged participation in the research by involving them and seeking input in all steps of the research process (Jurkowski, 2008; McDonald, 2017; Rosner, 2015; Stack and McDonald, 2014).

There is also a growing focus on alternatives to guardianship, namely supported decision-making (SDM), which focuses on identifying the support needs related to decision-making for a person with ID and developing systematic plans for provisioning these supports without the need for the removal of legal rights. SDM refers to the relationships, practices, and agreements designed to support a person with a disability to make and communicate their decisions to others (Dinerstein, 2012). Utilizing SDM, people with ID can exercise their right to make their own legal decisions, including research participation, with the assistance of a circle of trusted individuals they have selected, rather than relying on the final word of a legal guardian. An individual's family members, community supports, and/or friends may constitute a supportive network that can assist them to engage fully in the decision-making process. Studies show that individuals with ID feel most comfortable utilizing such "trusted gatekeepers" to help them navigate the informed consent/assent process, not to make decisions *for* them (McDonald et al., 2013).

Emerging tools such as the Supported Decision-Making Inventory System (SDMIS) can be used to identify specific support needs related to decision-making and to build the individualized supports needed to enable participation in research and other life domains (Shogren et al., 2017). The SDMIS includes questions about capacities for decision-making, current decision-making demands in major life domains (e.g., financial, health, relationships, community living), and supports needed to participate in the decision-making process. It was designed to provide information to supporters that could lead to effective SDM arrangements consistent with emerging policy and practice. Other nations such as Sweden, Israel, and Ireland have established such legal alternatives to guardianship that enable people with disabilities to designate supporters that can participate in the decision-making process for legal and other complex decisions, potentially including research participation (Autistic Self Advocacy Network, 2017).

## Conclusion

Ethics protocols may not fully consider the unique supports for people with ID that can facilitate informed consent and research participation, often instead acting to deny access to research opportunities for people with ID (Lennox et al., 2005). Stringent ethical requirements continue to challenge researchers in the field of ID and limit the participation of people with ID in broader population-based research, but a supports-based and participatory framework in the context of research participation for people with ID and their families/guardians has the potential to increase productive research relationships (Iacono and Carling-Jenkins, 2012; United Nations, 2006) and contribute to the development of knowledge and the promotion of valued outcomes for people with ID and the broader community.

It is the researcher's responsibility to find ways to meaningfully inform participants with ID about the benefits and potential harms of research participation (National Academies of Sciences Engineering and Medicine, 2017). To promote ethical participation in research, moving toward individualized supports and SDM models for consent may be an important future direction. Participating in research is one way for people with ID to realize self-determination and autonomy (Shogren and Broussard, 2011; Shogren, 2013b). Alternative strategies to enabling informed consent/assent such as SDM have the potential to increase self-determination and participation in research for people with ID, and address requirements for ethical and inclusive research practices. Determining ways to embed effective supports into the process of developing consent/assent procedures, reviewing research protocols, and conducting research needs to be addressed by all stakeholders.

## References

Autistic Self Advocacy Network (2017). "The Right to Make Choices: International Laws and Decision-Making by People with Disabilities. Part 5: Guardianship and Supported Decision-Making Law," http://autisticadvocacy.org/wp-content/uploads/2016/02/Easy-Read-OSF-5-Guardianship-and-SDM-Laws-v3.pdf (accessed February 26, 2019).

Beadle-Brown, J., Leigh, J., Whelton, B., Richardson, L., Beecham, J., Baumker, T., and Bradshaw, J. (2016). "Quality of Life and Quality of Support for People With Severe Intellectual Disability and Complex Needs," *Journal of Applied Research in Intellectual Disabilities*, 29/5: 409–421.

Brooker, K., van Dooren, K., Tseng, C. H., McPherson, L., Lennox, N., Ware, R. (2015). "Out of Sight, Out of Mind? The Inclusion and Identification of People With Intellectual Disability in Public Health Research," *Perspectives in Public Health*, 135/4, 204–211.

Cameron, L. and Murphy, J. (2007). "Obtaining Consent to Participate in Research: The Issues Involved in Including People With a Range of Learning and Communication Disabilities," *British Journal of Learning Disabilities*, 35/2: 113–120.

Cook, T. and Inglis, P. (2012). "Participatory Research With Men With Learning Disability: Informed Consent." *Tizard Learning Disability Review*, 2, 92–101.

Dean, Evan E., Fisher, K. W., Shogren, K. A., and Wehmeyer, M. (2016). "Participation and Intellectual Disability: A Review of the Literature." *Intellectual and Developmental Disabilities*, 54/6, 427–439.

Dewing, J. (2002). "From Ritual to Relationship: A Person-Centred Approach to Consent in Qualitative Research With Older People Who Have Dementia." *Dementia*, 1: 157–171.

Dinerstein, R. D. (2012). "Implementing Legal Capacity Under Article 12 of the UN Convention on The Rights of Persons With Disabilities: The Difficult Road From Guardianship to Supported Decision-Making." *Human Rights Brief*, 19/2, 8–12.

Ferguson, L. and Murphy, G. H. (2014). "The Effects of Training on the Ability of Adults With an Intellectual Disability to Give Informed Consent to Medication." *Journal of Intellectual Disability Research*, 58/9: 864–873.

Fisher, C. B. (2003). "Goodness-of-Fit Ethic for Informed Consent to Research Involving Adults With Mental Retardation and Developmental Disabilities." *Mental Retardation and Developmental Disabilities Research Reviews*, 9/1, 27–31.

Foe, G. and Larson, E. L. (2016). "Reading Level and Comprehension of Research Consent Forms." *Journal of Empirical Research on Human Research Ethics*, 11/1, 31–46.

Glen, K. B. (2015). "Supported Decision-Making and the Human Right of Legal Capacity." *Inclusion*, 3: 2–16.

Grady, C. (2015). "Enduring and Emerging Challenges of Informed Consent." *New England Journal of Medicine*, 372/9: 855–862.

Hammel, J., McDonald, K. E., and Frieden, L. (2016). "Getting to Inclusion: People With Developmental Disabilities and the Americans With Disabilities Act Participatory Action Research Consortium." *Inclusion*, 4/1: 6–15.

Hammel, J., Magasi, S., Heinemann, A., Whiteneck, G., Bogner, J., Rodriguez, E. (2008). "What Does Participation Mean? An Insider Perspective From People with Disabilities." *Disability and Rehabilitation*, 30/19, 1445–1460.

Iacono, T. and Carling-Jenkins, R. (2012). "The Human Rights Context for Ethical Requirements for Involving People With Intellectual Disability in Medical Research." *Journal of Intellectual Disability Research*, 56/11: 1122–1132.

Iacono, T. (2006). "Ethical Challenges and Complexities of Including People With Intellectual Disability as Participants in Research." *Journal of Intellectual & Developmental Disability*, 31/3: 173–179.

Iacono, T. and Murray, V. (2003). "Issues of Informed Consent in Conducting Medical Research Involving People With Intellectual Disability." *Journal of Applied Research in Intellectual Disabilities*, 16/1: 41–51.

Jurkowski, J. M. (2008), "Photovoice as Participatory Action Research Tool for Engaging People With Intellectual Disabilities in Research and Program Development." *Intellectual and Developmental Disabilities*, 46/1: 1–11.

Klitzman, R. (2012). "Institutional Review Board Community Members: Who Are They, What Do They Do, and Whom Do They Represent?" *Academic Medicine: Journal of the Association of American Medical Colleges*, 87/7: 975–981.

Krahn, G. L., Walker, D. K., and Correa-De-Araujo, R. (2015). "Persons With Disabilities as an Unrecognized Health Disparity Population." *American Journal of Public Health*, 105/S2: S198–S206.

Kramer, J. (2018). "Engaging Family Members and Guardians in Community Life Engagement: Barriers, Successes, and Strategies Webinar," https://www.communityinclusion.org/ (accessed February 26, 2019).

Lennox, N., Taylor, M., Rey-Conde, T., Bain, C., Purdie, D. M., and Boyle, F. (2005). "Beating the Barriers: Recruitment of People With Intellectual Disability to Participate in Research." *Journal of Intellectual Disability Research*, 49/4: 296–305.

McDonald, K. E. (2017). "On the Right Side of History: Community-Based Participatory Research and People with Developmental Disabilities." *Current Developmental Disorders Reports*, 4/1: 11–13.

McDonald, K. E. and Kidney, C. A. (2012). "What is Right? Ethics in Intellectual Disabilities Research." *Journal of Policy and Practice in Intellectual Disabilities*, 9/1: 27–39.

McDonald, K. and Patka, M. (2012), "'There is No Black or White': Scientific Community Views on Ethics in Intellectual and Developmental Disability Research." *Journal of Policy and Practice in Intellectual Disabilities*, 9/3: 206–214.

McDonald, K. E. and Raymaker, D. M. (2013). "Paradigm Shifts in Disability and Health: Toward More Ethical Public Health Research." *American Journal of Public Health*, 103/12: 2165–2173.

McDonald, K. E., Kidney, C. A., and Patka, M. (2013). "You Need to Let Your Voice be Heard': Research Participants' Views on Research." *Journal of Intellectual Disability Research* 57/3: 216–225.

McDonald, K. E., Schwartz, N. M., Gibbons, C. M., and Olick, R.S. (2015). "'You Can't be Cold and Scientific:' Community Views on Ethical Issues in Intellectual Disability Research." *Journal of Empirical Research on Human Research Ethics*, 10/2: 196–208.

McDonald, K. E., Conroy, N. E., Kim, C. I., LoBraoico, E. J., Prather, E. M., Olick, R. S., and Panel Project ETHICS Expert (2016a). "Is Safety in the Eye of the Beholder? Safeguards in Research With Adults With Intellectual Disability." *Journal of Empirical Research on Human Research Ethics*, 11/5: 424–438.

McDonald, K. E., Conroy, N. E., and Olick, R. S. (2016b). "Is It Worth It? Benefits in Research With Adults With Intellectual Disability." *Intellectual and Developmental Disabilities*, 54/6: 440–453.

McDonald, K. E., Conroy, N. E., Olick, R. S., and The Project ETHICS Expert Panel (2017). "What's the Harm? Harms in Research With Adults With Intellectual Disability." *American Journal on Intellectual and Developmental Disabilities*, 122/1: 78–92.

Maulik, P. K., Mascarenha, M. N., Mathers, C. D., Dua, T., and Saxena, S. (2011). "Prevalence of Intellectual Disability: A Meta-Analysis of Population-Based Studies." *Research in Developmental Disabilities*, 32/2: 419–436.

Millar, D. S. (2007). "'I Never Put it Together': The Disconnect Between Self-Determination and Guardianship—Implications for Practice." *Education and Training in Developmental Disabilities*, 42/2: 119–129.

National Academies of Sciences Engineering and Medicine (2017). *Fostering Integrity in Research*. Washington, DC: The National Academies Press.

National Core Indicators (2016). *Chart Generator 2014–2015*. Cambridge, MA: National Association of State Directors of Developmental Disabilities Services and Human Services Research Institute.

National Guardianship Association (2018). "What is Guardianship?" https://www.guardianship.org/what-is-guardianship/ (accessed February 26, 2019).

Office for Human Research Protections (2009). "45 CFR 46: Code of Federal Regulations, Protection of Human Subjects," https://www.hhs.gov/ohrp/regulations-and-policy/regulations/45-cfr-46/index.html#46.409 (accessed February 26, 2019).

Rosner, I. D. (2015). "From Exclusion to Inclusion: Involving People With Intellectual Disabilities in Research." *Tiltai*, 72/3: 119–128.

Shogren, K. A. (2013a), "Considering Context: An Integrative Concept for Promoting Outcomes in the Intellectual Disability Field." *Intellectual and Developmental Disabilities*, 51/2: 132–137.

Shogren, K. A. (2013b). "A Social–Ecological Analysis of the Self-Determination Literature." *Intellectual and Developmental Disabilities* 51/6: 496–511.

Shogren, K. A. and Broussard, R. (2011). "Exploring the Perceptions of Self-Determination of Individuals With Intellectual Disability." *Intellectual and Developmental Disabilities*, 49/2: 86–102.

Shogren, K. A., Luckasson, R., and Schalock, R. L. (2015). "Using Context as an Integrative Framework to Align Policy Goals, Supports, and Outcomes in Intellectual Disability." *Intellectual and Developmental Disabilities*, 53: 367–376.

Shogren, K. A., Wehmeyer, M. L., Uyanik, H., and Heidrich, M. (2017). "Development of the Supported Decision Making Inventory System." *Intellectual and Developmental Disabilities*, 55/6: 432–439.

Sigstad, H. M. H. (2014). "Characteristic Interviews, Different Strategies: Methodological Challenges in Qualitative Interviewing Among Respondents With Mild Intellectual Disabilities." *Journal of Intellectual Disabilities*, 18/2: 188–202.

Slaughter, S., Cole, D., Jennings, E., Reimer, M. A. (2007). "Consent and Assent to Participate in Research From People With Dementia." *Nursing Ethics*, 14: 27–40.

Stack, E. and McDonald, K. E. (2014), "Nothing About Us Without Us: Does Action Research in Developmental Disabilities Research Measure Up?" *Journal of Policy and Practice in Intellectual Disabilities*, 11/2: 83–91.

Swaine, J., Parish, S. L., Luken, K., and Atkins, L. (2011). "Recruitment and Consent of Women With Intellectual Disabilities in a Randomised Control Trial of a Health Promotion Intervention." *Journal of Intellectual Disability Research*, 55/5: 474–483.

Tamariz, L., et al. (2013). "Improving the Informed Consent Process for Research Subjects With Low Literacy: A Systematic Review." *Journal of General Internal Medicine*, 28/1: 121–126.

Thompson, J. R., Bradley, V. J., Buntinx, W. H. E., Schalock, R. L., Shogren, K. A., Snell, M. E., and Wehmeyer, M.L. (2009). "Conceptualizing Supports and the Support Needs of People With Intellectual Disability." *Intellectual and Developmental Disabilities*, 47: 135–146.

US Office for Human Research Protections (2018). "OHRP Guidance: Vulnerable Populations," https://www.hhs.gov/ohrp/regulations-and-policy/guidance/vulnerable-populations/index.html (accessed February 26, 2019).

United Nations (2006). "Convention on the Rights of Persons with Disabilities (CRPD)," http://www.un.org/disabilities/documents/convention/convention_accessible_pdf.pdf (accessed February 26, 2019).

# 4
# Research Cohorts
## Diverse Research Subjects, Similar Remedies to Errors in Consent

*Deborah R. Barnbaum*

### Introduction

Albert Jonsen's definition of "research subject" in his spoken testimony to the 1977 National Commission for the Protection of Human Subjects of Biomedical and Behavioral Research is cited by Zachary M. Schrag:

> A subject is one who falls within the power of an investigator such as that person's life, health, well-being, reputation, dot, dot, dot, whatever other qualities we consider important can be adversely affected and who, cannot for some reason, defend themselves (Schrag, 2014, p. 132).

Schrag endorses Jonsen's definition—a definition the Commission ultimately rejected—because it taps into two salient facts that we simultaneously know and fear. Research subjects are *at risk*, and they *lack power*. Heidi Li Feldman takes up where Schrag leaves off: Research subjects are at risk because they are separate persons than investigators, persons with distinct intentions, hopes, wishes, and experiences (Feldman, 2014). This separateness is the point of informed consent, according to Feldman, in that informed consent restores autonomy to research participants by recognizing this separateness of persons. It is the separateness of persons, and not primarily the risks of research, that necessitate informed consent. "I contend that whatever methods a researcher uses, whatever the degree of risk posed by these methods, whatever kind of possible harms involved, the question of a subject's autonomous participation remains the same" (Feldman, 2014, p. 301). This separateness of persons is an essential characteristic of all persons, those with cognitive impairments and those without.

This chapter starts from three key observations drawn from the aforementioned claims: (1) all research subjects are both at risk and lack some degree of power; (2) all persons, including typically developing, typically developed, and those with cognitive impairments, have distinct intentions and wishes; and (3) autonomous choice to participate in research is paramount. Does it follow that a research participant with cognitive impairments, who may be presumed to have less autonomy by virtue of those impairments, is in an even more compromised position when it comes to offering consent than a typically developed research participant?

Alan Wertheimer's answer to the above question might be, "Maybe, but not by much." Wertheimer calls into question the existence of the "ideal consenter" who is fully able to consent to all aspects of research participation. This "ideal consenter" would have all information needed in order to make an informed choice and would be able to make rational choices that both served the best ends, and the best means to the agent's ends, based on an understanding of that information; would act on authentic intentions based on the agent's own second-order desires; and would be free of internal and external constraints. These three conditions—the understanding needed to make rational decisions, intentional choice, and freedom from constraints—are Beauchamp and Childress's (2013) three necessary conditions for being autonomous. Beauchamp and Childress hold that that there are four principles of biomedical ethics: respect for autonomy, beneficence, nonmaleficence, and justice. Autonomous agents have understanding, exercise intentional choice, and are not impaired by constraints when making decisions, and that healthcare providers have an obligation to both respect autonomous choices, as well as foster the conditions that promote autonomy. Similar to the "ideal consenter," whose existence is rightly called into question, Beauchamp and Childress's notion of autonomy is at best an ideal. No agent has this level of perfect autonomy. Hence, Beauchamp and Childress endorse a sliding scale in which autonomy comes in degrees, just as the components of autonomy—authentic intention, understanding, and freedom from constraints—come in degrees. In the real world "most actual prospective subjects are vulnerable to a range of decisional deficiencies or impairments that render them unable to protect their own interests or advance their aims" (Wertheimer, 2011, p. 20). Onora O'Neill points out that informed consent makes it possible for individuals to choose autonomously, but this does not necessarily guarantee anything about "self-mastery, or reflective endorsement, or self-control, or rational reflection, or second-order desires," or many other presumed hallmarks of autonomy (O'Neill, 2002, p. 37). Wertheimer argues we need to face up to the inherent paternalism in the research enterprise. Policies such as the Common Rule[1] are constructed, in part, to protect groups of individuals by promoting their good when their autonomy is compromised—a stance that Wertheimer dubs "group soft paternalism." Otherwise "competent" research subjects enter studies based on less-than-autonomous or authentic consent all the time.

While this chapter focuses on the autonomy protections of informed consent, and the limits of consent, autonomy is, of course, not the only value that requires protection in human subjects research. Beauchamp and Childress's other principles—beneficence, nonmalefience, and justice—are cited as justifications for a positive ratio of benefits

[1] The Common Rule is the set of regulations that guides the protection of human research subjects as adopted by 14 United States governmental agencies. It was part of the National Research Act of 1974, which created rules for research at the Department of Health and Human Services (which includes the National Institutes of Health), and adopted by 14 additional agencies in 1991. A revision of the Common Rule, which extends to 15 agencies, as well as the Department of Health and Human Services, was adopted in July 2018 and fully implemented as of January 2019. See https://www.hhs.gov/ohrp/regulations-and-policy/regulations/finalized-revisions-common-rule/index.html.

over risks, for minimizing risks to all research participants, and for just and fair subject selection. Virtues of researchers, such as integrity, honesty, and objectivity, also contribute to an ethical research process. The fact that this chapter focuses on autonomy and informed consent in no way implies that autonomy is the sole, or even preeminent, principle when protecting research participants. Some have argued that autonomy, far from first among equals, is secondary to other considerations in research ethics (Litton and Miller, 2005; Miller and Brody, 2003). Given that informed consent is the subject of this chapter, however, and that informed consent is consistently cited as a means of protecting autonomy, questions of autonomy will be of special consideration here.

There are, of course, many ways in which autonomy may be compromised: disease status may compel research participation for some persons desperate for a cure; a controlled living environment such as a prison or nursing home may limit voluntariness; interminable "informed consent" documents laden with technical terms can erode rather than promote understanding. The distinctions between legal competence to make a decision, and decision-making capacity, and the elements of each, have been discussed in detail elsewhere (DuBois, 2008; Grisso and Appelbaum, 1998). This chapter's focus is on the *cognitive* aspects of autonomy. My argument is that typically developed persons, as well as persons with cognitive impairments, labor under cognitive difficulties when choosing to participate in research. It is widely assumed that the ability to make autonomous decisions may be compromised for those diagnosed with cognitive impairments. My contention is that cognitive barriers to autonomous decision-making have been understated in so-called typical individuals; as such, the gulf between the ability of typical individuals to make autonomous decisions about research participation and the ability of persons with cognitive impairments to make decisions about research participation is not as great as we think. In some cases the best way to address this gulf is to act more paternalistically towards typical individuals. However, in most cases what is called for is to act *less paternalistically towards cognitively impaired individuals*. My views are in keeping with those of Donald L. Rosenstein and Franklin G. Miller, who argue that many individuals who have mental disabilities that may affect decision-making capacity (DMC) nonetheless "are quite capable of providing informed consent for research participation. Furthermore, impaired DMC represents just one of several ways in which research subjects can be 'vulnerable.'" (Rosenstein and Miller, 2008, p. 438).

Rosenstein and Miller rightly observe that the complexities of decision-making are not well understood either in typically developing persons or in persons with cognitive impairments. Furthermore, given the fact that decisional impairment, like autonomy, is best understood on a sliding scale—determined by factors such as the degree of impairment, the decision the person is being asked to make, and the persons who are doing the asking—there is not a one-size-fits-all analysis as to which persons are competent to make which decisions. "[Decision-making capacity] is more accurately conceptualized as a skill set that varies along a continuum from incapacitated to fully capacitated" (Rosenstein and Miller, 2008, p. 439). My discussion here does not pertain to those who are fully incapacitated such that they would require surrogate decision-makers to enroll in research, or research advanced directives, as those cases have been discussed at length elsewhere (Grisso and Appelbaum, 1998; Cantor, 2005; DuBois, 2008; Chapter 3 in this volume). Rather, my focus is on individuals with mild or moderate cognitive impairments—those often afforded the opportunity to offer assent while requiring the legal permission of a guardian or representative, but may in fact be able to *consent* to participation themselves. Persons with cognitive impairments deserve the respect and dignity to make decisions, just as their typically developed peers do.

In earlier work (Barnbaum, 2008) I called the move towards greater respect and dignity for persons with autism "autistic integrity." Autistic integrity includes the right of adults with autism to live their lives without being forcibly cured, being compelled to live according to the social norms of persons who are neurotypical. The call for autistic integrity came from an entirely different argument, however: *Once autism and the unique lives of persons with autism is understood*, it follows that paternalism on the part of neurotypical individuals towards persons with autism is morally wrong. Here I begin by *first discussing persons who are typically developed*, examining the cognitive errors typically developing persons make when choosing to be research participants. Once the cognitive errors on the part of persons who are typically developed are reviewed it becomes clear that the differences among persons who are typical and persons who have cognitive impairments is not that great. The conclusion—that paternalism is unwarranted—is nonetheless the same. We allow typically developed individuals to make decisions that are not adequately informed, but we don't leap to paternalistic interference to correct perceived mistakes.[2] Persons with cognitive impairments deserve the dignity of choice, without the paternalistic over-reach that erodes their personhood.

## Three cognitive constraints: the therapeutic misconception, unrealistic optimism, and a lack of appreciation

It would be prohibitive to catalogue all of the ways in which persons with typically developed cognitive capacities are subject to cognitive constraints when offering informed consent to research participation. Furthermore, it would be prejudicial to assume that all typically developed persons share the same deficits in understanding. As with persons with cognitive impairments—individuals with their own unique strengths and weaknesses—there is no single profile of typically developing persons. Here I examine three well-known cognitive constraints that affect decision-making among typically developed persons.

[2] A classic example is the "right to folly," which gives persons who have the mental capacity to make their own decisions the right to make "bad" choices. For a discussion of this right see American Bar Association/American Psychological Association Assessment of Capacity in Older Adults Project Working Group, 2008. *Assessment of Older Adults with Diminished Capacity: A Handbook for Psychologists*. Washington DC: American Bar Association Commission on Law and Aging and American Psychological Association, pp. 10–11.

The therapeutic misconception is a well-documented phenomenon in which research participants mistakenly believe that enrolling in research will convey direct benefit. According to Paul Appelbaum and Charles Lidz, the therapeutic misconception can be manifest in one of two ways:

> (1) an incorrect belief that the patient/participant's individualized needs will determine assignment to treatment conditions or lead to modifications of the treatment regime (TM1), or (2) an unreasonable appraisal of the nature or likelihood of medical benefit from participation in the study, due to misperception of the nature of the research enterprise (TM2) (Appelbaum and Lidz, 2008)

According to this characterization, a therapeutic misconception may manifest either as a mistaken belief that research regimens are informed by the individual patient's treatment needs, or a mistaken belief that the nature of research is to benefit research participants. Appelbaum and Lidz examine survey data, as well as anecdotal evidence, that demonstrate the prevalence of the therapeutic misconception. In one of many examples, they cite Cassileth et al. (1982), who recount one survey in which only 5% of respondents said that direct medical benefit was a generic reason to participate in medical research, and yet 52% of respondents said *their own participation* would be driven by their desire to get the best medical care.

A cognitive error closely related to the therapeutic misconception is referred to by Horng and Grady (2003) as "therapeutic misestimation," in which research subjects either underestimate the risk, or overestimate the benefit, of research participation. Participants laboring under therapeutic misestimation have a misunderstanding of the odds of either success or failure of their participation: "Research participants may interpret probability data differently and [that] participants may be predisposed to interpret probability data in their own favor" (Horng and Grady, 2003, p. 13). Therapeutic misestimation is distinct from the therapeutic misconception in that participants who suffer from therapeutic misestimation have an understanding of the *nature* of research participation; however, they do not appreciate the odds of receiving benefit or harm by virtue of their participation.

Finally, Jansen et al. describe "the possibility that optimistic expectations for benefit are tied to a bias that distorts, or has the potential to distort, how patients process information about the potential risks and benefits of clinical trials" (2011, p. 1). They refer to this undue expectation of a positive outcome as "optimistic bias" or "unrealistic optimism." Unlike with therapeutic misestimation, participants with unrealistic optimism understand the odds of receiving benefit or harm when serving in research, they just do not think those odds apply to them. Jansen et al. do not see unrealistic optimism as a cognitive mistake so much as a bias that causes people to reframe the information that they are given, but in such a way as to "compromise the informed consent in clinical trials... by interfering with the ability to apply information realistically" (Jansen et al., 2011, p. 5). Even when participants understand the objective of research, their role in a study, and the odds associated with the chance of benefit, some participants nonetheless assume the best case scenario as a result of their participation (Swekoski and Barnbaum, 2013). They believe that they *will* get the experimental therapy. They believe that the experimental therapy *will* cure them.

Jansen (2014) refers to therapeutic misconception, therapeutic misestimation, and unrealistic optimism as examples of "therapeutic error." These errors are the result of mindsets—"cognitive orientations that help us to solve certain tasks" (Jansen, 2014, p. 26). Jansen believes that participants undergo a shift from a deliberative mindset, during which they make a choice to serve as a research subject, to an implementation mindset once they have accepted the role as a research subject. The implementation mindset—the mindset that agents adopt after having chosen a certain goal so as to affect the execution of that goal—often disposes agents to unrealistic optimism. This mindset sets people up for success, fostering persistence and an expectation that they will achieve their goal. It makes sense that once an agent decided to take a course of action that the mind would shift towards an optimistic bias that the agent's objectives would be obtained. "Mindset theory thus reveals an interesting way by which one's cognitive orientation mediates risk perception," according to Jansen (2014, p. 27). Since the implementation mindset is characterized by unrealistic expectations for success this may account for all of the aforementioned versions of therapeutic error.

A final example of a cognitive error in informed consent is offered by Grisso and Appelbaum (1998)—the concept of "appreciation." Appreciation is a two-pronged concept, characterized by both the acknowledgment of the patient or participant's circumstances, as well as the acknowledgement of the consequences of those circumstances and the treatment or research options presented to the individual. Appreciation is not mere awareness of facts; rather, "sometimes it is used to refer to understanding that goes beyond a factual grasp of consequences to an experiential sense of what the consequences would 'really' entail" (Grisso and Appelbaum, 1998, p. 43). Hence, appreciation mirrors Beauchamp and Childress's notion that autonomy is not merely about having the information available to make a rational decision, but requires makes a decision based on a *understanding* of that information. As summarized by Rosenstein and Miller, appreciation:

> ... is generally understood as the extent to which subjects understand the relevance of the research activity to their particular circumstances. For example, knowledge that a clinical trial includes both a placebo and an active medication arm demonstrates "understanding." In contrast, a full awareness that one may actually receive a placebo and as a result forgo other available treatment is an example of "appreciation" (2008, p. 443).

DuBois says that appreciation "requires that potential participants not only understand the relevant information but believe it and relate it to their own situation" (2008, p. 79). Jansen holds that unrealistic optimism could compromise appreciation, because this bias could interfere with the processing of information and the way participants relate it to their own situations. To elaborate, Grisso and Appelbaum present three requirements that characterize a failure of appreciation: (1) the belief must be substantially irrational, unrealistic, or a considerable distortion of reality; (2) the belief must be the consequence of impaired cognition or affect; and (3) the belief must be relevant to the treatment (or, in this case, research participant) decision. The second of these requirements is of the greatest interest here. While it is possible that a failure of appreciation could emerge from impaired cognition, false beliefs about treatment or research participation can result from other circumstances other than impaired cognition, such as denial or depression. In other words, typically developed persons who are otherwise autonomous may suffer from a lack of appreciation when offering informed consent. The safest non-paternalistic stance is to assume capacity to consent from all persons, but to nonetheless verify this capacity by judiciously probing for cognitive constraints, lest one of these constraints results in a person being taken advantage of.

## Addressing cognitive constraints and the lessons for persons with cognitive impairments

Wertheimer's view is that thwarting research participation by otherwise autonomous participants on the basis of a therapeutic misconception is too restrictive. Doing so may place a greater burden on subjects to comprehend information than they would wish, it may restrict freedom of choice to participate in research that may benefit the subjects, and requiring participants to "comprehend" all aspects of a study places too great a burden on researchers (Wertheimer, 2011, p. 104). Despite the fact that Jansen recognizes unrealistic optimism may affect the ability to process information, this recognition does not constitute a reason not to enroll persons with unrealistic optimism in research. Rather, she urges researchers to "pay more attention to how patient-subjects apply information to themselves and to become more aware of the social-psychological factors that might impair decision-making in this context" (Jansen, 2011, p. 7). This same recommendation applies when failures of appreciation appear to cloud the judgment of otherwise cognitively able persons. Working closely with research participants to understand why they make the choices they make—as part of an ongoing consent process, without paternalistically steering their choices—is an essential part of respecting participants' autonomy. Here Jansen echoes Howell and Shogren (Chapter 3) that the burden of making a consenting process clear to a potential participant falls squarely on the shoulders of researchers.

Wertheimer's view is that consent to research is like consent in other realms—often imperfect, not necessarily a guarantee that the person consenting will benefit, and subject to extensive background conditions that in many cases render the consent itself less morally transformative than we expect. The moral transformation that takes place when consent is offered is part of a large complex of protections that collectively contribute to the moral permissibility of research. In the research context, for example, the elaborate mechanisms in place to protect research subjects include institutional review boards, data safety monitoring committees, institutional protections, and even the integrity of researchers.

Jansen reaches similar conclusions to Wertheimer, for different reasons. On the one hand, if mindset theory is correct, then the deliberative phase, during which informed consent to participate in research takes place, may not be burdened with the therapeutic errors that characterize the implementation phase in which the participant serves as a research subject. This assumes, of course, that participants are genuinely deliberating about the choice to participate in research prior to consent—that their minds are not already made up. On the other hand, it may be the case that the therapeutic errors made by trial participants are merely exacerbated by the implementation mindset. Or, more troubling for Jansen, voluntariness of continued participation may be compromised by the unrealistic optimism that characterizes the implementation mindset. Jansen endorses what she calls a *diachronic deliberative model* of informed consent, in which consent is recognized as an ongoing process and not a one-time event of writing a signature, and in which investigators encourage participants to revisit their goals in serving in research so as to engage the deliberative mindset. Notably, while she thinks that these mindsets can compromise informed decision making, Jansen does not make any type of paternalistic move here. Subjects should be induced to engage a deliberative mindset when revisiting the benefits and risks of continuing in research, but it is their choice to continue to participate or not.

When dealing with the typically cognitively developed subject, the remedies to the aforementioned cognitive errors are straightforward: more education; consent documents and a consent process that take into account varying levels of comprehension and appreciation; creating a consent environment that decreases anxiety and helps to restore a sense of empowerment; patience and respect. Paternalistically preventing the typically developed subject from participating in research, because we are afraid they will fall prey to a therapeutic misconception, therapeutic misestimation, unrealistic optimism, or a failure of appreciation, is not a solution that respects the agency of that research participant. But these same remedies—more education, consent documents, and a consent process crafted to take into account the capacities of the individuals consenting, reducing anxiety while increasing empowerment, patience, and respect—are just as applicable to persons with mild or moderate cognitive impairments as they are to typically developed participants. There may be some instances in which greater care should be taken to ensure that a person with cognitive impairments is not unduly compromised in their efforts to offer informed consent. For example, the MacArthur Competence Assessment Tool for Clinical Research (MacCAT-CR), developed by Grisso and Appelbaum, and endorsed by Rosenstein and Miller, is one possible means of assessing appreciation in persons with cognitive impairments recruited to participate in research. DuBois (2008) also endorses this instrument.

There are substantive ways in which the consent process itself may be improved. Heerman et al. (2016) describe an enhanced informed consent process that involves writing consent forms at below an eighth-grade reading level, explaining any health-related jargon in the consent form, developing visual aids to facilitate comprehension, and using open-ended teach-back methods to gauge understanding among prospective participants. Graphic presentations of elements of the research, such as the timeline for participation, concepts such as randomization, and the types of interventions that participants will undergo, may further facilitate comprehension. Palmer et al. (2012) report that visual aides are superior to text when explaining the relationship among component concepts. For example, when explaining the two arms of a study, and what participants can expect each arm, a graphic that illustrates two distinct paths, and the interventions that happen as participants travel along each path, is helpful. Additional time may be needed to craft consent forms that speak to individuals with cognitive impairments that adequately address their concerns and comprehension levels. Consent should be obtained in an environment that puts potential participants at ease, and is devoid of distractions that may compromise understanding. Investigators should have expertise communicating to diverse individuals. For example, Heerman et al.'s methodology included four hours of training, four to six hours of mock practice sessions, and certification from the project coordinator for individuals who obtained consent from prospective participants. The four hours of training was not merely dedicated to understanding aspects of the study, but also to ensuring that the individuals procuring consent knew the value of consent.

The above processes merely scratch the surface of interventions that can facilitate better understanding of research participation. It should be clear that these recommendations should not be restricted to persons with cognitive impairments, or to those without cognitive impairments—these methods can facilitate autonomous consent for everyone. *All participants*, including those with mild or moderate cognitive impairments, should be equally represented in research and treated with equal levels of dignity. Autonomy may come in degrees, as Beauchamp and Childress's sliding scale notion implies, but all persons deserve that whatever degree of autonomy they *do* have should be recognized.

## Objections: proving too much, or historically tone-deaf?

I am advocating for more representation of persons with cognitive impairments in research, based on the claim that their "imperfect" consent is not so different from the "imperfect" consent of typically developed persons, and the remedies to address these imperfections are similar in both cases. Some might object to this argument on the grounds that, if it is the case that the remedies to imperfect consent are similar for both persons who are cognitively typical and persons who are cognitively impaired, then there is no reason for researchers to use typically developing individuals in research when a population of persons with cognitive impairments is available. Imagine a hospital located across the street from a residential home for persons with developmental disabilities. The hospital has contracted to recruit five participants for a multi-site trial of a new flu vaccine. Why, if any barriers to autonomous decision-making exist in both populations, should the local principle investigator (PI) go to the time and trouble of recruiting from the primary care clinics at the hospital when the residential home is so convenient?

This objection appears to miss the point of my claims. I am not claiming that the barriers to autonomous decision-making are *identical* in the cognitively typical and cognitively impaired populations. Both may have barriers to autonomous decision-making, and those barriers may be more or less compromising to autonomy. The local PI, in the earlier example, is making the same mistake in recruiting people out of the residential home as an investigator who chooses any convenience sample, or who would consciously choose to enroll children too young to either consent or assent, because relying solely on the consent of their parents or guardians is quick and easy. The fact that there are similar barriers to autonomous decision-making in both populations, or that the remedies to these barriers are similar, is not an excuse to use a convenience sample of persons with cognitive impairments in research. The use of convenience samples raises questions of justice and fair subject selection in any research study. In this case those injustices are further exacerbated by the known compromises in the autonomy of the residential patients—not just compromises in virtue of their cognitive abilities, but in virtue of living in what may be a restrictive environment.

A related objection may be to downplay the role of consent from any research participant, whether cognitively impaired or not.[3] While current, highly legalistic informed consent documents have received their share of derision over the years, Feldman is right to recognize the separateness of persons, each with different intentions, hopes, and wishes, as the basis of requesting consent. Consent, imperfect as it is, is the best means of recognizing, and protecting, the autonomy of each person, by acknowledging that uniqueness.

A second concern is that research on persons with cognitive impairments is distinct from research on cognitively typical persons because there is a history of abuse of individuals with cognitive impairments in the research setting. Consider the violations at Willowbrook State School in which children with cognitive impairments were intentionally infected with viral hepatitis (Shamoo and Resnik, 2009, DuBois 2008). Although the children at Willowbrook were significantly more impaired than persons with mild or moderate cognitive impairments discussed in this chapter, the lessons of that terrible event still stand. Abuses such as Willowbrook loom large when we consider the ethics of human subjects research, uttered in the same breath as abuses such as the Tuskegee syphilis study or the misuse of prisoners in medical research, as recounted in Allen M. Hornblum's (1998) *Acres of Skin: Human Experiments at Holmsburg Prison*. However, the lesson from Tuskegee and the long history of abuse of prisoners was *not to disallow* persons of color or prisoners in research. Rather, the lesson is to look to better risk/benefit ratios, better subject protection, fairer subject selection, and *more autonomous decision-making* on the part of potential participants, *not less*. It would be a grave injustice for the lesson of Tuskegee to be that persons of color should be paternalistically shielded from serving as research subjects, both because such a prohibition risks

[3] This possibility was suggested by an editor of this volume.

infantilizing persons of color, and because it limits the generalizable knowledge gained from research on underrepresented individuals. Similarly, the fact that there have been historical violations of persons with cognitive impairments in research is not a reason to fall back on paternalism; rather, it is a sentinel warning to allow for *greater* autonomous decision-making, not *less*.

## Conclusion

Elsewhere I have argued adults on the autism spectrum should not be forcibly cured, were a cure to become available. I term my position a call for "autistic integrity"—allowing adults on the autism spectrum to live out their lives without being forced into an existence foreign to the only one they have ever known (Barnbaum, 2008; see also Chapter 5, this volume, for a discussion of research on persons with autism). My position requires expending more resources in the neurotypical community, to better serve persons who are neurodiverse. Paternalistically expecting that persons who are neurodiverse would prefer the life of persons who are neurotypical is a mistake. Persons who are neurodiverse deserve the dignity that comes from being recognized as separate persons, and the freedom to live out their lives in the way that they choose.

In a similar vein, here I argue it is a mistake to paternalistically restrict persons with cognitive impairments from serving as research subjects. Are these two claims in a similar vein, some may ask? After all, "autistic integrity" eschews forcing treatment on persons who are neurodiverse, whereas the other case has to do with researchers' obligations to protect autonomy, and the rights of persons with cognitive impairments to have the dignity of choice that comes with informed consent. The similarity comes from taking the preferences and desires—the separateness of persons—seriously in both cases. A person on the autism spectrum who is happy with her life should be granted the dignity of that happiness being recognized and respected. A person with mild or moderate cognitive impairments, when faced with the choice to participate in research, should be granted the dignity of his preferences being recognized and respected. When persons with mild or moderate cognitive impairments are presumed unable to offer informed consent routinely expected from typical persons, we sell short the cognitive capacities of those with impairments, while at the same time over-selling the cognitive capacities of the typically developed persons. Typically developed persons fall prey to cognitive errors when choosing to serve as research subjects, but the response to those mistakes is not to paternalistically bar persons who are cognitively developed from research participation. The lesson from the troubling history of research violations has never been to prohibit entirely some individuals from being able to be research subjects. Rather, the response is to offer more education, clearer consent forms, and a more robust consenting process. In other words, the research community may expend more resources to engage persons with mild and moderate cognitive impairments in research, but researchers owe persons with cognitive impairments their right to autonomy and the agency to make choices. Feldman's separateness of persons, as spelled out in the introduction to this chapter, demands typically developed persons are accorded the respect and dignity that comes from making their own choices, based on their own intentions, hopes, wishes, and experiences. Persons with cognitive impairments are owed nothing less.

## References

Appelbaum, P. S. and Lidz, C. W. (2008). "The Therapeutic Misconception," in *The Oxford Textbook of Clinical Research Ethics*, Emanuel E.J., Miller, F. G., and Reidar, L., eds. New York: Oxford University Press, Chapter 58.

Barnbaum, D. R. (2008). *The Ethics of Autism: Among Them But Not of Them*. Bloomington, IN: Indiana University Press.

Beauchamp, T. R. and Childress, J. F. (2013). *The Principles of Biomedical Ethics*. New York: Oxford University Press.

Cantor, N. L. (2005). *Making Medical Decisions for the Profoundly Mentally Disabled*. Cambridge, MA: MIT University Press.

Cassileth, B. R., Lusk, E. J., Miller, D. S., Hurwitz, M. S. (1982). "Attitudes Towards Clinical Trials Among Patient and the Public." *Journal of the American Medical Association*, 248: 968–970.

DuBois, J. M. (2008). *Ethics in Mental Health Research: Principles, Guidance, and Cases*. New York: Oxford University Press.

Feldman, H. L. (2014). "What's Right about the "Medical Model" in Human Subjects Research Regulation," in *Human Subjects Research Regulation: Perspectives on the Future*, Cohen, G. and Fernandez Lynch H, eds. Cambridge, MA: MIT University Press, pp. 299–312.

Grisso, T. and Appelbaum, . S. (1998). *Assessing Competence to Consent to Treatment: A Guide for Physicians and Other Health Professionals*. New York: Oxford University Press.

Heerman, W. J., White, R. O., Hotop, A., Omlung, K., Armstrong, S., Matheiu, I., Sherwood, N.E., and Barkin, S.L. (2016). "A Toolkit to Enhance the Informed Consent Process for Community-Engaged Pediatric Research." *IRB: Ethics & Human Research*, 38/5: 8–14.

Hornblum, A. M. 1998. *Acres of Skin: Human Experiments at Holmsberg Prison*. New York: Routledge.

Horng, S. and Grady, C. (2003). "Misunderstanding in Clinical Research: Distinguishing the Therapeutic Misconception, Therapeutic Misestimation, and Therapeutic Optimism." *IRB: Ethics & Human Research*, 25/1: 11–16.

Jansen, L. A. (2014). "Mindsets, Informed Consent, and Research." *Hastings Center Report*, 44: 25–32.

Jansen, L. A., Appelbaum, P. S., Klein, W. M. P., Weinstein, N. D., Cook, W., Fogel, J. S., and Sulmsasy, D. P. (2011). "Unrealistic Optimism in Early-Phase Oncology Trials." *IRB: Ethics & Human Research*, 33/1: 1–8.

Litton, P. and Miller, F. G. (2005). "A Normative Justification for Distinguishing the Ethics of Clinical Research from the Ethics of Medical Care." *The Journal of Law, Medicine, and Ethics*, 33/3: 556–574.

Miller, F. G. and Brody, H. (2003). "A Critique of Clinical Equipoise: Therapeutic Misconception in the Ethics of Clinical Trials." *Hastings Center Report*, 33/3: 19–28.

O'Neill, O. (2002). *Autonomy and Trust in Bioethics*. Cambridge: Cambridge University Press.

Palmer, B. W., Lanouette, N. M., and Jeste, D. V. (2012). "Effectiveness of Multi-Media Aids to Enhance Comprehension of Research Consent Information: A Systematic Review." *IRB: Ethics & Human Research*, 34/6: 1–15.

Rosenstein, D. L. and Miller, F. G. (2008). "Research Involving Those at Risk for Impaired Decision-Making Capacity," in *The Oxford Textbook of Clinical Research Ethics*, Emanuel E.J., Miller, F. G., and Reidar, L., eds. New York: Oxford University Press, Chapter 41.

Schrag, Z. (2014). "What is This Thing Called Research?" in *Human Subjects Research Regulation: Perspectives on the Future*. Cambridge, MA: MIT University Press, pp. 285–298.

Shamoo, A. E. and Resnik, D. B. (2009). *Responsible Conduct of Research*. New York: Oxford University Press.

Swekoski, D. and Barnbaum, D. (2013). "The Gambler's Fallacy, the Therapeutic Misconception, and Unrealistic Optimism." *IRB: Ethics & Human Research*, 35/2: 1–6.

Wertheimer, A. (2011). *Rethinking the Ethics of Clinical Research: Widening the Lens*. New York: Oxford University Press.

# 5

# Autism, Autonomy, and Research

*Kenneth A. Richman*

## Introduction

Autistic individuals (*autists*) differ from non-autistic individuals (most of whom can be called *neurotypicals*) in ways that raise specific ethical challenges for recruiting autists to participate in research. Autism is associated with processes relevant to informed consent, such as understanding the intentions and predicting the behaviors of others, and appreciating the practical and social implications of decisions. In this chapter, I introduce the aspects of autonomy relevant to informed consent for participation in research, identify overlap between the functions that can be challenged in autism and the functions required for informed consent, and discuss the ethical and practical implications of this overlap. I then examine additional issues that arise when we consider not just participation in research in general, but autists participating in research on autism.

Autists can have widely varying experiences of everyday life. A great many autists find their autism to be a neutral or positive part of who they are; others experience substantial challenges. Autists with profound difficulties commonly have complex neuropsychological profiles that can involve intellectual disability, alexithymia, anxiety, or other factors. This chapter focuses on differences autistic individuals have by virtue of their autism, setting aside the impact of other features that may coexist. It will not apply to autists who are non-verbal or who have very limited observable orientation toward others.

## Autonomy and consent

Respect for autonomy is put into action by enrolling individuals in research only when they have given valid informed consent. The elements of informed consent are described variously but include at least the three key components identified in the Belmont Report: information, comprehension, and voluntariness (National Commission, 1979, p. 6).

Perhaps the most significant feature of autonomy is how fragile it is. Information is reduced through poor or incomplete disclosure. Comprehension can be reduced through factors that limit taking in and appreciating the information, such as lack of education, intellectual disability, or anxiety. Voluntariness can be reduced by a sense of duty to authority figures or anyone who may have control over one's health care, undue influence by family members, poor impulse control, or other factors.

Operationalizing their understanding of autonomy for informed consent, Beauchamp and Childress identify threshold elements (preconditions), information elements, and consent elements. For informed consent to be possible, the threshold elements of competence and voluntariness must be satisfied. The information elements require disclosure, "recommendation (of a plan)," and understanding of the previous two. Beauchamp and Childress identify decision and authorization as the consent elements (Beauchamp and Childress, 2016, p. 124).

Despite continued emphasis on the consent document itself, it has become expected to speak of consent for research as a process and not just a signature. Central to this process is *dialogue* between provider and patient (for treatment), or investigator and participant (for research) (Lidz et al., 1988). Through this dialogue, the professional is expected to provide not only any information that is specifically requested, but also whatever a reasonable person in the other's place would want to know (Herring et al., 2017). Gently and carefully applied, this "process" approach holds promise of smoothing over some of the roughness of simply presenting information and asking for a yes or no response. Community advisory boards and public consultation are other ways to address the complications of the consent process (Fisher and Wallace, 2000).

To put autism-specific challenges in context, we should note that all research participants are at risk of reduced autonomy. To start with, much research is aimed at understanding precisely those conditions that reduce autonomy. Furthermore, we know that people often see researchers as authority figures. Research subjects are thus characteristically at risk of coercion (even if unintended). However, this does not mean that they can never make choices that should be honored under a duty of respect for autonomy.

## Autism and related challenges

We have seen several essential elements of informed consent: information (disclosure), comprehension (understanding), voluntariness, engaging in dialogue, deciding, and authorizing. Researchers are responsible for disclosing information. They also have a role in facilitating the other elements. How might autism affect an autist's comprehension, voluntariness, dialogue, deciding, and authorizing in the context of informed consent for research? Are any of these harder or just different for autists compared to others?[1]

[1] Multiple competing models have been offered to explain the neuropsychological mechanisms characteristic of autists. These cognitive models focus variously on theory of mind (Baron-Cohen, 1995), executive function (Leung et al., 2016), central coherence (Happé and Frith, 2006), empathy imbalance (Smith, 2009), or other features. Rather than choose one model or survey them all, I will make use of whatever theories connect to the competencies required for consent, taking each competency in turn.

## Comprehension

Comprehension requires that participants understand the research procedures and associated risks and benefits. Participants must understand the intention of the researcher(s), who will be implementing and shaping the meaning of the research activities. Difficulties with theory of mind tasks, such as understanding what the researcher or recruiter intends to get out of the interaction (Baron-Cohen et al., 1985), are known features of autism that can reduce understanding.

Atypically low executive function in "cognitive flexibility" among autists (Russo et al., 2007) could also reduce understanding. Autists are known to have "a need for sameness, a strong liking for repetitive behaviours, lack of impulse control, difficulty initiating new non-routine actions and difficulty switching between tasks" (Robinson et al., 2009, p. 362). Because autism research often takes place in healthcare settings and involves healthcare providers (Pellicano et al., 2014), low cognitive flexibility may make requests for research participation unexpected and hard to comprehend. Indeed, earnest medical researchers report difficulties getting neurotypical patients to see how research differs from the health care they usually receive in medical settings (Miller, 2000). We would expect it to be even harder for autists to direct attention to the specific character of research if they do not have regular experience participating.

Higher-order executive functions, such as "reasoning, problem solving, and planning" (Diamond, 2013), depend on executive function in other domains. This could affect an autist's ability to appreciate the steps involved in participating. One could agree to participate without realizing how this might be disruptive or uncomfortable. Knowing what to expect can be especially important for the many autists who experience atypically strong sensitivity to sensory input (American Psychiatric Association, 2013).

## Voluntariness

With or without support and assistance, participants should be able to do these things or refrain from them by their own choice, without being forced or unduly influenced. This falls under a broader concept of *authenticity*.

It is important to recognize that autism is not a mental illness like depression or schizophrenia. Autism does not interfere with people expressing their authentic selves; autism is integral to an autist's self (Sinclair, 2012).

At the same time, being autistic in a mostly neurotypical society can make it difficult to act on authentic preferences. Autists who are not entirely independent may depend on a "gatekeeper"—someone, such as a parent, guardian, or physician, who can paternalistically block access or veto decisions. It may be difficult for neurotypical gatekeepers to accept choices as authentic or autonomous when those choices do not make sense to them. For instance, a choice may involve a preference for sameness or avoidance of uncomfortable sensory experience (perhaps even the smell of the researcher), which a gatekeeper cannot make sense of or even recognize. Lack of insight on the part of a gatekeeper can limit free exercise of authentic choices.

Autists may be especially vulnerable to "oppressive socialization" (Sisti and Stramondo, 2015, p. 68). For instance, autistic children receive strong encouragement to fit in and do what is "expected" (Richman, 2015), which can make authentic action appear off limits. In addition, autists' relatively strong emotional empathy (Smith, 2009) may make the prospect of disappointing others particularly uncomfortable. These factors can reduce voluntariness.

## Dialogue

Participants should be able to engage in pragmatic conversational exchanges to ask for and receive information relevant to the proposed research (Lidz et al., 1988). This directly connects with the diagnostic criteria for autism, which include "Persistent deficits in social communication and social interaction" (American Psychiatric Association, 2013, p. 50). These can involve "failure of normal back-and-forth conversation," "failure to initiate or respond to social interactions," and "poorly integrated verbal and nonverbal communication" (American Psychiatric Association, 2013, p. 50). In more neutral language, differences between autists and researchers may make it hard for autists to get researchers to understand their information needs, and researchers may be challenged to determine whether participants' questions have been answered.

## Deciding

Deciding requires considering different options and choosing one (Kalis and Meynen, 2014). Those who cannot think of alternatives or who are unable to make up their minds cannot give valid consent.

Evidence suggests that autists tend to find it harder to think of options and alternatives, an executive function called generativity (Robinson et al., 2009). This could be thought to limit the ability to choose (Kalis and Meynen, 2014). However, autists are perfectly capable of having clear preferences, and the decision required during the consent process usually involves only two options—consenting to participate or declining to participate. Thus, there is no good reason to suggest that autism reduces ability to decide about research participation.

## Authorizing

Authorizing is about expressing one's decision and giving permission for research participation to proceed. This involves social communication, and hence may be subject to difficulties akin to those affecting dialogue. Researchers have responsibility to be sure that participants actually intend to authorize participation before proceeding.

## Addressing these challenges

Based on the analysis presented, autism can pose challenges to obtaining sound informed consent for research. It can pose barriers to understanding, make it harder for gatekeepers to recognize unexpected decisions as authentic, make it harder for autists to hold onto their own preferences in the face of real or perceived expectations from others, and make dialogue with researchers more difficult.

The challenges identified for obtaining ethically sound informed consent from autists for research in general are not much different from the challenges of working with any research participant. People mistake research for treatment, do not understand procedures, feel pressure to agree, and do not know how to ask for the information they need. However, as noted in the previous section, the cognitive functions required for overcoming these challenges can be atypically low for autists. Autists are more likely than neurotypicals to face these difficulties and to need support in addressing them.

With autists, these challenges are also embedded in an atypical framework for processing information. Thus, researchers need to take extra care both to deliver and to receive information. Unlike with neurotypicals, researchers cannot rely on non-verbal communication, assumptions of common knowledge, or conversational implicature. Because many autists often attend to details more than overall import (Happé and Frith, 2006), documents and discussion should highlight key points clearly. Where necessary, a family member or caregiver could help determine what additional information is relevant to specific autists. For example, the need to change from street clothes to an examination gown for a procedure might not be obvious to an autist, and might be much more stressful for some autists than for neurotypical participants. Autists may also need more time to "process, plan, respond" (Buckle, 2016).

Social stories are often used with young autists to prepare them for new situations, and would be an appropriate tool for the context of recruitment for research.[2] A social story for research informed consent might include statements such as "tomorrow I will go to the hospital to see Dr Smith. Dr Smith does many things at the hospital. On some days, she examines patients and helps them live healthy lives. On other days she does research. When she does research, she is not trying to help or hurt anyone. Instead, she is a scientist gathering information." To explain that participation is voluntary, a social story might read "I can say 'yes' or 'no' to Dr Smith when she asks whether I want to be part of her research. If I say 'no,' she will be happy and it will be OK. If I say 'yes,' she will

[2] Beresford and colleagues provide a sample social story for children whose parents have given permission for their participation (Beresford et al., 2004). Their social story includes a few details that might not be important to neurotypical participants, such as the color of the car the interviewer will park outside the participant's house. It describes how to request to stop or take a break from the research interview, but assenting to the research interview is assumed.

be happy and it will be OK. Dr Smith wants me to make my own choice." Most adults won't need such simple language, but it could be offered as a helpful supplement.

Researchers should be prepared to answer very specific questions that could not have been anticipated. An autist might be concerned that participation will disrupt a specific plan or involve exposure to something anxiety-producing. Because variation from what is expected can be especially stressful for autists, researchers must be truthful about any variables or unknowns.

Researchers should be careful when requesting authorization from autists. Leading questions may elicit inauthentic agreement (National Autistic Society, 2017). Other questions may be interpreted more narrowly or more broadly than intended. For instance, "do you think you might like to participate?" could be heard as "can you imagine a possible situation in which you would like to participate?" rather than "do you want to participate now?"[3]

Guardians, non-custodial family members, or carers (those who can serve as "appropriate adults" (The National Autistic Society, 2017)) can insulate participants from perceived pressure to comply with requests from researchers, but they can also be coercive themselves. These appropriate adults could make it difficult for a vulnerable person to decline participation, perhaps because of their own concern that refusal will make it harder for the vulnerable person to get services. Alternatively, those who believe in a right to participate in research (e.g., Shaw, 2014) might object to these "appropriate adults" impeding access to research participation that a vulnerable person would otherwise have authentically chosen. When requesting informed consent, researchers should consider what conditions offer the best balance between support and authenticity: researcher and participant; researcher and participant with appropriate adult; participant and appropriate adult without researcher; or participant alone in a quiet space with a consent form.

Researchers should allow extra time not just for understanding, but also for deciding and authorizing after appropriate dialogue. Researchers should accept "stimming," which could include hand flapping or vocalizations, without assuming it indicates distress or inattention (Stevenson, 2018). They should ask whether autists are comfortable, and offer to adjust room lighting, turn off screens, and so on, to reduce stress and distraction due to sensory issues. These measures can facilitate authentic decision-making.

A researcher's overall attitude toward these challenges is important. Celia B. Fisher suggests "Conceptualizing consent impairments as a product of the relationship between the person and the consent context" rather than focusing on deficits or differences in the participant (Fisher, 2003, p. 27). Fisher is writing about "adults with mental disorders," but the idea can be applied more broadly: challenges will be relational not unilateral. Indeed, while it is common to think of autists as having a one-sided deficit in understanding the thoughts and feelings of others, researchers should recognize

[3] Consider this passage intended to help police understand autism: "... asking, 'Has your laptop got anything on it about plans for any terrorism acts?' is likely to elicit agreement, as a web browser or a text editor could be used to plan anything." (National Autistic Society, 2017).

the "double empathy problem" (Milton, 2012): neurotypical researchers are as likely to have difficulty understanding autists as vice versa.

Furthermore, researchers should understand that they have an obligation to obtain consent but autists have no obligation to give it. While autists should do their part, bridging any gap in understanding is not their responsibility.

## "Identification" and autistic participation in autism research

The discussion thus far has been about consent for research in general. When autists are recruited to participate in research on autism, specific issues arise. Participation in autism research is complicated by the potential mismatch between the goals of researchers (who are often oriented toward curing or preventing autism), and the goals of autists (many of whom find research aimed at cure or prevention profoundly offensive (Autistic Self Advocacy Network, 2018)).

Parents and caregivers may experience this as a real tension. Placed Janus-like between the perspectives of researchers and the perspectives of the autism community, parents and other gatekeepers can feel torn between, on the one hand, embracing the uniqueness of a son or daughter, and, on the other hand, choosing to participate in research in hopes of maximizing the autist's typical function or contributing to cure and prevention. This tension is likely to hit hardest when children are young, parents are still finding their identities in the autism community, and a child's trajectory is uncertain.

This potential mismatch might not seem significant if we consider consent as agreement to participate without regard to how data will be used. However, people are often concerned about how their actions contribute to larger projects. Given that the significance of research is generally defined by the professional researchers who craft the protocols and interpret the data, a robust notion of consent requires that participants understand and accept what they are contributing to.

Hans Jonas offers an ideal conception of this understanding and acceptance in his classic paper "Philosophical Reflections on Experimenting with Human Subjects" (1969). Jonas argues that consent for participation in research is most fully autonomous when the participant can adopt the researcher's goals for the research as her own. On this picture, full consent requires "such authentic identification with the cause [the aims of the research] that it is the subject's as well as the researcher's cause—whereby his role in its service is not just permitted by him, but *willed*" (Jonas, 1969, p. 237).[4]

In this light, autism research may look very different from research on cancer. In cancer research, participants might have unrealistic hopes of benefiting from participating, but they almost certainly have the same overall orientation toward cancer. Even if quite confused about what is going on, they will, in a general way,

[4] Jonas is aware that this ideal of identification is highly restrictive. To satisfy it, researchers would do best to recruit only other researchers, for clearly the research community is the best place to find people who can truly identify with the goals of research (Jonas, 1969, p. 234).

identify with the researcher's goal of reducing the impact of cancer rather than seeing cancer as normal human variation that should be accepted or embraced. In contrast, an autist who agrees to research participation without understanding could end up contributing to an end she would find abhorrent. While full identification (rational convergence (Matthews et al., 2018)) may be much too strong a criterion for valid consent, the scientific goals of research should at least not be anathema to the participants.[5]

These complications do not arise simply because some autists reject categorizing autism as a disorder or do not want to change. Unlike with most conditions attended to by the healthcare establishment, many thoughtful, educated autists and autism allies have argued persuasively that standard outcome measures and assessments may not capture appropriate goals for autism interventions. Autists may have different ideas of the good life, well-being, and health (Rodogno et al., 2016). They may find efforts to make their behavior typical or "normal" to be more disabling than their autism (Milton and Moon, 2012). Studies designed with prevention and cure in mind, and even studies that merely apply standard assessments of behavior and quality of life, may be profoundly out of line with the values of participants. The responsibility to obtain valid informed consent therefore requires that the orientation of the research be made explicit in the consent process.

In this respect, the researcher–participant relationship has parallels with friendships and intimate relationships. If the parties unknowingly want very different things from the relationship, one of them will appear vulnerable and ill-used. There are, of course, non-traditional relationships in which each party agrees to participate with the knowledge that the other party values different aspects of the interaction. With disclosure and understanding, these can be permissible. For instance, it could be permissible to enroll participants who do not especially embrace the study goals, but value test results that become available through participation. Someone else might choose to participate as a form of constructive engagement, hoping to broaden the researchers' perspectives. Given the asymmetry of the researcher-participant relationship in traditional research, these types of participant motivation need not be known to the researcher as long as there is sufficient disclosure from the researcher and understanding by the participant. An exception would be when a participant's motivations threaten to subvert the validity of the data.

There are circumstances, however, when it would be difficult to justify this kind of asymmetric consent. Participants whose settled values oppose those of the research cannot give informed consent without behaving inconsistently or without integrity. If an autistic participant who is committed to a neurodiversity perspective agrees to participate in research oriented toward prevention and cure, consent would be inauthentic and therefore questionable. Researchers who are aware of this happening might have an obligation not to accept such participants in their studies, or at least to pursue further

[5] Note that the concept of therapeutic optimism or unrealistic hope of benefit does not apply when the research is intended to contribute to prevention, "cure," or conformity and the participant does not see these as providing benefit to anyone.

dialogue. If it should happen that commitment to neurodiversity is correlated with factors relevant to obtaining a representative sample of the population, these considerations suggest a dilemma between obtaining authentic consent from all participants and recruiting a population sample that supports valid data and conclusions.

One way to address or even avoid these value conflicts is to implement inclusive or participatory research methods. In community-based participatory research (CBPR), researchers work with members of the community being studied at all stages, including setting the research question. CPBR has been applied in a variety of settings (Fadem et al., 2003). Damian Milton is one researcher leading efforts to develop participatory autism research (Milton et al., 2018). Discussion of specific participatory research methods is outside the scope of this chapter, which assumes a more traditional approach. However, we can see how truly participatory approaches are likely to improve the quality of consent by reducing the chance of discordance between research goals and the values of participants, and by facilitating robust review of consent procedures by those who can appreciate the needs of participants.[6]

## Conclusion

In research ethics, respect for autonomy is operationalized in the process of informed consent. The informed consent process involves some abilities, such as dialogue and understanding the intentions of the researchers, that can be more challenging when researchers recruit autists compared to when they recruit neurotypicals. This chapter reviewed these abilities, and suggested ways to provide meaningful support to promote autonomy in autists and help researchers meet their responsibilities. Beyond these more general challenges, we explored the issue of the participant's identification with the goals of the study and raised concerns about the permissibility of enrolling participants whose values clash with the intended outcomes of the research design.

Anyone who can be supported to make autonomous decisions about research participation should be so supported. This discussion provides some insight into how to do that for autists, and may be helpful for the general population, as well. We have some data about priorities of autists for research (Pellicano et al., 2014). The issues discussed here suggest that additional empirical research on attitudes and procedures around informed consent involving autists could help us develop and validate best practices.

## Acknowledgements

This work builds on a project supported by the Miriam Foundation of Montreal. I am indebted to the volume editors for helpful insights in response to earlier versions.

[6] This chapter was developed in light of previous engagement with autists, and using sources written by autists, but without direct input from any autist reviewer or collaborator.

## References

American Psychiatric Association (2013). *Diagnostic and Statistical Manual of Mental Disorders (DSM-5)*. Washington, DC: American Psychiatric Publishing.

Autistic Self Advocacy Network. (2018). "Position Statements," http://autisticadvocacy.org/about-asan/position-statements/ (accessed August 2018).

Baron-Cohen, S. (1995). *Mindblindness: An Essay on Autism and Theory of Mind*. Cambridge, MA: MIT Press.

Baron-Cohen, S., Leslie, A. M., and Frith, U. (1985). "Does the Autistic Child Have a 'Theory of Mind'?" *Cognition*, 21/1: 37–46.

Beauchamp, T. L. and Childress, J. F. (2016). *Principles of Biomedical Ethics*. New York: Oxford University Press.

Beresford, B., Tozer, R., Rabiee, P., and Sloper, P. (2004). "Developing an Approach to Involving Children With Autistic Spectrum Disorders in a Social Care Research Project." *British Journal of Learning Disabilities*, 32/4: 180–185.

Buckle, L. (2016). "From the Committee to the Laboratory: Autistic Collaboration," https://drive.google.com/file/d/0B83m4GMhHY23TXREYWVxUjFDMm8/view (accessed August 2018).

Diamond, A. (2013). "Executive Functions." *Annual Review of Psychology*, 64: 135–168.

Fadem, P., Minkler, M., Perry, M., Blum, K., Moore, L., and Rogers, J. (2003). "Ethical Challenges in Community-based Participatory Research," in Minkler, M. & Wallerstein, N., eds. *Community-based Participatory Research for Health*. San Francisco, CA: Jossey-Bass, pp. 242–262.

Fisher, C. B. (2003). "Goodness-of-fit Ethic for Informed Consent to Research Involving Adults With Mental Retardation and Developmental Disabilities." *Developmental Disabilities Research Reviews*, 9/1: 27–31.

Fisher, C. B. and Wallace, S. A. (2000). "Through the Community Looking Glass: Reevaluating the Ethical and Policy Implications of Research on Adolescent Risk and Sociopathology." *Ethics & Behaviour*, 10/2: 99–118.

Happé, F. and Frith, U. (2006). "The Weak Coherence Account: Detail-focused Cognitive Style in Autism Spectrum Disorders." *Journal of Autism and Developmental Disorders*, 36/1: 5–25.

Herring, J., Fulford, K., Dunn, M., and Handa, A. (2017). "Elbow Room for Best Practice? Montgomery, Patients' Values, and Balanced Decision-Making in Person-Centred Clinical Care." *Medical Law Review*, 25/4: 582–603.

Jonas, H. (1969). "Philosophical Reflections on Experimenting With Human Subjects." *Daedalus*, 98/2: 219–247.

Kalis, A. and Meynen, G. (2014). "Mental Disorder and Legal Responsibility: The Relevance of Stages of Decision Making." *International Journal of Law and Psychiatry*, 37/6: 601–608.

Leung, R. C., Vogan, V. M., Powell, T. L., Anagnostou, E., and Taylor, M. J. (2016). "The Role of Executive Functions in Social Impairment in Autism Spectrum Disorder." *Child Neuropsychology*, 22/3: 336–344.

Lidz, C. W., Appelbaum, P. S., and Meisel, A. (1988). "Two Models of Implementing Informed Consent." *Archives of Internal Medicine*, 148/6: 1385–1389.

Matthews, D. J., Fins, J. J., and Racine, E. (2018). "The Therapeutic 'Mis' Conception: An Examination of its Normative Assumptions and a Call for its Revision." *Cambridge Quarterly of Healthcare Ethics*, 27/1: 154–162.

Miller, M. (2000). "Phase I Cancer Trials. A Collusion of Misunderstanding." *Hastings Cent Report*, 30/4: 34–43.

Milton, D. E. M. (2012). "On the Ontological Status of Autism: The 'Double Empathy Problem.'" *Disability & Society*, 27/6: 883–887.

Milton, D. and Moon, L. (2012). "The Normalisation Agenda and the Psycho-emotional Disablement of Autistic People." *Autonomy: the Critical Journal of Interdisciplinary Autism Studies*, 1/1.

Milton, D., Ridout, S., Kourti, M., Loomes, G., Martin, N., Murray, D., Stewart, C., Beardon, L., and Booth, J. (2018). "The Participatory Autism Research Collective," https://participatoryautismresearch.wordpress.com/ (accessed August 2018).

National Autistic Society (2017). "Autism: A Guide for Police Officers and Staff," https://www.autism.org.uk/products/core-nas-publications/autism-a-guide-for-criminal-justice-professionals.aspx (accessed August 2018).

National Commission for the Protection of Human Subjects of Biomedical and Behavioral Research (1979). "The Belmont Report," https://www.hhs.gov/ohrp/regulations-and-policy/belmont-report/read-the-belmont-report/index.html (accessed August 2018).

Pellicano, E., Dinsmore, A., and Charman, T. (2014). "What Should Autism Research Focus Upon? Community Views and Priorities From the United Kingdom." *Autism*, 18/7: 756–770.

Richman, K. A. (2015). "Autism, the Social Thinking Curriculum, and Moral Courage." *Power and Education*, 7/3: 355–360.

Robinson, S., Goddard, L., Dritschel, B., Wisley, M., & Howlin, P. (2009). "Executive Functions in Children With Autism Spectrum Disorders." *Brain and Cognition*, 71/3): 362–368.

Rodogno, R., Krause-Jensen, K., & Ashcroft, R. E. (2016). "'Autism and the Good Life': A New Approach to the Study of Well-being." *Journal of Medical Ethics*, 42/6: 401–408.

Russo, N., Flanagan, T., Iarocci, G., Berringer, D., Zelazo, P. D., & Burack, J. A. (2007). "Deconstructing Executive Deficits Among Persons With Autism: Implications for Cognitive Neuroscience." *Brain and Cognition*, 65/1: 77–86.

Shaw, D. (2014). "The Right to Participate in High-Risk Research." *The Lancet*, 38: 1009–1011.

Sinclair, J. (2012). "Don't Mourn for Us." *Autonomy: the Critical Journal of Interdisciplinary Autism Studies*, 1/1.

Sisti, D. & Stramondo, J. (2015). "Competence, Voluntariness, and Oppressive Socialization: A Feminist Critique of the Threshold Elements of Informed Consent." *International Journal of Feminist Approaches to Bioethics*, 8/1: 67–85.

Smith, A. (2009). "The Empathy Imbalance Hypothesis of Autism: A Theoretical Approach to Cognitive and Emotional Empathy in Autistic Development." *The Psychological Record*, 59/3: 9.

Stevenson, P. (2018). "Stim Your Heart Out," https://www.stimyourheartout.com/ (accessed August 2018).

# SECTION 2
# CHALLENGES

# 6

# Disability, Vulnerability, and the Capacity to Consent

*Stephanie Patterson and Pamela Block*

Traditionally, and particularly from the perspective of non-disabled people, the disabled community is considered a "vulnerable" population.[1] Merriam-Webster's dictionary defines the word *vulnerable* as "capable of being physically or emotionally wounded: open to attack or damage" (Merriam-Webster, 2018), and it naturally conjures up visions of helpless babies, neglected animals, children being bullied, and elderly people being abused. The word pulls on our heartstrings, our righteous sensibilities, and our beliefs about the right to be safe and protected. When used to describe (and label) an entire group, it suggests individuals that require "utmost care, specific ancillary considerations and augmented protections" (Shivayogi, 2013).

It cannot be denied that there are members in many communities, some with disability, who need specialized attention and require cautious and thoughtful concern. From an early age, children learn about manners, caring for others, and kindness within their families and social groups. Awareness, sensitivity, and safeguards are important throughout life as individuals interact on a one-to-one basis with each other. It is just a normal part of social experiences. Significant boundaries and safety measures become crucial, however, when individuals interact outside their personal circles with agencies, organizations, governmental facilities, and scientific and educational institutions.

In such circumstances, many people feel intimidated and vulnerable, regardless of whether they are disabled or not. For example, it can be frightening and dehumanizing to become involved with the court system or social services. Although there are continued attempts to address issues like providing individualized customer service and person-centered programs, such entities, by their very nature and the sheer number of customers, are not designed to serve and safeguard individuals. Applying for benefit programs, pursuing higher education, or registering for a driver's license include the experience of being one among many. Though intimidating, eye-opening, and sometimes humbling, these interactions do not entail a high level of actual risk.

This is not the case, however, with participating in research studies. In light of the numerous atrocities that have been committed in the name of research, such as experiments on Nazi Concentration Camp prisoners (Lifton, 1986) and purposely choosing to leave participating African Americans in the Tuskegee Syphilis Experiment uninformed about risks and benefits (Smolin, 2012), it is easy to see why very specific and stringently enforced restrictions to protect *vulnerable* human subjects must be maintained. Such research falls into a hazardous category and can hold significant dangers for anyone involved. Participants cannot automatically assume that the purpose of the research is worthwhile, the researchers are honorable, and that the outcomes will not be harmful to individuals or society.

But does having a disability automatically and categorically render a person vulnerable in such circumstances? Regulations concerning research with human subjects routinely place individuals with disability into the examples of vulnerable populations, especially those with cognitive or intellectual disability diagnoses. Such a practice causes researchers and disability advocates to take long pause. Can it not be argued that when disabled people—those who "are substantially limited in one or more major life activity" (ADA.gov, 2013), or are considered to have visible or invisible mobility, sensory, cognitive, intellectual, or communication impairments—are in fully accessible environments, they are no more at risk for abuse in participating in non-medical research than non-disabled people? Are not the abilities of individuals with the aforementioned diagnoses extremely varied, ranging from either no or merely slight difficulties in decision-making to the complete inability to give informed consent of any kind? Unquestionably, there are some people who cannot make safe and appropriate decisions in certain circumstances, but, clearly, this is not true for everyone. Consequently, inadvertently grouping such subjects into one rank of incapacity is neither accurate nor helpful; and such labeling and discrimination against minority groups is actually both disrespectful and harmful.

Even for people who can exercise full autonomy—the ability to make decisions on one's own—there is no guarantee against being taken advantage of or harmed. According to vulnerability studies scholar Alyson Cole, "Vulnerability is a condition of life . . . It is both universal and particular, constant and yet temporally and contextually varied" (Cole, 2016). Being protected or shielding oneself from harm when making decisions can depend on many factors and circumstances. For example, when deciding whether or not to participate in non-medical research, how, when, and where the delivery of information about risks and benefits is conducted can easily affect anyone's ability to comprehend crucial details needed to make appropriate choices. Full autonomy and invulnerability are not mutually exclusive.

In second author Block's experience and discussions she has had with other researchers and self-advocates, getting approval for people with intellectual and cognitive disabilities to participate or collaborate in research can be complicated. Block was told in the early 2000s by a community member of an institutional review board (IRB) at Brown University, where she was a research assistant professor, that it was not ever possible to be completely sure that individuals with traumatic brain injury (TBI) were capable of consent. It was this psychiatrist's opinion that typical instruments to determine consent, like the Mini-Mental Status Exam (Tombaugh and McIntyre, 1992), were not sufficient to ensure capacity to consent. His inclination was not to allow people with a TBI to participate in the research. Block, along with her research coordinator, who herself had a TBI, had to reason with the IRB staff to gain permission. How strange that this research coordinator, who acquired her master's degree subsequent to her

TBI, be considered capable of running the research but not capable of consenting to participate in it.

A complicated compromise was negotiated between Block and the objecting psychiatrist with a very elongated and simplified version of the consent form developed specifically for anyone with TBI. This experience was not unique. Other researchers have told Block of IRBs not allowing them to engage in collaborative research with people with intellectual disability. They might be research subjects, but not colleagues and collaborators. Others, similar to Block's experience, had difficulties getting their IRBs to even accept the possibility that it could be determined that people with intellectual disability could be capable of consent. Certainly, spoken language and literacy are privileged in the consenting process, though some creative studies involving non-speaking people with dementia have been approved. These studies used drawing and body language to determine consent or assent (Bartlett, 2012). What of individuals with intellectual disability that want to initiate their own research? Must they always be under the shadow of someone without a diagnosis in order to get their research approved?

Sweeping and stereotyping generalizations about people with disability affront the ethical principle of justice—the moral standard of fairness—that assures the "equitable distribution of benefits and burdens to individuals" (Feinsod and Wagner, 2008) within a group, especially as it relates to the autonomy and civil rights of people with disability across many categories. The vulnerable/invulnerable categorization often "produces rigid social hierarchies" and "serves to stigmatize and regulate groups (usually through idioms of risk and self-management)." Taken to the extreme, it can even be considered a mechanism of discipline (Cole, 2016). It is impossible to assure personal autonomy when the very instruments used to establish capacity are discriminatory and in violation of individual civil rights.

The issue becomes more complex because assuring the practice of treating non-disabled and disabled people similarly is not the goal. If considering personal autonomy is truly the task at hand, owing to the wide range of diversity, the concept of "disability justice," as outlined by Mia Mingus (2011), demands "moving away from an equality-based model of sameness and "we are just like you" to a model of disability that embraces difference, confronts privilege, and challenges what is considered "normal" on every front. In this way, disability justice focuses not just on independence, but also the central interdependence that both disabled and non-disabled people experience in the world.

Formulated by disability studies theorists and activists (Ben-Moshe et al., 2014; Burch, 2014; Erevelles, 2002, 2011; Mingus, 2010; Nishida, 2016), a disability justice concept of interdependence acknowledges power disparities and includes an understanding of gender, race, and social status, in addition to disability. Questioning the notion of "independence" as a goal, disability justice fundamentally centers disability experience and expertise as an important component of the ability of disabled people and non-disabled people to work together collectively to support each other. With this in mind, a better approach and simple solution to assuring that no one is harmed by participating in research is maintaining a focus on the *capacity to consent* and the *power to resist manipulation*. These factors are a more helpful dividing line than a disability or impairment category.

## Are disabled people vulnerable?

The term "vulnerable' is used repeatedly in regard to research, but "little consensus exists on what it actually means in the context of human subject protection ... " (Coleman, 2009). This lack of consensus becomes particularly important when noting that as a group and without regard to their circumstances, individuals with disability are considered "at risk" research participants. A person's diagnosis is highly personal and individualized, making the use of the term "physical," "cognitive," or "intellectual" disability completely misleading. Even more pertinent, an individual's abilities and experience under a particular diagnosis classification cannot be assumed or generalized. Personal experiences of a disabling condition cannot be pigeon-holed, making reliance on generalized and uniform rules unfair and illogical.

Any type of standardized test or diagnosis can be scrutinized when it comes to an individual's actual experience. For example, the accuracy of homogenous categorizations of intelligence have been under assault since the 1970s (Benson, 2003); and the diagnosis of autism was broadened to autism spectrum disorder in 2013 because "There is a great range of abilities and characteristics of children with autism spectrum disorders—no two children appear or behave the same way. Symptoms can range from mild to severe and often change over time" (American Psychological Association, 2018). This diversity and individualization of experience can be applicable to people with cognitive disabilities, cancer, quadriplegia, and so on. The list is endless. There is no "one size fits all." If this is true when it comes to diagnosis, how can it not be true when determining vulnerability?

Another troubling assumption is that having a diagnosis inherently reduces a person's capacity to consent and increases their likelihood of incurring stigmatization, stereotyping, and prejudice. The presence of possible discrimination does not automatically and categorically reduce a person's capacity to consent or predispose an individual to "harm" from a research study's unethical practices. There are a host of invisible disabilities that are not apparent to even the most skillfully trained eye. For example, sensory and communication impairments, and seizure and autoimmune conditions, in addition to "cognitive disorders" such as TBI, learning and intellectual disabilities, and dementia. But even in these instances, people are not automatically susceptible to harm by research.

People with all types of disabilities may experience different kinds of precarity in their lives, including the lack of access, resources, opportunities for employment, and education, than the general population, but that has nothing to do with their personal capacity to consent. It is more an environmental and attitudinal issue. The simple act of any kind of categorization for this minority group is demoralizing and infantilizing. Traditionally, examples of vulnerable groups that require protection have included pregnant women, children, and prisoners (those with a history of risk for abuse and potential harm), but this caution is mainly warranted for groups that have been exploited in the past or in biomedical research where actual physical health may be at risk.

In December 2017, the Public Health Awakened network, a project of Human Impact Partners, wrote a letter to Acting Secretary of the Department of Health and Human Services (HHS), Eric Hagan, with a cc to Brenda Fitzgerald, Director, Center for Disease Control and Prevention. The letter expressed concern over the fact that, according to the *Washington Post*, HHS staff were directed to omit words like "evidence-based," "transgender," and "vulnerable" when preparing the President's Fiscal Year 2019 budget. Asserting that "words matter," Public Health Awakened stated that in order for federal agencies to achieve the goal of public health, accurate terms must be used (Adams, 2017). The concern for such omissions is tangible and should be addressed. History reveals many unfortunate examples of unethical research on human subjects. But, from another point of view, there are also concerns about routinely *including* a term such as "vulnerable" when referring to people with disability.

Rather than protecting disabled people, it can be argued that the "vulnerable" label actually *causes* what is known as "pathogenic vulnerability," a condition where harm is inflicted by injustice and repression stemming from systems that are devised to alleviate these situations (Biros, 2018). Instead of helping the disabled community, these classifications can actually make things worse. Continuing to write laws with such language perpetuates myths that have long since been eradicated by the 1990 Americans with Disabilities Act (ADA). It is a decided step backwards to continue adding such phrases and concepts into current legislation. Rather, new legislation should reflect the present belief that individuals with disability are citizens that fully participate in adult life experience. Otherwise the obsolete notion that people with disability are liabilities will re-emerge.

It is never appropriate to assume automatically anything about a minority group. In any policy development, interactions, or even thoughts about minority groups, it is wise to be vigilant against stereotyping and automatic responses. Routine responses to situations involving marginalized groups often lead to inaccurate assumptions and discrimination, regardless of whether or not it is intentional.

## Case-by-case basis

"Justice can be considered the engine for autonomy" (Feinsod and Wagner, 2008). People have the right to make their own decisions about their activities, their interests, and their participation in scientific or research pursuits. To repeatedly and consistently place disabled individuals within groups considered vulnerable is shortsighted and discriminatory. Certainly, there are individuals whose conditions render them vulnerable, but to systematically classify all disable people as vulnerable does not make sense. Since every disability experience is based on unique impairments, and the ADA, in its spirit and its crafting, has assured that each person and each situation must be handled on a "case-by-case" basis, it is not logical to assume that every individual with disability is unable to act independently, make competent decisions, or protect themselves from harm.

It is inaccurate to believe that having a physical disability (or mobility, sensory, or communication disability or impairment) or even a cognitive or intellectual disability automatically and unequivocally renders a person at high risk for abuse if participating in non-medical research. There is nothing inherently vulnerable in the state of being physically disabled or even cognitively disabled that would render an individual incapable of autonomous decision-making—these decisions must be made on a case-by-case basis. People may be rendered vulnerable by tangible and intangible influences such as poverty and ignorance, stress, exhaustion, and alcohol or substance use. When resources and information are lacking, or people are pushed or push themselves beyond their limits, they may be impaired and have difficulty making mature and empowering choices. Assuming that people with disability are easy prey for coercion and manipulation continues the practice of infantilizing this minority group.

## A change in focus and next steps

In the fall of 2016, there was a Notice of Proposed Rule-Making from the office for Human Research Protections of the United States Department of Health and Human Service soliciting comment on proposed changes to the Common Rule. It was intended to improve rules protecting human subjects (https://www.hhs.gov/ohrp/regulations-and-policy/regulations/nprm-home/index.html). In a response to this call, and encouraged by the Stony Brook University IRB officer Judy Matuk, second author Block sent out a call to disability studies and disability activist groups on social media for commentary with regard to the proposed changes. This solicitation generated a series of rich online discussions from which Evans and Block (2016) then compiled a list of comments. The compilation presented views of disability scholars and activists about why people with disability should not be classified as inherently vulnerable. People providing comments noted that it is counterproductive to designate people with physical, cognitive, or intellectual disability as fundamentally vulnerable or susceptible to unethical research. Research must consider individual vulnerability, consent protocols, and overall best practices in the context of the individual's daily sociocultural framework. This includes personal assistance services, augmentative and alternative communication, and other supports.

A better research concern, rather than vulnerability, is the provision of access by reviewing the research methods and practices being used. These should be clearly stated in simple language so that all prospective participants, regardless of intellectual or cognitive disability, can understand what the study entails. This, in addition to providing appropriate and necessary accommodations, will prevent abuse, manipulation, and/or mistreatment. A focus on diagnoses or sweepingly global categories is fruitless, providing neither accurate nor helpful information. It is disrespectful to both children and disabled adults to group them together, as if all of their needs were similar. Their needs are not. In fact, the practice limits the ability to serve either group appropriately. If researchers conducting a study are concerned that disabled participants are at risk of being misrepresented, then that vulnerability extends to the entire participant pool being jeopardized by harm, not just those individuals. Trying to categorize neatly the experience of disability by the use of umbrella terms is not only non-productive, but quite often harmful. "Researchers have an obligation to design and implement research that mitigates inherent vulnerability and works to eliminate pathogenic vulnerability" (Biros, 2018). Assuring that research study practices maintain the ethical principle of nonmaleficence, selecting potential research participants must be non-discriminatory and inclusive.

The focus on *capacity to consent* and *power to resist manipulation* are more helpful dividing lines, not disability or impairment categories. Consent and autonomy are the most important criteria when identifying participants for research. Using mechanical and perfunctory disability labels/categories needlessly excludes human subjects and reduces the chance for research on disabled people. The questions then are (1) how do we assure the autonomy of people with disability when the current criteria to establish capacity and obtain consent may be discriminatory or even in violation of civil rights; and (2) how can we navigate this process justly to assure capacity to consent across the many categories of disability experience?

Currently, the criteria for determination of capacity include:

- ability to understand information about treatment;
- ability to appreciate how that information applies to individual situations;
- ability to reason with that information;
- ability to make a choice and express it (Tunzi, 2001).

Having a disability can subject a person to vulnerability, but mainly in terms of limited access and restrictive environments. This has nothing to do with the individual personally. Even if capacity to consent is impaired, it is still not an all-or-nothing situation. Not being able to make some choices about care does not mean that a person cannot be involved at all. Changing federal regulations defining "vulnerable populations" is an excellent step toward a more *just* system. The focus must be kept on *the ability to consent* and the *power to resist manipulation.*

In response to the comments and discussions initiated by the HHS to contemplate proposed federal policy revisions, the Department made the following recommendation:

> In agreement with the majority of comments, the final rule no longer includes pregnant women or "handicapped" or physically disabled individuals as examples of populations that are potentially vulnerable to coercion or undue influence. The final rule uses the term "individuals with impaired decision-making ability" to replace the term "mentally disabled persons." (Federal Policy for the Protection of Human Subjects, 2017)

Disabled people, even those with diagnoses of cognitive or intellectual disability, should not automatically be considered vulnerable or of "impaired decision-making ability." The new phrasing does not stigmatize people with particular diagnoses and puts the responsibility on the researcher to ensure all their participants have the ability to make decisions prior to participation in research. Disabled people have rights in deciding their own care and whether or not to participate in research. Federal officials understand this and the changes will be enacted in January 2019. The next step is to educate providers, researchers, and the general public.

## References

ADA.gov (2013). "Americans with Disabilities Act of 1990, as Amended," http://www.ada.gov/pubs/adastatute08.htm (accessed February 28, 2019).

Adams, M. (2017). "Letter to Secretary Hargan," https://publichealthawakened.com/wp-content/uploads/2017/12/LetterToHHSFromHealthProfessionals_2017.12.22.pdf (accessed February 28, 2019).

American Psychological Association (2018). "What Is Autism Spectrum Disorder?" https://www.psychiatry.org/patients-families/autism/what-is-autism-spectrum-disorder (accessed February 28, 2019).

Autism Speaks, Inc. (2018). "DSM-5 diagnostic criteria," https://www.autismspeaks.org/what-autism/diagnosis/dsm-5-diagnostic-criteria (accessed February 28, 2019).

Bartlett, R. (2012) "Modifying the Diary Interview Method to Research the Lives of People With Dementia." *Qualitative Health Research*, 22/12: 1717–1726.

Ben-Moshe, L., Chapman, C., and Carey, A. (2014). *Disability Incarcerated*. New York: Palgrave MacMillan.

Benson, E. (2003). "Intelligent Intelligence Testing," http://www.apa. org/monitor/feb03/intelligent.aspx (accessed February 28, 2019).

Biros, M. (2018). "Capacity, Vulnerability, and Informed Consent for Research." *Journal of Law, Medicine & Ethics*, 46/1: 72–78.

Burch, S. (2014). "'Dislocated Histories': The Canton Asylum for Insane Indians." *Women, Gender, and Families of Color*, 2/2: 141–162.

Cole, A. (2016). "All of Us Are Vulnerable, But Some Are More Vulnerable Than Others: The Political Ambiguity of Vulnerability Studies, an Ambivalent Critique." *Critical Horizons*, 17/2: 260–277.

Coleman, C. (2009). "Vulnerability as a Regulatory Category in Human Subject Research." *The Journal of Law, Medicine & Ethics*, 37/1: 12–18.

Erevelles, N. (2002). "(Im)material Citizens: Cognitive Disability, Race and the Politics of Citizenship." *Disability Culture Education*, 1/1: 5–25.

Erevelles, N. (2011). *Disability and Difference in Global Contexts: Enabling a Transformative Body Politic*. New York: Palgrave Macmillan.

Evans, C. and Block, P. (2016). "Proposed Human Subjects Language Changes: Are Physically Disabled People an Automatically and Categorically 'Vulnerable Population?'" http://pamelablock.blogspot.com/2016/04/ (accessed July 27, 2017).

Federal Policy for the Protection of Human Subjects (2017). Federal Register, 82/12, https://www.govinfo.gov/app/details/FR-2017-01-19/2017-01058(accessed July 27, 2017).

Feinsod, F. and Wagner, C. (2008). "The Ethical Principle of Justice: The Purveyor of Equality." *Managed Health Care Connect*, 16/1.

Lifton, R. (1986). "The Nazi Doctors: Medical Killing and the Psychology of Genocide," http://phdn.org/archives/holocaust-history.org/lifton/contents.shtml (accessed February 28, 2019).

Merriam-Webster. (2018). "Vulnerable," https://www.merriam-webster.com/dictionary/vulnerable (accessed February 28, 2019).

Mingus, M. (2010). "Reflections on an Opening: Disability Justice and Creating Collective Access in Detroit," https://inciteblog.wordpress.com/2010/08/23/reflections-from-detroit-reflections-on-an-opening-disability-justice-and-creating-collective-access-in-detroit/ (accessed September 7, 2016).

Mingus, M. (2011). "Changing the Framework: Disability Justice," https://leavingevidence. wordpress.com/2011/02/ (accessed July 27, 2017).

Nishida, A. (2016). "Neoliberal Academia and a Critique From Disability Studies," in Block, P., Kasnitz, D., Nishida, A., and Pollard, N. eds. *Occupying Disability: Critical Approaches to Community, Justice, and Decolonizing Disability*. New York: Springer, pp. 145–158.

Shivayogi, P. (2013). "Vulnerable Population and Methods for Their Safeguard." *Perspectives in Clinical Research*, 4/1: 53–57.

Smolin, D. M. (2012). "The Tuskegee Syphilis Experiment, Social Change, and the Future of Bioethics." *Faulkner Law Review*, 3/2.

Tombaugh, T.N. and McIntyre, N.J. (1992). "The Mini-Mental Status Examination: A Comprehensive Review." *JAGS*, 40: 922–935.

Tunzi, M. (2001). "Can the Patient Decide? Evaluating Patient Capacity in Practice." *American Family Physician*, 64/2: 299–308.

# 7

# Research Ethics Board/Institutional Review Board Variability and Other Ethical Challenges in Multi-Site Research Involving Participants on the Autism Spectrum

*Mackenzie Salt*

## Introduction

Research involving participants from "vulnerable populations"[1] can be challenging for a number of reasons; one of these challenges can be recruitment. Depending on the nature of the study, the population being studied, the geographical location where the study is being conducted, and the inclusion and exclusion criteria being used in the study, it can be difficult to recruit enough participants to be able to run the study. Expanding participant recruitment to multiple sites or running the study in multiple sites can address this difficulty. In Canada, research ethics boards (REBs) are guided by principles and procedures put forth in the Tri-Council Policy Statement: Ethical Conduct for Research Involving Humans (TCPS2). Regarding multi-site research, the TCPS2 states that "institutions are accountable for research conducted under their auspices, irrespective of the location where it takes place" (Canadian Institutes for Health Research et al., 2014, p. 102). The TCPS2 also states that institutions are allowed to establish alternative models or arrangements for research ethics review but that "the ultimate responsibility for approving alternative research ethics review models for potential use by REBs and researchers remains with their individual institutions" (Canadian Institutes for Health Research et al., 2014, p. 102). This creates variability between REBs as they may or may not have specific models of ethics review to address multi-site studies and different REBs may interpret the guidelines in the TCPS2 differently. In this chapter, I discuss the issues that I encountered with the multi-site ethics review process that I went through for my doctoral research, and I provide recommendations for researchers who find themselves in similar situations. These issues include logistical costs

[1] The term "vulnerable" has come under scrutiny as being vague, among other criticisms (Racine and Bracken-Roche, 2019). Also, the definition of what constitutes a vulnerable person varies between different sets of research ethics guidelines (Bracken-Roche et al., 2017). I use the term "vulnerable" in this chapter in line with the TCPS2 definition, which is discussed later in this chapter. However, owing to the nature of the study, an observed issue with regard to the concept of vulnerability was that an REB conflated vulnerability and lack of capacity to consent.

of multiple REB applications, the reluctance of people to participate based on negative experiences in past research studies, and especially conflicting interpretations of the TCPS2 between REBs. The concepts that created conflicts between REBs that are discussed in this chapter are vulnerability, the ability to give consent, how vulnerability and ability to consent should be assessed, and the level of risk of a study. While the information in this chapter most closely applies to my experiences doing my doctoral research in Canada and interacting with REBs, I suspect it may be helpful to researchers elsewhere interacting with institutional review boards (IRBs).

## Background

During my doctoral research, I encountered issues with recruitment. At the time, I was studying communication between adults with autism spectrum disorder (ASD) and between adults with ASD and neurotypical (NT; typically developing, people without ASD) adults.[2] The study consisted of video-recorded conversational sessions among adults with ASD or between adults with ASD and NT adults that would be transcribed and analysed. For this study, I was looking for a homogenous group of research participants to aid in the analysis of the results and detecting trends; however, ASD is widely acknowledged as heterogeneous in its presentation (Emerich et al., 2003, p. 256). I was looking for "high functioning"—meaning people with ASD who do not have a comorbid cognitive delay (Sanders, 2009, p. 1562)—verbal adults with ASD. I also sought to match both NT participants and ASD participants by their level of education, as well as their cultural background. These participation criteria made it difficult to recruit ASD participants for this study. As part of the screening process, a test—the Peabody Picture Vocabulary Test, Fourth Edition (PPVT-IV)—was administered to each participant to assess verbal IQ as a proxy measure for whether participants had a cognitive delay and to assess their overall language ability. Questionnaires were also given to participants to collect demographic information. After several months of active recruitment, I could not find enough participants who met the criteria for my study; I then decided to expand recruitment to other sites.

At my primary institution, there were two REBs: one for medical research, and another for non-medical research. As my study was not medical in nature, it was reviewed by the non-medical REB, which will henceforth be referred to as REB Alpha.[3] The study,

[2] In this chapter, I use person-first language, such as "person with autism," and identity-first language, such as "autistic person," interchangeably. The use of person-first language is controversial in many disability communities, including the ASD community (Collier, 2012), with many people with ASD preferring the identity-first, "autistic person," over person-first language (Sinclair, 2013). While some style guides have prescribed that authors use person-first language, it has been argued that inconsistent use of person-first language, namely using person-first language for referring to people with disabilities, while using identity-first language for people without disabilities, can have the effect of increasing stigma for people with disabilities (Gernsbacher, 2017). Therefore, to put people on equal footing in this chapter, and to respect the fact that not all people prefer one type of language to the other, I use both types of language to refer to both disabled persons and persons without disabilities.

[3] REBs discussed hereafter will be identified with the names of Greek letters to allow them to remain anonymous and protect the privacy of their members.

while complex, was classified as being of minimal risk to the participants as the participants were having conversations with other people, which is in itself no more risky than talking to people during the course of a regular day. All transcripts and video tapes were anonymized after collection to protect the participants' privacy. Upon completion of the ethics review process, I began to actively recruit participants for this study, using posters and emails. I was looking for six participants in total. In three months of active recruiting, I had screened four participants with ASD who were recruited through institution Alpha. These participants were either members of institution Alpha or had personal relationships with members of the institution. After completing the screening process for these participants, only two were eligible to participate. At that point, I wanted to expand my recruitment strategy to include other nearby institutions, including higher education, healthcare, and government institutions. Each institution had its own REB; however, several were integrated with the medical REB at my primary institution. If I had gone to the medical REB, I would have been cleared by three institutions. When I was seeking to expand my recruitment, I asked the non-medical REB whether I could seek clearance from the integrated medical REB; however, I was informed that the two REBs were mutually exclusive and that my project did not fit under the mandate of the integrated medical REB. For those reasons, I had no choice but to approach each of the constituent REBs individually. I was informed by REB Alpha that for this process to go as smoothly as possible, it would be best to submit paperwork to each REB consecutively. The rationale behind this was that if different REBs had different opinions on any particular point, it would not then warrant starting a protocol change procedure at another institution while they still may be reviewing the original submission.

## Seeking other sites

The first REB I went to after my primary institution was that of a government agency, hereafter referred to as REB Beta, which I thought may have some participants who could meet the inclusion criteria of the study. REB Beta required a full board review and, in addition to the materials I submitted to REB Alpha, I was required to complete the TCPS2 Course on Research Ethics (TCPS2: CORE). Upon completion of the review, REB Beta informed me that they would have given the study their ethics clearance, but did not due to not having any potential participants within the age range for inclusion in the study.

The next REB I approached for clearance to recruit participants was REB Gamma, an educational institution. Like REB Beta, REB Gamma required that I undergo a full ethics review as opposed to an expedited review, but they stipulated that in terms of recruitment that I would only need to submit documentation and procedures that would specifically affect participants recruited from their institution. Thus, I did not have to submit any of the paperwork related to recruitment of participants at other sites. The ethics application was approved without modification.

REB Delta was at a healthcare institution. REB Delta, along with REB Epsilon, which is described in the next paragraph, was also part of the integrated REB at my primary institution that handled ethics applications for medical research. REB Delta accepted the clearance of REB Alpha without further review and issued their approval based on the review done by the previous REB.

REB Epsilon was part of a higher-education institution. REB Epsilon informed me that my protocol would have to undergo a full board review. Also, unlike the previous REBs, I was required to submit all documentation that had already been submitted to all of the other REBs, including recruitment protocols for other sites, for review. REB Epsilon also requested copies of email communications between myself and the other REBs, including any questions I was asked and my responses. This was to avoid redundancy and to ensure I was not being asked questions by REB Epsilon that I had been asked by other REBs and had answered already. Also, as with REB Beta, I was required to submit a TCPS2: CORE certificate of completion. Lastly, unlike the other REBs, I had to provide a research proposal separate from the required methodology and other related ethics documentation.

Other sites were approached for recruitment that did not have REBs and these usually fell into one of three categories: sites that were happy to distribute my recruitment materials once they had been cleared by REB Alpha; sites that declined to distribute the recruitment materials regardless of REB clearance as they felt I would not be able to recruit participants from them for various reasons; and sites that declined to distribute recruitment materials regardless of REB clearance because they did not want to associate themselves with research. I found that the last two categories of sites were somewhat related. Several of the sites in the last two categories that I approached expressed that they would not distribute recruitment materials for any sort of research studies because they had created a safe space for people with ASD and that some of their members had had bad experiences with research in the past and were distrustful of researchers. Some sites felt that their members would be unlikely to participate owing to their feelings about participating in research and thus did not want to distribute the materials, and encouraged me to look elsewhere. I had not originally realized that this sentiment was present or prevalent among adults in the ASD community. I am an adult with ASD; I was diagnosed as a teenager almost 20 years ago but was not aware of or took part in any research studies until I was a graduate student, so my experience was very different from those of the participants in my study. This demonstrates the heterogeneity of ASD. There is an expression in the ASD community, "if you have met one person with autism, you have met one person with autism," and this applies not just to symptomatology, but also to experience. When I asked each of the participants with ASD in my study, almost all of them had had bad experiences with research to the point that I moved the location where the conversational sessions, and some of the screening sessions, were to take place. I selected another location in the community that was not affiliated with my primary institution. While this is not an issue with REBs per se, it is related to other REB issues that are discussed later in this chapter.

## Ethics protocol issues with multi-site research

In general, there are several issues that arise in multi-site research with reference to REBs and IRBs and have been previously identified and described. Multi-site studies can take a long time to be cleared (Greene and Geiger, 2006, p. 785; Racine et al., 2010, pp. 12–14), and they can incur substantial costs over and above the cost of conducting a single site study (Gold and Dewa, 2005, pp. 292–293; Greene and Geiger, 2006, p. 785). Of particular interest to researchers working with vulnerable populations is the fact that different REBs may interpret parts of the TCPS2 guidelines (or other ethical guidelines or legislation relevant as appropriate in other jurisdictions) differently. This creates a situation whereby one ethics board may apply a judgment to one section of a protocol, and another ethics board may apply a completely different, possibly contradictory, judgment to that same section of a protocol. This is important to researchers working with vulnerable populations because principles like autonomy in the TCPS2, defined as "the ability to deliberate about a decision and be able to act on that deliberation" (Canadian Institutes for Health Research et al., 2014, p. 6), and vulnerability, defined as "a diminished ability to fully safeguard one's own interests in the context of a specific research project" (Canadian Institutes for Health Research et al., 2014, p. 210), are not always clear cut in every research study. The TCPS2 presents, rightly, that autonomy can change and circumstances can create vulnerability where one might not assume that vulnerability exists, so REBs and researchers should consider this in their ethics protocols. When multiple REBs disagree on the interpretation of autonomy or vulnerability in a given study, it creates a conflict that can seem to be a difficult conflict to address for the researcher. Several of these conflicts are addressed in the next section.

## REBs in conflict

The first conflict that arose between REBs with this study was between REB Alpha and REB Gamma. REB Gamma suggested a change to the methodology of running the conversation sessions; namely, to use dyads of participants in the conversation sessions instead of triads. This was not an ethical issue per se but a methodological one. There were several reasons why I chose triads over dyads. The primary reason was that conversational turn structure was one of the aspects of communication that I was studying and dyadic conversations can create an artificial turn structure (speaker 1, speaker 2, speaker 1, speaker 2, etc.). This structure is not necessarily as natural as a conversation between three or more people as participants in these larger groups may have to jockey for a conversational turn. Also, I had designed the study such that each participant never interacted with another participant more than once and each participant would participate in two sessions so the sessions were balanced and this would avoid familiarity as a confounding variable. When this was explained to REB Gamma, the methodology suggestion was withdrawn and the original methodology was approved. Having already run at least one session under the original methodology as approved by

REB Alpha this suggestion would have altered the design of the study such that I would have had to recruit more participants and I would have had to run additional sessions to create a balance with the new paradigm.

As stated previously, I was looking for “high functioning” participants with ASD. This was to be primarily assessed using the PPVT with each participant. A standardized score of 70, being a proxy for a verbal IQ score of 70, was set as a criterion for participation based on a general consensus of the ASD research community that “high functioning” classification can be used when a person with ASD has an IQ over 70 (Klin, 2006). In the feedback I received from REB Epsilon, I was asked “There is concern among REB members that some of the ASD participants, particularly from Epsilon, may be vulnerable or not competent to consent. Is a Peabody Picture [Vocabulary] Test score of greater than 70 considered high functioning? Generally [people with] IQ scores under 80 are considered vulnerable or unable to consent. Can you explain the scoring and justify using >70 as an indicator of high functioning?” The first concern I had with this question was the notion that participants with IQ scores under 80 would be considered unable to consent. To exclude automatically participants with an IQ under 80 goes against the spirit of the TCPS2. On the issue of consent, the TCPS2 says that:

> In keeping with the principle of Justice, those who lack the capacity to decide on their own behalf must neither be unfairly excluded from the potential benefits of research participation, nor may their lack of decision-making capacity be used to inappropriately include them in research. REBs and researchers should be aware of these ethical considerations and seek to find a balance between them for the benefit of prospective participants who lack decision-making capacity. (Canadian Institutes for Health Research et al., 2014, p. 43)

In terms of evaluating decision-making ability, the TCPS2 does not use IQ as a criterion. Decision-making capacity is defined in the TCPS2 as “the ability of prospective or actual participants to understand relevant information presented about a research project, and to appreciate the potential consequences of their decision to participate or not participate” (Canadian Institutes for Health Research et al., 2014, p. 42). In fact, the TCPS2 also states that decision-making capacity “may vary according to the complexity of the choice being made, the circumstances surrounding the decision, of the point in time at which consent is sought. The determination of capacity to decide whether or not to participate in research, then, is not a static determination” (Canadian Institutes for Health Research et al., 2014, p. 42). Therefore, following the TCPS2, the question is not “does the participant have a high enough IQ to consent?” but “does the participant understand the information presented as part of the study and can they appreciate the potential consequences of participating or not?” My response to REB Epsilon was a long one and covered several topics. First, I explained the PPVT in more detail and explained how I was using it to not only assess baseline verbal IQ, as previous versions of the PPVT have been shown to correlate strongly with verbal IQ scores on other tests (Emerson et al., 2010, p. 580), but also to assess overall structural language ability. Therefore, I was not using the PPVT solely to determine the capacity of a participant to consent: I was also using it as a potential variable. The final part of my response to REB Epsilon has been reproduced here: "I am also using screening questionnaires to establish functional criteria [for capacity to give consent]. If the person with ASD is doing things [such as] living independently, working at a job without a support worker, pursuing higher education, I would consider them able to consent as they are already making important life decisions and this study does not have substantial risks that would be comparable to the life decisions such as the preceding. Also, all participants would have a minimum of a high-school education." This response was informed greatly by my own experience as an adult with ASD. There are many stereotypes and assumptions made about people with ASD and, as noted earlier in this chapter, "if you have met one person with autism, you have met one person with autism." This is why I wanted to focus on using functional criteria rather than just score cut-offs to determine whether the participants had the ability to consent. This response was accepted by REB Epsilon.

Another issue arose with REB Epsilon. The question from REB Epsilon was: "It is possible that participants will have well-functioning days and lower functioning days. Have you considered having a specialized professional available should any issues or conflict arise during the Conversational Sessions?" As an integral part of this study, I did not tell participants what topics to discuss or avoid. The goal was to observe conversation develop as naturally as possible. Having a professional on hand, or resources available for people who have engaged in focus groups or interviews on sensitive topics, is fairly common. The professional in question could be someone who deals with those topics regularly and has special training, such as in the case of a genetics counsellor being available for participants of studies about heritable conditions. In the case of my sessions, it was impossible to predict what sort of professional would be necessary. Also, given the distrust that some of my participants already had toward my primary institution based on their previous experiences as research participants, I felt that it would be best that if they were upset that they would talk to someone already in their support system whom they trusted, rather than an outsider, in order to minimize potential harms. Additionally, the conversational sessions were designed to be as natural as possible, and therefore replicate as closely as possible an everyday social interaction and therefore not present any more harm than a social conversation with a stranger in public.

I found it interesting that the question was phrased as it was, using the phrasing about levels of functioning, when it would have been much more straightforward and far less marked to ask about participants' bad days or good days, especially given the previous comment about what it means to be a "high functioning" person with ASD. In addition to the previous issue with REB Epsilon, I believe that these may have been due to the experiences the REB had had with participants with ASD in clinical studies in the past. REB Epsilon generally dealt with clinical or healthcare-related studies previously, and this may have shaped their perceptions as to how a person with ASD functions. I responded to REB Epsilon as follows: "As an experienced researcher, I will make a judgement about the participants' willingness and comfort. If they seem anxious, I will offer to reschedule when doing the verbal re-consent ... The risks of these conversational sessions are no greater than those present in everyday life. It is impossible to foresee what kind of professional would be appropriate for each participant." REB Epsilon accepted this response to their inquiry and soon after approved the protocol.

## Ethical problems overview and advice to researchers

As demonstrated in the previous section, a number of problems can occur for researchers conducting multi-site research studies involving vulnerable populations. REBs may disagree on capacity to consent of the participants, the extent of the vulnerability of participants, and the level of risk of the study.

Disagreements between REBs can also definitely slow things down for researchers. In my case, because REB Alpha had already approved my study, and some sessions had already been conducted with the participants that I had managed to recruit before expanding recruitment to other sites, these disagreements were particularly difficult to address. I did not want to be treating participants unequally, or have to go back and change the study and start all over again from the beginning, potentially leading to further recruitment problems. To ensure that all participants were treated equally, once I began the REB processes at other sites, I did not run any research sessions until all of the REB review processes at all of the sites that I approached were completed. In addition, I made sure that those participants who had already consented to the study and/or had already participated in part of the study were given the most up-to-date consent forms and I asked them to re-consent to the study. This was suggested by REB Alpha, but they emphasized it was not necessary. I decided to go ahead and re-consented each participant to ensure fairness amongst all of the participants. In addition, because only one of the ethics boards recognized another, every time I had to do an amendment, I had to do it three times, once for each of three different REBs, and this took time as well. For other researchers considering doing multi-site research, especially with vulnerable populations, I would suggest you look for integrated ethics boards whereby the ethics clearance of one REB is recognized without further review by a number of other sites. I would also suggest seeking REB approval at all of the sites that you are considering first if possible. While it may be slower to get started, once your recruitment and study begin, you will not need to take a long hiatus in the middle to get approval at another board. In all, approval from REB Alpha took two months from submission to approval. After another two months of recruiting, I then started applying to the other sites to recruit. From when I applied to REB Beta until I received approval from REB Epsilon took four and a half months.

As the TCPS2 gives guidelines without specific examples, REBs may interpret the guidelines differently. REBs consist of various people with varying amounts of experience in different areas and they use that experience to help them with reviewing research ethics protocols. This can mean that REBs with a background in one research area may have preconceived notions about a particular vulnerable population. This can cause the REB to over- or underestimate the vulnerability and/or capacity to consent of research participants. If this sort of issue comes up, you may need to advocate for your research participants. As a researcher, you know your participant population and your study better than anyone else does. If an REB is requesting that you make changes that you feel may not respect the autonomy or the capacity to consent of your research population, you should respond to them and let them know your concerns. REBs and researchers need to work together to create and maintain respect for human dignity in research, as expressed in the core principles of the TCPS2: respect for persons, concern for welfare, and justice (Canadian Institutes for Health Research et al., 2014, p. 16).

Lastly, the actions that you take as a researcher may affect your participants and other researchers in the future. As stated previously in this chapter, several of the participants who would eventually participate in my study had had bad experiences in the past with research and were reluctant to participate at first. Unfortunately, these were not isolated incidents and I later found out that this was a salient and common experience for many adults with ASD who I tried to recruit for my study. The participants who were reluctant to participate were young children when they first participated in research at a university or a hospital and they did not feel that they themselves or their contributions were respected. Some participants informed me that they would not come to the campus of my primary institution to be screened for the study because they had had such bad experiences with research in the past. They described to me being volunteered by their parents to participate in studies even though they did not want to, not being compensated by the researchers involved, and not having their questions answered or otherwise being ignored by the researchers involved. For some of my participants, these things happened between 15 and 25 years ago at various institutions, but it created such a feeling of distrust with them that they were reluctant to participate in or go near places of research as adults. When participants have these kinds of experiences, it reflects badly on not just the original researcher or their institution, but also research as a whole: all researchers, all institutions. It can take quite a lot of work to build that trust back when it has been lost.

## Conclusion

In closing, multi-site studies can have additional ethical challenges when involving vulnerable populations. These challenges include dealing with disagreements between REBs on various ethical principles, including consent, vulnerability, and risk. Researchers can mitigate some of these challenges through planning and proactive engagement with REBs. In cases of disagreements between REBs, researchers should also take on the role of educator and advocate, standing up for their participants and educating the REB members about that community.

## References

Bracken-Roche, D., Bell, E., Macdonald, M.E., and Racine, E. (2017). "The Concept of 'Vulnerability' in Research Ethics: An In-depth Analysis of Policies and Guidelines". *Health Research Policy and Systems*, 15/1: 8.

Canadian Institutes for Health Research, Natural Sciences and Engineering Research Council of Canada and Social Sciences and Humanities Research Council of Canada (2014). "Tri-Council Policy Statement: Ethical Conduct for Research Involving Humans," http://www.pre.ethics.gc.ca/eng/policy-politique/initiatives/tcps2-eptc2/Default/ (accessed February 28, 2019).

Collier, R. (2012). "Person-first Language: Noble Intent but to What Effect?" *Canadian Medical Association Journal*, 184/18: 1977–1978.

Emerich, D.M., Creaghead, N.A., Grether, S.M., Murray, D., and Grasha, C. (2003). "The Comprehension of Humorous Materials by Adolescents With High-functioning Autism and Asperger's Syndrome." *Journal of Autism and Developmental Disorders*, 33/3: 253–257.

Emerson, E., Einfeld, S., and Stancliffe, R. (2010). "The Mental Health of Young Children With Intellectual Disabilities or Borderline Intellectual Functioning." *Social Psychiatry and Psychiatric Epidemiology*, 45/5: 579–587.

Gernsbacher, M.A. (2017). "Editorial Perspective: The Use of Person-first Language in Scholarly Writing May Accentuate Stigma." *Journal of Child Psychology and Psychiatry*, 58/7: 859–861.

Gold, J. L. and Dewa C. S. (2005). "Institutional Review Boards and Multisite Studies in Health Services Research: Is There a Better Way?" *Health Services Research*, 40/1): 291–308.

Greene, S.M. and Geiger, A.M. (2006). "A Review Finds That Multicenter Studies Face Substantial Challenges but Strategies Exist to Achieve Institutional Review Board Approval." *Journal of Clinical Epidemiology*, 59/8: 784–790.

Klin, A. (2006). "Autism and Asperger Syndrome: An Overview." *Revista Brasileira de Psiquiatria*, 28: s3–s11.

Racine, E. and Bracken-Roche, D. (2019). "Enriching the Concept of Vulnerability in Research Ethics: An Integrative and Functional Account." *Bioethics*, 33: 19–34.

Racine, E., Bell, E., and Deslauriers, C. (2010). "Canadian Research Ethics Boards and Multisite Research: Experiences From Two Minimal-Risk Studies." *IRB: Ethics & Human Research*, 32/3: 12–18.

Sanders, J.L. (2009). "Qualitative or Quantitative Differences Between Asperger's Disorder and Autism? Historical Considerations." *Journal of Autism and Developmental Disorders*, 39/11: 1560–1567. Sinclair, J. (2013). "Why I Dislike "Person First" Language." *Autonomy, the Critical Journal of Interdisciplinary Autism Studies*, 1/2).

# 8

# Bridging Worlds

## Can Anthropology Be a Communication Therapy?

*Leonardo Carbonieri Campoy*

### Introduction: playing as a method of research

For my PhD in anthropology, I conducted ethnographic fieldwork in a child neurologist's volunteer project for autistic children and their families in a large Brazilian city. This child neurologist, a recently graduated young woman, started the project (housed in the city's public university) with the aim of offering care to low income families who had difficulties accessing health services in Brazil. With her permission, I joined her consultations between 2013 and 2015, observing her examine children, determine diagnoses, and talk to families about autism, schools, and therapies. Consultations were once in a week, on Wednesday afternoons, with an average of eight children per day. During my fieldwork, I probably participated in around 800 consultations, distributed among around 150 children, who often returned every 3 months, and sometimes after longer periods of time. All children had been diagnosed as autistic. Most were boys and their conditions, or what the doctor called symptoms, varied enormously in terms of severity and impairment.

When the family entered the doctor's office and noticed me for the first time, the neurologist would explain my presence—as an anthropologist working on his doctoral research—and asked if they accepted my presence during the appointment. The families not only accepted my presence, but also encouraged their children to interact with me. A lot of interaction with the kids was generated in all kinds of ways: from subtle hellos, handshakes, and kisses on the cheeks to playing and games on the play mats. I was not only doing my fieldwork, but also becoming a friend to almost every child who attended the project. Moms and dads started to say that, two or three days before the consultation, their children—at least the ones that had verbal communication—asked if they were going to meet their buddy—me—at the consultation.

I was not expecting this interaction with the kids. Moreover, it was not my goal, since my research was projected as an anthropology of autism, not of autistic children. The question that guided my research was how autism is clinically diagnosed, in other words, how psychiatric and neuroscientific knowledge was clinically enacted (Mol,

2003) by a doctor authorized to decide that some kids are autistic and others are not. My attention was initially focused on the work of the doctor and then, with all the interaction with the kids, all I was doing was laying down on the play mats with dinosaurs and hot wheels, following the child's lead in some game. Just playing.

Instead of stalling the interaction, I went along with it. Interacting with the children gave me another entry into autism, counterpointing the doctor's actions and words. It showed me that their lives go beyond what the diagnosis determines. In the context of the consultations, a moment controlled and led by the doctor, interacting with the children indicated to me that the medical language could not grasp the totality of who they were and how they related to the world.

Here is an example featuring a three-year-old boy with, in the doctor's words, "severe autism and no verbal communication." While his father had lately been saying that his son had been demonstrating a "strange habit of climbing on anyone's lap," he began to climb my legs and fight for space with my notebook. I dropped it, accepted him, and he laughed. I started to play with him, rocking his body back and forth, up and down, and he laughed even more. We stayed like this for a while.

After they left the room, the doctor said, "did you notice he wasn't playing with you"? I answered, "Really? It seemed to me he was having a good time, laughing and, yes, playing with me!" She then said "Yes, having a good time, but he wasn't socializing, he was using you as an object of his own will, it was not an interaction."

Going through several situations like this one throughout the research showed me that, in order to understand how autism is diagnosed, I would need to interpret how medicine articulates very specific concepts of socialization and communication. After all, it is by identifying socialization and communication deficits that an autism diagnosis is determined.

Following the Diagnostic and Statistical Manual of Mental Disorders, 5th Editon (DSM-5), the neuropediatrician understands autism as a disability and as a disorder. In another words, autism is faced as a sensory and mental disorder that has to be addressed as a problem, an individual and public problem. I highlight this point because the debates around autism as a difference or as a disease, aroused globally by the neurodiversity movement in recent decades (Ortega, 2009), did not appear at all in the consultations that I observed. I don't know if families were aware of the neurodiversity movement. My guess is that the vast majority of them were not, since they had very little access to information about autism besides the consultations. The doctor was very practical around the issue. She recognized the legitimacy of the neurodiversity argument, but, as a clinician, as she said in one of our conversations, "it is not my problem to decide if it is identity or disease, I leave that for researchers, my problem is helping and caring for them, and their families came up to me because their sons have difficulties."

It is beyond the scope of this chapter to explore the construction of the diagnosis of autism (Campoy, 2017). Suffice to say that, as a methodology of research, the analysis profoundly relies on the interactions that I had with diagnosed children in the context of consultations. Without planning, I ended up interacting with diagnosed children as a methodology of research on autism.[1] I let the children engage me in their actions by understanding that, in this way, I would have more ethnographic perspectives on how they communicate and socialize, two fundamental aspects of an autism diagnosis according to medical knowledge.

Here, I want to draw upon the ethical issue raised by the interactions. Engaging with the children made me realize that they socialized and communicated a lot but not in the way that medicine or even some parents expected them to do. By my interpretation, these kids did not have socialization and communication deficits. Rather, the problem is that health professionals and some parents do not understand their specific ways of socialization and communication. The ethical question raised was: what should I do with this perspective? I was there in the consultation room as a researcher, as an anthropologist, not as a therapist. I felt somewhat unethical in relation with the doctor, families and their children, as if I was receiving but not giving back, just like Tim Ingold has put it:

> Disguised as social scientists we enter this world either by stealth, feigning invisibility, or under false pretenses by claiming we have come to learn from teachers whose words are heeded not for the guidance they have to offer but as evidence of how they think, of their beliefs or attitudes. Then, as soon as we have filled our bags, we cut and run. This, in my estimation, is fundamentally unethical. It is to turn our backs upon the world in which we live and to which we owe our formation (2013, pp. 5–6).

Going into the world and collecting evidence on how people think, believe, and act, and shortly after run away from those experiences is fundamentally unethical, according to Ingold. To no longer do anthropology in this way, the author proposes to establish a relation of correspondence with the world (Ingold, 2013, p. 7), understood as a posture that, before talking about the world, thinks and acts with the world. Ingold's proposal is that, by means of a sensory-cognitive immersion, the anthropologist opens his discipline to creations that can be made by a "going along with the world," not only in terms of concepts and theories, but especially of practices. In a more purposeful relationship with the world, anthropology can do more than produce verbal texts written in a scholastic tone. It can immerse itself in different creative fields and hence suggest other forms of anthropological production. With art as his interlocutor, Ingold organizes his proposition:

> If there are similarities between the ways in which artists and anthropologists study with the world, then could we not regard the artwork as a result of something like an anthropological study, rather than as an object of such study? We are already used to the idea that the results of anthropological research need not be confined to written texts. They may also include photographs and films. But could they also include drawings, paintings or sculpture? Or works of craft? Or musical compositions? Or even

[1] In a sense, just like it happened with Corsaro (2003, 2017), engaging with children as a result of a position of atypical adult in their own environment. In his case, the school; in mine, the consultation.

> buildings? Conversely, could not works of art be regarded as forms of anthropology, albeit "written" in non-verbal media? (Ingold, 2013, p. 8).

If certain art practices can suggest new forms of anthropology, can research with autistic children do so as well? Can interactions with diagnosed children and interlocutions with their parents and health professionals also be results of anthropological research?

Inspired by Ingold's critique and proposition, I found a way of dealing with the ethical question raised by my research. What to do with knowledge that I was realizing could be useful in some way to my interlocutors, to the child neurologist, parents and of course the children? Besides a text, an interpretation of autism, could my research also produce an action of care for autistic children, their families, and for their doctor as well? Couldn't my research represent a kind of anthropological therapy in the context of Brazilian child psychiatry? To elaborate the affirmative answer, I developed a case based on the consultations.

## The boy who sings and doesn't speak

Seven years old, tall for his age, fine blond hair with a bowl haircut, and an almost icy-white skin, this boy always entered the office alone with his mother, a woman in her mid-thirties working as a janitor in a common public school attended by the child. In the four visits I observed, she seemed tired from work, from dealing with the child, and the marriage with the boy's father that was about to end. She said in one of the appointments that the father did not accept the diagnosis—she said: "he thinks the child is just being lazy or because of the freedom I give the boy"[2]—and also no longer seemed to accept her as his wife—"we're separating, he doesn't want this anymore; neither do I, it's hard." And the boy remained placid, light, radiating a seemingly unshakable calmness mixed with a complete lack of concern as to what was happening around him. His eyes wandered without focusing on any single object or person in the doctor's office. He never hugged the neurologist nor looked at me or asked for his mother's lap, a common action by children in this clinic. Upon entering the room, he walked in slow steps across the space, as if levitating, or he would lay down on the mat, without interfering with any of them or, at most, contemplating the turning wheels of the miniature trucks.

In the first visit, as he was laying on the carpet without having issued any vocal sound, I quickly and quietly ask neurologist: he doesn't speak, right? She answers: no, he doesn't speak.

However, a few minutes later, a child's voice resembling a church choir takes over the room, singing in very accurately articulated English and correctly following the scale of musical notes: *twinkle, twinkle little star, how I wonder what you are, up above the world so high, like a diamond in the sky, twinkle, twinkle, little star, how I wonder what you*

[2] Direct quotations like this one are the author's translations from Portuguese.

*are*. Quite possibly with a surprised look on my face I exclaimed: he sings marvelously! Both women looked at me with an expression of surprise as they were seeing someone realize what was more than familiar to them. They stopped talking for a while as we enjoyed the delight emanating from this unexpected performance of an American lullaby classic. I interrupted the boy's aria by asking his mother: "How did he learn this?" She replied, "On the computer, he's always on this video website, clicking on the figures on the side, other videos, and stays there for hours watching and listening to the same songs". "He does this all by himself?", I asked. "Yeah, all by himself, he sings all day, different songs, all of them in English, I can't understand anything," she replied.

I turn to the doctor and ask: "Did you know this?" And she says she didn't. She knew he singed, but not how he learned it.

She continued: "But it's interesting, his cognition is very good, apparently with no impairments. He knows how to learn in his own way, he memorized the figures in the videos and the songs and reproduces them exactly as he hears them. He has great memory; he just doesn't know how to talk or communicate."

His mother woefully added: "Exactly, that's my biggest problem, I never know what he wants! He doesn't speak! I give him milk, he vomits, I give him rice and beans, he refuses, he doesn't want meat, he doesn't want chicken. I don't know what he wants! That's my biggest problem, to understand what this boy wants!"

Like a well-rehearsed dramatic play, the tension in the mother's last sentence was the cue for the boy to soften the narrative, breaking the growing distress in the conversation, but leaving doubts in abeyance: *twinkle, twinkle little star, how I wonder what you are*.

The doctor's claim that by singing the boy is not communicating means that, for her, the child has not mastered English as a tool to "bond" with another, he does not use YouTube as a communication device, or that he's singing for someone to listen to him. Rather, he would have memorized from accessing the website and listening to the songs, reproducing his memories at random without any communicative function. His singing would be the execution of something that mainstream medicine defines as stereotypy, a constant repetition of a behavior with no apparent significant connection with the context.

Likewise, the mother, distressed by not understanding what the child wants, cannot be labeled as an insensitive person unable to perceive the autistic child's apparently heterodox attempts at communication. How to know what the boy wants to eat, one of the main difficulties at home, if he only sings in English, a foreign language to her? How could she know he has severe lactose intolerance—as gastrointestinal tests have confirmed—if he did not indicate any refusal of dairy products? The doctor's assessments and the mother's anguish make sense according to their perspectives and it would be an exaggeration to interpret them as exclusively normalizing.

On the one hand, an anthropological point of view cannot disregard that the boy displays *some* linguistic ability when using the computer and singing songs in English. The computer, YouTube, English, and music are entry and exit vehicles between the boy and the world. We do not know if he is indeed saying something with meaning, if his playing around with electronic content and his musical performances seek to convey, to the extent of the possibilities of an autistic child, a message to another person duly recognized by the boy. On the other hand, he is certainly responding to the world, in his own particular way, according to his abilities. In this case, he received the world and returned some reaction; he interrogated the world as he deemed appropriate and possible.

Stemming from these inductions, the plausibility of the doctor's and the mother's perceptions and the acknowledgement of some sort of language in the boy, we could say that the problems—his, his mother's, and the doctor's—lies in the communication between these three actors. The child suffers from the symptoms of his autism, the mother is in anguish for failing to deal with it as she would wish, and the doctor wants to help the mother in caring for the child, but even though they live in the same house and meet regularly in the clinic it seems that their languages do not share a vocabulary. They talk and listen, but do not seem to fully understand each other, the mother, the doctor, and the boy.

The problem lies in the relationship between the three. The doctor's language remains essentially a medical language. As simple as her words may be, her treatment empathetic and caring, she is still seen by the mother as a professional who masters a fairly esoteric knowledge, prescribing substances and interpreting exams. How to perceive the child practically, how to be attentive to his particularities on a day-to-day basis, how to establish communication channels between mother and child: the doctor is unable to provide the mother with answers to these questions, whether in theory or in practice. Anchored in contemporary neuroscience, she pinpoints the child's developmental needs, arguing that the autistic brain needs specially equipped environments to trigger behavioral changes. The doctor was unable to direct the mother to translate this medical recommendation into her daily life with the child.

In turn, even if the mother may intellectually comprehend that she must commit herself to her son, how could she adequately interpret him in order to change his daily environment into a constant practical construction of understandable communications? How could this woman, apparently worn out by her work as janitor and dismayed by the dissolution of a marriage with a man unable to accept the autistic condition of his child, find within her an altruistic inclination toward the child to change and develop him?

The second medical appointment was identical to the first: the deadlocks regarding food selectivity, intertwined with the mother's anguish and the doctor's care, the sound of the boy's recital. In the third consultation, which began identically to the previous ones, I decided to speak. Attentive not to disrupt any explanation or deliberation during the conversation between the two, I turned to the mother and asked, "Have you ever thought about enrolling him in music therapy? Your son sings very well, he has a proper notion of musical notes, and it's surprising that he learned all this by himself, alone on the computer, as you have mentioned. I don't believe it's a natural gift, nothing of the sort, but I believe we could say it's an interest of his, something in music, in computers, and even in the English language draws his attention, and in some way he is expressing himself through these interests. And who knows, maybe in music therapy he'd interact more based on his interest in music, he could perhaps further stimulate his communication through music therapy. It may not work, but then again it might."

As I closed my mouth I immediately looked at neurologist in fear of a reprimand for having exceeded my observer status, but instead she continued my argument by saying, "It's true, music therapy may be an excellent stimulus for him, no doubt, whether you'll see positive results depends on many factors, but it's worth a try. A university professor contacted me, she's setting up a class for autistic children to work with her students. Single sessions would be ideal, but it's a start, right? Do you think you can take him there to the university?" "I think so, I'll figure it out," the mother responded. "I'll talk to her, it's not certain, but if it works out I'll let you know." "I hope it works out," the mother concluded, "maybe it will help me to understand what this boy wants."

Unfortunately, it did not work out, as we learned in the fourth and final consultation. The constant shortages of service, which defined the neurologist's office, once again became an issue, now in the almost immediate filling of the university professor's music therapy class. Sorry to hear the news and not being able to afford a private therapist for the child, the mother uttered "Maybe someday, right?"

In any case, this boy's situation was essential for me to reflect upon how anthropology may act on children's mental health beyond the production of written articles. The music therapy suggestion arose from my impression that, differently from what the mother believed, her son was, indeed, expressing himself.[3] Music was the language used by the child to let the world enter into him and to situate himself in the world. If the mother could build from this observation, she might be able to stimulate the child's communication and to better understand what he wants, her greatest difficulty as a caregiver/nurturer. Apparently, she did not perceive her relationship with the child in such a way. Moreover, the neurologist's requests for the mother to commit herself to the child's condition did not seem to translate itself into practical effects on the family's everyday life. Both seemed oblivious to the fact that this commitment could be translated into a perception of the child's musical affinities. Therefore, could these impasses in languages and translations be, if not solved, at least better understood by an expert in relationships and differences? In other words, could my suggestion for music therapy be more productive for the mother, the neurologist, and especially for the child if not uttered as a sudden intrusion during a neurologist appointment, but rather as a session with an anthropologist?

## Anthropology as care practice

At least the way I conceive it, anthropology is a discipline capable of perceiving and demonstrating realities that are not apparent. Through ethnography, movements and conditions that define the contexts under scrutiny, usually overlooked by the actors

[3] Besides autism, I also conduct research on music, heavy metal specifically. The methods and perspectives of music therapy were no stranger to me at the time when I began attending the doctor's appointments.

involved, are identified, indicated, and openly enunciated by researchers in anthropology. The nature of anthropological knowledge is constituted by reports and analyses that uncover the importance of what is conceived by dominant discourses as irrelevant, illusory, or doomed to disappearance.

My ethnography of a neuropediatric clinic of autism illustrates precisely this type of perspective. Experiencing the relations among health professionals, diagnosed children, and their families, I noticed dimensions and aspects of biomedicine, care, autism, childhood, and kinship that shape the reality of this clinic, but which are not perceived by the people involved or are simply disregarded.

One of these aspects is precisely what I related in the case of the boy who sings and does not speak. The lack of meaningful communication the boy supposedly presented governed, in fact, all communication in the office, between physician, mother, and child. It was like everyone was there speaking, but, at the same time, they did not really communicate with each other.

It is necessary to further continue this analysis, investing in the anthropological interpretation of this form of communication between physician and patient, trying to understand how medicine often constructs the diagnosis and the lines of care and treatment in the context of poor communication taking place in consultation rooms. Likewise, in an alliance with autism advocacy movements, it is also necessary to insist on the view of autistic expressions as meaningful languages; that is, that they significantly communicate some action and/or reaction to the world,[4] even if they seem, from a commonsense view of communication, unassimilable noise or declarations without goals. Autism does not take away communication from children.

However, the purpose of this chapter is to ask what to do with these analyses and anthropological observations. Having accompanied the cases of so many children and families in conditions of suffering due to the impasses caused by what is described as autism made me understand that anthropology can participate in their care. The anthropological understanding of the relations between children, their families, and health professionals can help to alleviate the suffering of the former and qualify the work of the latter with considerations about translations, languages, and differences. If anthropology can indicate practical ways to alleviate suffering, why wait to act until families and health professionals discover and read our analyses if we ourselves can reach them? According to my ethnographic experiences, I fully share Wilkinson and Kleinman's suggestion that the social sciences must change their conceptions of human suffering by including practical intervention in their critical agenda:

> This all involves a strong commitment to the development of social science as a field of social care and caring practice. There has to be more than an expression of intellectual interest and emotional concern here; there must also be an application to "work that sustains life". [...] Under the effort to promote social possibilities for people's recovery,

[4] Deligny (2015) offers elucidating clues to thinking the language of the autistic child as one without representation.

> regeneration, and healing, it challenges us to forge alliances and working partnerships with colleagues outside our immediate spheres of expertise and nationhood. [ . . . ] It aims to make social science transformative in aspiration: both a caregiving and world changing activity (2016, pp. 19-20).

Forging such alliances and partnerships with colleagues outside our immediate spheres of expertise, such as healthcare professionals, does not presuppose that we should suppress our criticisms and accept the cultural dominance of contemporary biomedical discourse. Instead, it is precisely because of the criticism that we should participate in actions to promote care, well-being, and health. Human suffering is too serious to be left only in the hands of health professionals and policy-makers. If social sciences in general indicated, throughout the twentieth century, what was wrong in caring for people and people suffering, why not now, in the twenty-first century, suggest changes and participate in the implementation of a different kind of care? Anthropology, in particular, may well supplement the molecular orientations of thought, so grounded in the Western view of the biomedical individual, with practices more sensitive to social and cultural differences.

## Anthropology as communicational therapy?

Given what has been discussed thus far, I agree with other researchers that autism undermines the expectations that parents had when the child was born, of raising children and establishing a family (Bagatell, 2010; Cascio, 2012; Grinker, 2007; Silverman, 2012). This is not merely a sabotage of the "dreams" that parents harbored for their child. In my research, I observed that autism goes beyond, undermining the notion that parents had of what it means to be a person by living together with a child diagnosed as autistic.

From an anthropological perspective, one can affirm that autism denatures what was taken for granted by parents or, if one prefers, it presents a major problem to the relationship between nature and nurture as known by the parents, as Rapp and Ginsburg (2011) have shown. What was expected to naturally happen in the development of the child, with autism, it doesn't. Therefore, what should one do in face of autism's criticism to the fundamentals of personhood and kinship held by the parents?

The official forum for this matter is the health service. Here, the danger to the parents, at least from an anthropological point of view, is normalization: forcing the body toward some notion of normality. Apparently, many health professionals in Brazil articulate these responses together with the parents, subscribing to substances and therapies so mechanically and thoughtlessly that they may only point to the physical and behavioral disciplining of the strange body. As for our neurologist, she understands that this is not the best way to care for an autistic child.

Like many other health professionals, she understands that the starting point should be the individualities of the child in order to develop their potentials. What Mol (2008) calls "learning how to live with the disease" translates itself into the neurologist consultation as a disregard for normality standards in favor of the child's individuality. The commitment she asks from the parents should be based on the awareness of these individual needs to establish therapeutic interventions—professional and/or amateur—best suited to each child. Knowing how to live with the disease is, therefore, accepting that the child's individuality is indelibly autistic in order to develop their skills and competencies as a unique subject. However, as empathic as the physician may be, her language is limited to guiding the parents toward a commitment. It is the parents' task to understand what she understands by commitment and to translate these guidelines into practical realities with their children.

Anthropology as a kind of communication therapy would operate therein, performing an apparently crucial and essential translation of languages that intersect in the relationships between health professionals, parents, and the child. Whether with professionals closer to a normalizing model or with physicians such as our child neurologist, more inclined to the individual needs of the diagnosed patients, the main motto behind an anthropological therapeutic intervention would be the translation of the medical and the autistic child's language to the parents.[5] The chief idea would be to have parents as mentees to help them interpret what health professionals want them to do with their children, and, second, and most importantly, that they may become able to describe the children for themselves. From these translations parents could be helped to use all therapies, ideas, tools, and daily practices—in short, everything available to them to communicate and interact with their children.

Devoid of any epistemological obligation to the health sciences, while also being critical of normative paradigms, anthropology may help parents understand that for development to happen, more important than focusing on socialization deficits or mainstream therapies, the child's affinities, tastes, interests and inclinations have to be discerned, and attempts created toward bonding grounded in languages of the children themselves.[6] Thus, an anthropology applied to children's mental health would have convergent, as well as divergent, partnerships with health professionals, parents as advisees, and children as the protagonists of their interventions. This endeavor would entail not only office work, with dialogues between these three actors, but also fieldwork, in which the anthropologist participates in consultations with health professionals and everyday situations of the family, observing the relationship between parents and children to suggest descriptions and interventions.

[5] I am not alone here, since Hart (2014) and Chew (2013) have similar perspectives, but on different aspects, on the translation of autism.

[6] Suskind (2014) provides a beautiful and precious account of how perceptive parents are to the affinities of the children can trigger in the child impactful communicative developments. Noting that his son had a keen interest in Disney movies, Suskind and his wife staged dialogues and scenes with the child and his older brother at every possible moment, making a product of the cultural industry become a reality, at least from the perspective of the diagnosed child. According to Suskind's account, these dialogues were fundamental for the boy to gradually perceive the relationship between text and context and to move from the echolalia to a proper and meaningful speech according to specific situations. If Suskind's family was able to articulate this type of perception and invention without an anthropological orientation, less perceptive and inventive parents could rely on our knowledge to act similarly with their autistic children.

I recognize that many objections may be raised against an anthropology applied to children's mental health. One could say that a practical application would impoverish the diversity of anthropological perspectives, both in method and theory, transforming this multiplicity into a singular unit. It could also be argued that it has a potential hazard of reproducing colonialist attitudes inscribed in the history of anthropology, making use of controlling ideals to parents and children under the guise of aid. Without ignoring such dangers, which should certainly be considered if the proposal is effectively carried out, I underline the fact that the suggestion of a practical application of anthropology to children's mental health is inspired by ethical motives, and also by the possibilities that an anthropological perspective offers.

The desire to contribute to the care and development of the autistic child not only arises from my personal experience of the pain and courage found in the physician's clinic, but primarily from having experienced them as an anthropologist. By observing that the child neurologist's relational empathy could be increased if it were not so convincingly grounded in neuroscience, by understanding that the emotional dedication of parents could be more communicative if the child's alterity was considered, by observing that educators could further stimulate children to accept that intelligences are diverse and that therapists could be more effective if they did not so forcefully comply with the methods of their protocols. When establishing these perceptions that I experienced in the clinic, anthropological knowledge seemed useful not only as an alternative description of, but also as a significant intervention within, this reality. Or, rather, anthropological knowledge itself could enable us to perceive the importance of the residual in practices and discourses unique to autism. Anthropology is interested in what remains unexplained in the realities of health services. The importance of these residues have historically constituted anthropology's argumentative strength. When it comes to Western health services, at least in Brazil, these residues are still there. It is still important to intervene from these residues. Why can't anthropology of health services go beyond words and writings to suggest actions from these residues?

## References


Bagatell, N. (2010). "From Cure to Community: Transforming Notions of Autism." Ethos, 38: 33–55.

Campoy, L. (2017). Sociedade do Autismo, Etnografia de Vida. Rio de Janeiro: Federal University of Rio de Janeiro.

Cascio, A. (2012). "Neurodiversity: Autism Pride Among Mothers of Children With Autism Spectrum Disorders." *Intellectual and Developmental Disabilities*, 50/3: 273–283.

Chew, C. (2013). "Autism and the Task of the Translator," in Davidson, J. and Orsini, M., eds. *Worlds of Autism: Across the Spectrum of Neurological Difference*. Minneapolis, MN: University of Minnesota Press, Chapter 13.

Corsaro, W. (2003). *"We're Friends, Right?": Inside Kid's Culture*. Washington, DC: Joseph Henry Press.

Corsaro, W. (2017). *The Sociology of Childhood*. Thousand Oaks, CA: SAGE.

Deligny, F. (2015). *The Arachnean and Other Texts*. Minneapolis, MN: Univocal.

Grinker, R. R. (2007). *Unstrange Minds: Remapping the World of Autism*. New York: Basic Books.

Hart, B. (2014). "Autism Parents & Neurodiversity: Radical Translation, Joint Embodiment and the Prosthetic Environment." *BioSocieties*, 9/3: 284–303.

Ingold, T. (2013). *Making*. London: Routledge.
Mol, A. (2003). *The Body Multiple*. Durham, NC: Duke.
Mol, A. (2008). *The Logic of Care. Health and the Problem of Patient Choice*. London: Routledge.
Ortega, F. (2009). "The Cerebral Subject and the Challenge of Neurodiversity." *BioSocieties*, 4: 425–445.
Rapp, R. and Ginsburg, F. (2011). "Reverberations: Disability and the New Kinship Imaginary." *Anthropological Quarterly*, 4/2: 379–410.
Silverman, C. (2012). *Understanding Autism*. Princeton, NJ: Princeton University Press.
Suskind, R. (2014). *Life, Animated. A Story of Sidekicks, Heroes, and Autism*. Los Angeles, CA: Kingswell.
Wilkinson, I. and Kleinman, A. (2016). *A Passion for Society. How We Think About Human Suffering*. Oakland, CA: University of California Press, 2016.

# 9

# Challenges of Participating in Research About Living with Mild Cognitive Impairment Among Disabled Veterans

*Christine Schneider and Eva Kahana*

One regretful time in my life was after my dad was diagnosed with dementia. I knew already—the signs were there for many years. I watched the negative effect the diagnosis had on his self-confidence and instead of asking him how he felt—my Dad and I basically ignored it. We tried to pretend everything was normal. The worst thing was the fact that nothing was normal again. The way we interacted was socially awkward at times, overly critical at others, and I cannot imagine how my dad felt about this. Looking back now, I wish I would have sat down with him to discuss things honestly, asking his opinions. Unfortunately, I never had the chance. I am sure his last years could have been much less frustrating if I would have taken the time to get the answers, only he could provide: how living with mild cognitive impairment (MCI) in everyday life truly is. He died while I was a graduate student. I was a non-traditional student. After high school I joined the United States Navy and was ultimately released from duty with a disability. Since, I have received my health care at the Veteran's Administration Medical Center. These two groups—disabled veterans and people experiencing mild cognitive impairment are very important to me—for personal and professional reasons. Little research has been done in either of these areas because these populations are viewed as vulnerable and research inclusion is very difficult. I am now completing a study of veterans who were recently diagnosed with MCI. This chapter provides some of the findings, trials and tribulations of conducting an interview study of this group.

Christine Schneider

## Introduction

With average life expectancy increasing in the population, people are surviving long enough to experience mild cognitive impairment (MCI), or know someone who does. While caregiver burden has been extensively studied—the lived experience of "forgetting" from the care-getter perspective has been largely ignored (Kahana et al., 2010). One reason for the exclusion of individuals with cognitive difficulty or diagnosis from studies is the assumption that responses by such individuals may not be valid (Harris, 2002; Clare and Shakespeare, 2004). An unfortunate consequence of this is the absence of information that could elucidate the perspectives of the very people most affected: the patients who are living with the "forgetting experience."

Accordingly, older patients diagnosed with MCI may be viewed much like racial minorities, who have been excluded from research. The ethical problems raised by such exclusion have been increasingly recognized by scientists and have resulted in the emergence of the field of "recruitmentology" (Epstein, 2008). This field is focused on the ethical imperatives and challenges of recruiting underserved populations for research. We recognize that stigmatized and underserved groups may also demonstrate reluctance to be involved in research.

Problems in understanding the lived experience of forgetting among populations with MCI relate to major recruitment problems due to administrative, interpersonal, and personal reasons. This chapter provides insights about the barriers and facilitators of recruiting patients with MCI in the organizational context of the Veterans Administration Medical Center (VAMC) through referrals from clinical providers. We hope that identification of salient barriers can improve research participation rates of this vulnerable group, who can both offer and ultimately derive significant benefits through responsible research. Benefits of research based on perspectives of patients with MCI include education of both care providers and informal caregivers, so they can better offer support to this stigmatized and neglected patient group (Young, 2002). As noted in the preface regarding the first author's (CS) experience with her father, care of those with dementia could better meet ethical guidelines if carers could learn about the lived experience of patients and understand their perspectives.

Individuals in early stages of MCI often "know" that they are experiencing memory problems and fear that they are on a downward trajectory (Clare, 2004). This biographical disruption leads individuals to question their identity and their competence in future interactions (Bury, 1982; Gubrium, 1986). The views of people diagnosed with initial MCI can be accessed and are essential for our understanding of the experience of diagnosis and ethical management of the illness (Bedard, 2003; Clare, 2002). They afford a window of opportunity for researchers to try to understand the lived experience of MCI in its early stages.

The symptoms of MCI are manifested in forgetfulness (repeatedly asking the same things, not immediately remembering names of places or people) or confusion (how to react in some everyday situations, making decisions). Individuals experiencing MCI, and those with whom they interact, may be unsure how to act in previously routine social situations. These changes in routine interactions may produce a social "awkwardness," which affects day-to-day living for individuals and their loved ones.

Coping with uncertainty, potential decline, and struggling to remain independent may affect a person's ability to ask for, or receive, help when needed. It is also likely to produce psychological distress (Brown, 1995). Remaining socially engaged in everyday life and within social support groups is critical in order to maintain psychological well-being (Rook, 1987; Vandervoort, 1999). Other ways of reconstructing the self may include use of proactive coping strategies and an acceptance of symptoms and diagnosis

(Brown, 1995). These patient experiences and modes of coping can all affect the research process.

Barriers to recruitment have been identified as posing major challenges to clinical research (Sung et al., 2003). Older adults have been underrepresented in research, and challenges in recruitment for studying this group have been noted (Mody et al., 2008). This chapter illustrates the barriers to research participation by elderly veterans who have been newly diagnosed with MCI at an urban VAMC. It aims to add to understanding of diverse organizational, social, and individual factors that deter research participation and reduce insights that such research can offer for improving patient care. Research related to MCI poses added challenges based on stigma associated with experiencing MCI (Garand et al., 2009) and to caregiver resistance (Connel et al., 2001).

## The VAMC study

The goal of this qualitative study is to learn about patients' experiences after their diagnosis of MCI. Physicians and nurse practitioners from the geriatric and psychology clinics were asked to refer patients who have recently been diagnosed with MCI. Once identified, CS approached patients in the clinic to ask to obtain consent for participation in a semi-structured interview at the VAMC. Interviews take place either immediately following patients' clinic appointment or at another more convenient time at their request. The entire sample in this study to date is comprised of African American men aged 78–94 years. This is important because African Americans have been disproportionally affected by chronic illness and are more likely to develop dementia than white people in the US population (Thies and Bleiler, 2013; Hughes et al., 2017).

Recent literature has increasingly identified some common barriers and facilitators to recruitment of vulnerable populations and provides strategies to overcome barriers (Roberge et al., 2017; Liljas et al., 2017; Bartlett et al., 2018). However, such research, with few exceptions (Bartlett et al., 2018; Kolanowski et al., 2013), focused on vulnerable populations not specifically diagnosed with MCI. Research dealing with disabled veterans with MCI is even more limited. The current VAMC study not only provides insight into the lived experience of MCI, but also addresses this gap in published literature and the growing concern with problems recruiting veterans in health promotion and clinical research.

### VAMC administrative recruitment barriers

CS has both a personal and professional interest in the population of people with MCI, specifically older disabled veterans. In addition to having cared for her father who suffered from MCI, she had worked as a research assistant on previous studies at the VA and developed a strong desire to continue working with the disabled veteran population. In spite of her familiarity with bureaucratic structures of the military, as a veteran herself, she was surprised at the extremely complicated administrative process involved with getting this study approved.

Multiple institutional review boards (IRBs) are usually involved in Veterans Affairs studies, which results in a lengthy and time-consuming approval process. This study was approved in June 2016 by the VAMC, but was initially rejected by the university's IRB. An addendum was submitted and approved in January 2017. In the year and a half since the inception of the study, CS has approached over 150 patients to invite their participation, but has only been able to enroll 24, yielding 21 completed interviews to date.

Administrative IRB delays may be expected in studies with vulnerable populations. Disabled veterans are a group that is severely understudied. To address this issue, recommendations were put forth by the Office of Inspector General, US Department of Health and Human Services, in 1998. The final report suggests that duplication of review across multiple sites is inefficient and discourages researchers from initiating projects (Christian et al., 2002). Recent advances calling for a single review may serve to alleviate this problem in the future.

Especially relevant to this research is the VA Human Research Protection Accreditation Program (VAHRPAP). In 2001, the VAHRPAP, in partnership with the National Committee for Quality Assurance, created an independent external review board to increase human protections while streamlining the administrative process. In theory, the dual purpose of strengthening human protections for VA research participants and streamlining the IRB process was a great first step. In practice, it further perpetuated the overly bureaucratic structure. The research IRB for this project had to go through a total of four subcommittees before the study was approved.

## Recruitment barriers based on the IRB consent form

In addition to the time-consuming IRB approval process, the overly detailed and long consent forms serve as further major deterrents to recruitment. For this research, the final consent form approved by both the VA and the university was 14 pages long and reads like a contract. Although many patients expressed an interest in speaking with the researcher about their memory problems, after seeing the consent form some did not want to participate.

Patients reacted negatively to the consent form for various reasons. One patient suspected that signing the consent forms would force him to move to an assisted-living facility, since his daughter had recently encouraged him to join adult daycare. Because of the official letterhead of the VA consent template he was very nervous that the VA may be trying to "keep him." Another patient was concerned that he was signing a contract that would have lasting impact on his life or healthcare.

With the experience of memory loss, fear and suspicion are normal. However, limiting the length of the 14-page consent form, using a less formal letterhead, and conducting the interview outside the hospital setting may have facilitated recruitment. Less formal consents can still be meaningful (Ridda et al., 2010). A straightforward consent form, written in common language without the formal administrative pieces from each participating university/organization, would be less overwhelming and easier to comprehend, particularly for individuals with MCI.

## Recruitment barriers based on physician reluctance/rotation

The VAMC requested that patients be referred for participation through physicians or other medical personnel. Numerous times, the referral did not materialize. The attending medical personnel often assumed refusal without asking patients directly. They made comments like "he was really annoyed today," or "he would not be interested in something like that." This barrier to recruitment has also been documented in the literature. Hinshaw et al. (2001) found that attending clinicians, who are logical referral sources, may be reluctant to enroll their patients. Patients being treated in outpatient facilities, and particularly the VA, often encounter long waits and other stressful experiences. Many physicians aim to protect their patients from research that could add further stress.

Recruitment would have been greatly facilitated if the researcher could have talked with the patients directly and determine if they were in the right frame of mind or interested. There were occasions when the physician identified a patient to CS and gave her an opportunity to explain fully the study and ask the patient if he would be interested in being interviewed while waiting for his appointment. Each time the patient agreed to participate. Often patients wait and once their appointment is finally over they do not want to prolong their visit by spending more time with a researcher. Many patients only come to the VA clinic every 30–90 days, so the sample size was severely depleted as a result of not being able to approach patients in clinic in a more informal setting than the doctor's office.

Another barrier to recruitment relates to physicians' clinical rotation. New teams of physicians who practice in the clinics may be unaware of the research study. Flyers posted in clinic may go unnoticed by new physicians. This problem was alleviated when the researcher was able to utilize permanent medical care staff. While attending residents and physicians are on a rotation schedule, full-time registered nurses, licensed practical nurses, and other staff are permanent. Because some of these personnel have an actual patient list, they fall under the IRB approval to refer patients. However, it is not always clear to researchers who these full-time personnel are. Recruitment was facilitated in our study when CS was able to work with a nurse who met with patients regularly to fill their pill boxes to help with medicine adherence.

Utilizing the nurse's patient list helped our recruitment by approaching eligible patients while they were getting their medications refilled. Once the patient was checked in and had their vitals and chart updated the nurse let CS know that she would be going down to the pharmacy to refill medications and CS could talk with patients while they waited. It was a very comfortable environment and patients were often happy to talk. CS was able to recruit and complete interviews during this process. This situation created a very smooth and informal process with fewer power dynamics involved.

If a research project is able to meet all HIPAA (Health Insurance Portability and Accountability Act of 1996), Human Subjects Protections, IRB guidelines, and the referral design is written in the study protocol, all eligible patients should be referred to the research team. Awareness of the opportunity to participate in research can be beneficial to the patients. Many of the individuals CS spoke with indicated that they were glad to know that this type of research was available. One patient who agreed to participate appreciated talking with the researcher because he noted that it is hard to talk to family members about memory. Another patient who refused did not feel like he had any memory problems but told CS that he was happy to know that there are studies like this for when he needs it. When people know that they are not alone in dealing with MCI, it helps normalize their condition.

## Recruitment barriers based on patient reluctance

One recurring theme of patient reluctance to participate in the study was the frustration expressed at yet another set of memory "questions." Patients with cognitive diagnoses are accustomed to frequent memory tests for updates in clinical settings. They may fear negative consequences based on their cognitive ability. They know that physicians at the VAMC are responsible for referring patients for a driver's evaluation if cognitive testing is borderline. As one patient stated, "the last time I talked about my memory, they tried to take my car away!" To facilitate recruitment, CS had to reassure patients that they would not be tested on their memory; instead, they would have the opportunity to discuss their experiences of forgetting. The ability to reinforce that the study was independent of their medical care was beneficial for recruitment.

Some patients, who receive an MCI diagnosis while seeking care for physical health problems, may be unaware of their diagnosis, or may choose to minimize or even fully deny the existence of the problem (Mody et al., 2008). Some patients CS approached appeared to be completely unaware or denied having cognitive problems, even when below-average memory testing was repeatedly documented in their charts. Supporting this observation, Furimsky et al. (2008) found that early in the course of treatment for a newly diagnosed mental illness, many patients are still trying to understand the implications and treatment options related to their diagnosis. It may take time for patients to develop insight into their illness and accept the diagnosis. It is also possible that some patients are not fully informed about their diagnosis since that is not the primary concern of their physician regarding their health.

## Recruitment barriers based on caregiver/family/guardian influences

There may be both positive and negative influences of the family for enrolling participants. For example, one patient was really interested in participating in the study, but his daughter, who drove him to the VA appointment, was busy and did not want to wait.

Another patient did not want to participate, but his daughter suggested that we trick him into speaking with the researcher because it would benefit him. CS did not agree to this proposal but noted that she would try to connect again with the father at his next appointment. Even though he never did participate in the study, his daughter indicated that she talked with him a few times about how this type of study could help him.

Family members' attitudes to recruitment mattered because most eligible patients were no longer driving. Family members may work full-time and be unable to bring patients to study appointments, posing a significant barrier to enrollment and retention in clinical trials (van Stuijvenber et al., 1998). Both the patients' and families' acceptance of the diagnosis and treatment are critical to full participation in research studies. Ross et al. (1999) found that patients were less likely to participate in research if someone important to them was against it. This highlights the fact that strategies to improve recruitment must address barriers with both the patients and their families.

## Recruitment barriers based on missed appointments

Vulnerable populations, specifically veterans, are less likely to keep appointments and have higher no-show rates than other research participants (Kheirkhah et al., 2016). Both inclement weather and the lack of transportation can pose real barriers to research participation for older patients with MCI. Because many patients commute a long distance to receive their care at the VA, they make multiple appointments on the same day, resulting in patients spending hours in waiting rooms. There have been multiple times where a patient arrived for his initial appointment late, had a long wait, and was not willing to stay later to talk to a researcher about memory problems.

Liljas et al. (2017) illustrated another barrier to patients keeping VA appointments. Most VA patients are seen in the geriatrics clinic for their many chronic conditions. Their health may not allow them to attend scheduled appointments. VA appointments are often scheduled a month in advance. Reminder phone calls are usually made 48 hours before the scheduled appointment. Since many VA patients have no phone or are out of data, reminders from clinics can go unheard, resulting in forgetting about the appointment and appointments are missed.

## **Suggestions for improving recruitment**

Based on this study, we identified significant but addressable, barriers to enrolling participants from the VA. Barriers include multiple IRBs, numerous and lengthy consent forms, physician resistance, overbooking of appointments, lack of family support, and high no-show rates. While some of the individual and organizational barriers to recruitment may be difficult to overcome, in combination they result in excluding voices of patients in the healthcare system from being heard and deprive them of experiences of sharing their stories with the scientific community.

We have much to learn about the lived experience of forgetting. We need to hear the voices of patients, both in the general population, and among harder-to-reach populations—like veterans. We can only do so by eliminating bureaucratic barriers and making research participation attractive to both patients and their caregivers. VA hospitals can be a wonderful venue for research. They are research hospitals, they serve a broad cross-section of patients, and are able to facilitate recruitment for research studies.

Effecting changes to facilitate recruitment in these settings is possible. Caregivers and support networks are often overlooked as sources of assistance in recruitment. Diverse medical personnel who have access to the patient population should be invited to help. Research teams should have access to newly employed physicians to promote enrollment. It would be beneficial to gain access to locations outside of the VA for conducting interviews. Patient interviews should be scheduled on days where the participants may not experience stress due to multiple appointments and travel. Consent procedures should be streamlined to avoid institutional fear.

Elderly veterans who participate in research have a lot to offer the area of research on living with forgetting. In addition to contributing to a better understanding of the lived experience of MCI study participants may have a positive experience to have an opportunity to voice their concerns and strategies for coping with the challenges of MCI. They also appear to derive comfort from articulating their experiences. Elderly veterans who participated in this study had very positive reactions and provided valuable data that reinforces the need to overcome barriers to recruitment.

## Conclusions

Facilitating research recruitment of older adults with MCI is useful on many levels. It can achieve a better understanding of the perspectives of patients living with this increasingly prevalent and debilitating condition. Such understanding can contribute to improved clinical practice and policy development. Recent research indicates that older adults prefer advocacy by their physicians, rather than self-advocacy (Kahana et al., 2018). Learning about patient experiences and perspectives after a diagnosis of MCI is critically important for physicians and other healthcare providers to offer counseling and social support to this population. Similarly, it would be highly desirable for family members to receive education and guidance through support groups to develop a better understanding of needs and coping strategies of their loved ones, in order to be more effective caregivers. The first author's experience with her father's illness poignantly illustrates this unmet need.

The stigma produced from initial diagnoses of MCI affects how individuals perceive themselves and how others perceive them (Garand, et al., 2009). Research can lead to greater access for patients to positive informal and formal support from both healthcare providers and family members. Such support is critical to promote resiliency in persons diagnosed with MCI. Such individuals often experience frustration upon diagnoses because healthcare professionals offer few insights about their prospects and treatment options and do not share with them insights based on studies with other patients (Young, 2002).

We must stop assuming that people with MCI have a lack of awareness in all domains. Just because a person shows evidence of MCI, we should not assume that "awareness in one domain precludes awareness in others" (Clare, 2004). These hard-to-recruit participants have much to offer research to increase well-being for older adults in our society. Understanding the awareness process of cognitive problems, the implications of diagnosis, perceptions of social support, and coping strategies may increase well-being for individuals living with the daily experience of "forgetting." Accomplishing these goals will also serve the ethical imperative for inclusion of underserved populations.

## References

Bartlett, R., Milne, R., and Croucher, R. (2018). "Strategies to Improve Recruitment of People with Dementia to Research Studies." *Dementia (London)*, Jan 1 (Epub ahead of print).

Bedard M. (2003). "Validity of Self-Reports in Dementia Research: The Geriatric Depression Scale." *Clinical Gerontologist* 26: 155–163.

Brown, P. (1995). "Naming and Framing: The Social Construction of Diagnosis and Illness." *Journal of Health and Social Behavior*, 35: 34–52.

Bury, M. (1982). "Chronic Illness as a Biographical Disruption." *Sociology of Health and Illness*, 4: 167–182.

Christian, M. C., Goldberg, J. L., Killen, J., Abrams, J. S., McCabe, M. S., Mauer, J. K., and Wittes, R. E. (2002). "A Central Institutional Review Board for Multi-Institutional Trials." *New England Journal of Medicine*, 346: 1405–1408.

Clare, L. (2002). "We'll Fight it as Long as We Can: Coping With the Onset of AD." *Aging and Mental Health*, 6/2: 139–148.

Clare, L. (2004) "The Construction of Awareness in Early-Stage Alzheimer's Disease: A Review of Concepts." *International Journal of Geriatric Psychiatry*, 16: 879–885.

Clare, L. and Shakespeare, P. (2004). "Negotiating the Impact of Forgetting: Dimensions of Resistance in Task-oriented Conversations Between People With Dementia and Their Partners." *Dementia*, 3: 211–232.

Connell, C., Shaw, B., Holmes, S., and Foster, N. (2001). "Caregivers' Attitudes Toward Their Family Members' Participation in Alzheimer Disease Research: Implications for Recruitment and Retention." *Alzheimer Disease & Associated Disorders*, 15/3: 137–145.

Epstein, S. (2008). "The Rise of Recruitmentology' Clinical Research, Racial Knowledge, and the Politics of Inclusion and Difference." *Social Studies of Science*, 38/5: 801–832.

Furimsky, I., Cheung, A., Dewa, C., and Zipursky, R. (2008). "Strategies to Enhance Patient Recruitment and Retention in Research Involving Patients With a First Episode of Mental Illness." *Contemporary Clinical Trials*, 29: 862–866.

Garand, L., Lingler, J. H., Conner, K. O., and Dew, M. A. (2009). "Diagnostic Labels, Stigma, and Participation in Research Related to Dementia and Mild Cognitive Impairment." *Research in Gerontological Nursing*, 2/2: 112–121.

Gubrium, J, (1986). *Oldtimers and Alzheimer's: The Descriptive Organization of Senility*. Greenwich, CT: JAI Press.

Harris, P. (2002) *The Person with Alzheimer's Disease: Pathways to Understanding the Disease.* Baltimore, MD: The John Hopkins University Press.

Hinshaw, S., Hoagwood, K., Jensen, P. S., Kratochvil, C., Bickman, L., Clarke, G., et al. (2001). "AACAP 2001 Research Forum: Challenges and Recommendations Regarding Recruitment and Retention of Participants in Research Investigations." *Journal of the American Academy of Child Adolescent Psychology*, 43/8: 1037–1045.

Hughes, T., Varma, V., Pettigrew, C., and Albert, M. (2017). "African Americans and Clinical Research: Evidence Concerning Barriers and Facilitators to Participation and Recruitment Strategies." *Gerontologist*, 57/2: 348–358.

Kahana, B., Yu, J., Kahana, E., and Langendoerfer, K. B. (2018). "Whose Advocacy Counts in Shaping Elderly Patients' Satisfaction With Physicians' Care and Communication?" *Clinical Interventions in Aging*, 13: 1161.

Kahana, E., Kelley-Moore, J. A., Kahana, B., and Brown, J. A. (2010). "Social Dimensions of Late Life Disability," in Gueldner, S. and Wykle, M., eds. *Healthy Aging: Gerontological Education for Nurses and Other Health Care Professionals*. Sudbury, MA: Jones and Bartlett, pp. 457–468.

Kheirkhah, P., Feng, Qianmei, Travis, L., Tavakoli-Tabasi, S., and Sharafkhaneh, A. (2016). "Prevalence, Predictors and Economic Consequences of No Shows." *BMC Health Services*, 16: 13.

Kolanowski, A., Mulhall, P., Yevchak, A., Hill, N., and Fick, D. (2013). "The Triple Challenge of Recruiting Older Adults With Dementia and High Medical Acuity in Skilled Nursing Facilities." *Journal of Nursing Scholarship*, 45/4: 397–404.

Liljas, A., Walters, K., Jovicic, A., Manthorpe, J., Goodman, C., and Kharicha, K. (2017). "Strategies to Improve Engagement of 'Hard to Reach' Older People in Research on Health Promotion: A Systematic Review." *BMC Public Health*, 17: 349–357.

Mody, L., Miller, D. K., McGloin, J. M., Freeman, M., Marcantonio, E. R., Magaziner, J., and Studenski, S. (2008). "Recruitment and Retention of Older Adults in Aging Research." *Journal of the American Geriatrics Society*, 56/12: 2340–2348.

Ridda, I., MacIntyre, C.R, Lindley, R.I., and Tan, T.C. (2010). "Difficulties in Recruiting Older Adults in Clinical Trials: And Examination of Barriers and Soultions." *Vaccine*, 28/4: 901–906.

Roberge, E., Benedek, D., Marx, C., and Rasmusson, A. (2017). "Analysis of Recruitment Strategies: Enrolling Veterans with PTSD into a Clinical Trial." *Military Psychology*, 29/5: 407–417.

Rook, K. (1987). "The Negative Side of Social Interaction: Impact on Psychological Well-Being." *Journal of Personality and Social Psychology*, 46: 1097–1108.

Ross, S., Grant, A., Counsell, C., Gillespie, W., Russell, I., and Pescott, R. (1999). "Barriers to Participation in Randomised Controlled Trials: A Systematic Review." *Journal of Clinical Epidemiology*, 52: 1143–1156.

Sung, N., Crowley Jr, W, Genel, M., Salber, P., Sandy, L., Sherwood, L. M., Johnson, S. B., Catanese, V., Tilson, H., Getz, K., Larson, E. L., Scheinberg, D., Reece, E. A., Slavkin, H., Dobs, A., Grebb, J., Martinez, R. A., Korn, A., and Larson, E. L. (2003). "Central challenges facing the national clinical research enterprise." *JAMA*, 289/10: 1278–1287.

Thies, W. and Bleiler, L. (2013). "Alzheimer's Disease Facts and Figures." *Alzheimer's Dementia* 9: 208–245.

Vandervoort, D. (1999). "Quality of Social Support in Mental Health." *Current Psychology: Developmental, Learning, Personality, Social*, 18: 205–222.

van Stuijvenber, M., Suur, J., de Vos, S., Tjiang, G. C. H., Steyerberg, E. W., Derksen-Lubsen, G., and Moll, H. A. (1998). "Informed Consent, Parental Awareness, and Reasons for Participating in a Randomized Controlled Study." *Archives of Disease in Childhood*, 79: 120–125.

Young, R. (2002). "Medical Experiences and Concerns of People with Alzheimer's Disease," in Harris, P., ed. *The Person With Alzheimer's Disease: Pathways to Understanding the Disease*. Baltimore, MD: The John Hopkins University Press, pp. 29–46.

# 10

# Mediators of Inclusion

## Challenges to Including Adults with Mild Intellectual Disability in Qualitative Research

*Vanessa Cox, Treena Orchard, Pamela Cushing, and Elizabeth Anne Kinsella*

### Introduction

Researchers wishing to include people with cognitive impairments must grapple with how to ensure these participants are able to exercise autonomy, have free choice, and that they understand that their involvement is voluntary. Adults with mild intellectual disability (MID) are frequently excluded from qualitative research out of the belief that intellectual impairment hinders autonomy, rendering them child-like and in need of protection. Instead, professionals or family members often speak *for* them in qualitative research. This poses a significant problem for people with MID because it renders their valuable first-hand experiences invisible and reinforces the assumption that others are more equipped to make decisions for them and speak on their behalf. Addressing this important inequity is critical to developing evidence-based policy and programming based on their lived experience. To this end, critically oriented action research can be part of this shift in research that makes room for including adults with MID to speak on their own behalf (Scotland, 2012).

The purpose of this chapter is to discuss the methodological challenges of including adults with MID in qualitative research. The data for this chapter come from a larger, qualitative study that explored independence, social relationships, and sexuality among adults with MID, family caregivers, and support workers. We begin with a discussion of how sensitive topics, namely sexuality, intersect with vulnerability in research settings and everyday life for adults with MID. These complex intersections often produce concerns about the need to protect these adults from any harms or tensions regarding sexuality, which are often heightened in discussions about adults with MID in ways that are unique compared with other marginalized or vulnerable groups. We argue, however, that their vulnerabilities should not preclude their participation in research and the rare and valuable insights gained from the inclusion of these adults in our study demonstrates that it can be done. The next section describes the design and primary methods employed in the study, which is followed by our analysis of the themes regarding caregiver control over public and private spaces, challenges to research inclusion, and the experiences of adults with MID participating in the study. The chapter concludes with a discussion of the contributions our data make to the disability and sexuality research literatures, and provide several recommendations regarding study design and approach that will be valuable to other researchers who seek to include adults with MID in their scholarly work.

## 'Sensitive' topics and vulnerability

Sensitive topics in qualitative research are those that make participants, and sometimes researchers, uncomfortable to discuss, and they also include those that can pose certain kinds of ethical or cultural challenges to the safety and discretion of participants (Wellings et al., 2000). Sexuality, operationalized here as sexual identities, behaviors, and preferences, is a complex issue that is often considered sensitive, contentious, and as something more safely discussed in the private realm. However, sexuality does not only occur in the private realm and in its various forms it has long been used as a technique of political governance through part of larger social and state-mandated efforts to marginalize, contain, and discipline certain populations, as well as practices (Foucault, 1990; Weeks, 1998). Including members of vulnerable groups, who are often assumed to be easily coerced or exploited (Bracken-Roche et al., 2017; Iacono, 2006), in research studies that explore sexuality or other sensitive topics can be challenging to researchers (see Liamputtong, 2007). Institutional, social, and more intimate family forces can conspire to make this kind of work exceedingly difficult, prolonged, and circumscribed in focus, which has historically led many researchers to exclude these groups from participating altogether.

Adults with MID do not enjoy the same sexual freedoms and reproductive autonomy afforded to more powerful groups in society. This is exemplified in the eugenics movement of the early to mid-twentieth century, in which people with intellectual disability were forcefully sterilized or had legal limits placed on marriage (Kempton and Kahn, 1991; Simmons, 1982 Trent, 1994). Although these legal sanctions regarding the regulation of their sexual and reproductive behaviors have been lifted, these adults still experience social restrictions on their socio-sexual behaviors and in many realms related to the maintenance of their personal health and bodily autonomy (Abbot and Horwath, 2007; Foley, 2012; Kelly et al., 2009; Healy et al., 2009; Shakespeare et al., 1996; Seibers, 2008; Walker-Hirsch, 2007). These challenges are often attributed to fears of pregnancy and sexual abuse, as well as assumptions of child-like innocence and asexuality (Abbot and Horwath, 2007; Shakespeare et al., 1996; Seibers, 2008; Walker-Hirsch, 2007). Adults with MID also experience exclusion in the context of sexuality research, which then reinforces ablest assumptions that the sexualities of adults with MID are unimportant as compared to other groups in society. Including the lived experiences of adults with MID in sexuality research can expose the challenges to inclusion in social and sexual life faced by these adults, and can also illuminate the ways in which their sexual lives are similar to those without MID.

## Details of the study: purpose and methods

The purpose of the featured study was to explore how adults with MID exercise independence in the development and maintenance of socio-sexual relationships within the context of familial and social/care environments. These are issues that are woefully under-researched in the disability studies field and it is unclear how or if dependence on others affects the ability of people with MID to form and maintain social and sexual relationships. We also do not know the ways in which this dependency informs the social and sexual well-being of these adults. This was a qualitative study, which is well suited for gaining rich understandings of the meanings given to a particular phenomena, as the researcher is committed to seeing "through the eyes" of the participants (Snape and Spencer, 2003).

With respect to data collection, we conducted[1] individual, semi-structured interviews with 29 participants. Three participant groups were recruited: adults with MID (n = 15; seven women, eight men); support workers of an adult with MID (n = 8; six women, two men); and parents of an adult with MID (n = 6; all women). Gender divisions within each participant group were coincidental. The interview guides differed according to participant group, but all consisted of questions designed to explore the first-hand experiences of independence, socio-sexual relationships, and sexuality of adults with MID from the varying perspectives. The lead researcher used a relaxed, conversational style, probing deeper at times, and encouraging story-telling as examples. The interviews were held in locations chosen by the participant and included cafés in the community, the participants' homes, the lead author's university office, and a meeting room at a local agency. In addition to the interviews, descriptive and reflexive notes were recorded after each interview that describe the interview context and setting, as well as the feelings and emerging insights regarding the research interaction by the lead researcher.

Recruitment was purposive, as we sought to find participants that are experts in the phenomena under investigation (Beail and Williams, 2014). Therefore, for this research we aimed to recruit 20 adults with MID, eight parents of an adult with MID, and eight support workers of adults with MID. Support workers and parents were recruited by advertisements in community agency newsletters, as well as word of mouth from gatekeepers at these agencies and other participants. Finding adults with MID for the study required the help of community agencies to identify and inform potential participants who fit the inclusion criteria about the study, as flyers or advertisements may not have been effective for this population due to differences in literacy ability.

Data analysis was thematic and began with the lead author immersing herself in the data through, firstly, the transcription of the interviews and then multiple, active readings of each one. Initial ideas, or codes, were written down and then organized into themes that informed the overall study objectives, searching for patterns of frequency

[1] These were conducted by the first author as part of her doctoral research and the other authors include the primary supervisory and committee members.

and nuance within and between interviews and participant groups (Clarke and Braun, 2006; Beail and Williams, 2014; Taylor et al., 2016). Concepts central to critical disability theory and the theory of sexual citizenship also shaped the interpretation of our study data. For example, we focused on the ways in which others used deviations in cognitive capacity as justification for exclusion from social and sexual life (Shildrick 2012; Seibers, 2008). We also examined the ways in which autonomy and freedom of choice over sexual and reproductive matters were restricted (Richardson, 2000; Weeks, 1998) on account of these deviations. The study received approval from the authors' institutional research ethics board; this process took no longer than other projects seeking approval owing to the extreme care and diligence taken in crafting the ethics protocol. All names of participants used in this chapter are pseudonyms.

## Key findings

### Socio-sexual relationships: The roles of space and caregivers

One of the most significant study findings was the integral role of parents and/or support workers in mediating the social and sexual lives of adults with MID, primarily through control over access to public and private spaces. Most of the study participants with MID spent a significant amount of time in supervised, segregated spaces, such as day programs, employment classes, and sports activities such as Special Olympics. Participants valued these spaces in important ways and they were integral to making and connecting with friends and partners. Some of the adults, however, wanted more free time with friends, rather than the regulated activities that characterize these spaces:

I: Where do you meet most of your friends?
A: At work [day program/classes]. Yeah.
I: Do you ever see them outside of work?
A: Uh, I see some of them go bowling. Yeah some of my friends go bowling ...
I: Do you wish that you saw some of them more?
A: Yeah. Yeah ...
I: What do you think gets in the way of seeing them more?
A: Um, just my, my social life, like bowling and my weekends. I wish I could see them on the weekends.
I: What would you want to do with them on the weekends?
A: Um, I don't know. Maybe go to a movie, maybe? Yeah, go to a movie, just hang out.

Parents and support workers also reported that it was common for adults with MID to have limited opportunity to socialize outside of these structured activities. Parents and support workers attributed this to either a lack of ability and/or willingness on behalf of caregivers to support opportunities for independent socializing. These opportunities, particularly for those who do not live independently, are frequently mediated by their reliance on others, thus compromising autonomous participation in social activities, as well as participation in research. Reliance on others for transportation, scheduling, permission due to safety concerns, and caregiver rules has significant implications for the capacities of adults with MID to be included in research.

Some participants with MID had romantic partners but could only spend time with them within the context of structured, supervised spaces such as day program classes. This was more common among participants who lived in the parental home, and were associated with feelings of frustration during the interviews. Here is an excerpt from the interview with Nathan, a participant with MID in his early thirties who is not allowed to date officially, even though him and his girlfriend have been together for a number of years:

I: Do you see her outside the [day program], like do you go to her house, or does she go to your house?
N: I want to see her outside the [day program] but our moms haven't met yet.
I: Oh, OK.
N: We met each other, like I've met her mom and she's met my mom, but our moms haven't met yet. So that's why we haven't kind of done anything yet like dating.
I: So your mom likes to meet the mom of who you're dating before you can hang out?
N: Yeah. It's been a rule since the caveman days! [Laughs]
I: [Laughs]. How do you feel about that rule?
N: I don't really like it. I don't think I would meet my son's or daughter's parents, well you know what I mean ... um their girlfriend or boyfriends parents, like I'd just let them date!
I: Yeah, OK, how long have you had this girlfriend?
N: Um, we've been on and off but we've probably been together four years.

This excerpt demonstrates the level of control that parents are capable of wielding over the romantic relationships of the adults with MID that depend on them via restrictions on the spaces they may interact with partners. This ultimately leaves these adults with no choice but to navigate their romantic and sexual lives within a context of near-constant surveillance by others, restricting opportunities to engage in sexual behavior that are typically afforded more freely to adults without MID. An example of this challenge came from Chantelle, who, facing a lack of privacy at home and in day program activities, tried to be intimate with her partner by sneaking away to a locker room, and was ultimately reprimanded when caught by staff: "The staff caught us once and I'm like, 'Oh my God!' And then after, the staff is like, 'You guys shouldn't be doing that anyway, Chantelle ... '

## Challenges to research inclusion

One of the most pressing challenges to including adults with MID in the study was a lack of interest and support from community agencies. Only one of five agencies that work with adults with MID on a regular basis responded to requests to discuss gaining access to this population for recruitment purposes. The rationale behind agency disinterest remains unclear, as attempts to open up communication have been unsuccessful. While the participating agency helped immensely, to have had the support of the other agencies would have increased the number of adults with MID who could have been notified of the research opportunity. Having participants from various agencies would have also provided more opportunity to unpack some of the differences and similarities in the experiences of adults with MID who get primary support from other agencies. Additionally, because only one agency was involved, and support workers told their own service users about the study, adults with MID had an additional risk to their anonymity to consider on account of these caregivers being aware of who showed interest in participating. Ultimately, 19 adults with MID expressed interest in participating, but only 15 were interviewed in the end, which may have been influenced by this risk to anonymity.

A second issue that presented a challenge to including the adults with MID was that the lead researcher, at times, was regarded as a potential threat to the well-being of the adult with MID that they support. One example of this suspicion occurred while making plans over the phone to meet with an adult with MID, Miranda, who had expressed interest in the study. Miranda said that she would prefer to meet at her own home; her support worker then got on the phone and after a discussion about the study, the support worker stated, "You'll need a police check before meeting at the house," and said that she would call head office to find out if the lead researcher was permitted to do the interview there. The rationale for the support worker's interruption was not clear, but it reflects how Miranda's decisions in regard to participation are not entirely her own. The interview was ultimately held in Miranda's home, and no police checks were required.

A third challenge to the inclusion of adults with MID in the study was that, for a number of participants, the time and location of the interview had to coincide with the availabilities of their parents and support workers. In many cases, the lead researcher was passed by phone from the adult with MID to a caregiver to discuss the logistics of meeting. While this may be attributed, in part, to cognitive challenges associated with intellectual impairment, it also reflects, as with the previous example, the degree to which their availabilities are tied up in the schedules of those around them. For example, one support worker asked, "Can we do it in the morning so we can get groceries done by the end of my shift?" This interconnectedness between the caregiver and adult with MID's schedules demonstrates the power held by these caregivers to facilitate or constrain participation in research. Chantelle, a participant with MID, demonstrated the power that this reliance on her mother's availability has on her decision-making:

"I gotta ask my mom first before I make decisions because in case we might be busy and I don't even know about it."

Parents and formal caregivers also have the power to take control of certain aspects of their participation, particularly as it relates to privacy. This occurred during our study on more than one occasion. For example, one parent took the phone from her son, Vince, to organize where and when the interview would take place. Her preference was that it would be at their home. Even though the lead researcher requested privacy, throughout the interview Vince's mother hovered in an adjacent room, at times entering to clean. As a result, Vince was visibly uncomfortable discussing sexuality because his mother was within earshot. Sensing this and out of respect for him, the lead researcher did not probe for more information when it came to this more sensitive topic, and at times omitted questions, especially in regard to sexual behavior. Had Vince's mother allowed privacy for the interview, more of Vince's perspectives could have been elicited, which would have added to the depth and overall quality of the interview.

## Adults with MID reflect on research participation

Adults with MID played an active role in negotiating their participation in the study. This involved requesting additional information prior to giving consent, and consenting to some aspects of the study but not others. Each potential participant with MID and the lead researcher engaged in conversations prior to the lead researcher obtaining consent, during which time the details of the study were explained, from its purpose to its voluntary nature. Potential participants often asserted themselves by asking questions to clarify details that were unclear to them, and sought out the information they needed in order to make an informed decision. For example, one adult with MID called the lead researcher a few times before meeting to ask questions and seek clarification about what the study would involve. These questions included asking about where and how the interview would be written about, how the quotes would be anonymized, and who would hear the interview. The lead researcher brought an example of a qualitative journal article to the interview to show her a visual representation of the way it would be written, and the way quotes remove real names and specific identifiers. This collaborative process of ensuring consent was voluntary and fully informed for this participant demonstrates the capability of these adults to be active in this process of obtaining knowledge necessary to make an informed choice.

Participants with MID demonstrated an ability to be assertive in negotiating aspects of the study that they did not want to partake in. For example, Vicky originally said that she would be fine with audio-recording, but changed her mind about this before beginning. The lead researcher then recorded information during the interview with short jot notes, and wrote answers to the interview questions immediately after. This act demonstrated that she felt uncomfortable with this particular aspect of participation, but she was capable and assertive enough to decide this and communicate her altered decision. Similarly, a number of participants felt uncomfortable with certain questions, and communicated a desire to not answer either explicitly or implicitly. The following excerpt is an example of Jeff responding to probing in regard to whether or not he had wanted to have sex with his ex-girlfriend:

J: I'll just say, "not available."
I: Oh, OK, you'd prefer not to answer?
J: That's correct. I'll just say, "not available."

Even if participants did not communicate discomfort with the line of questioning in as explicit a way as Jeff did, there were participants who showed their discomfort in non-verbal ways, and the lead researcher noticed and changed topic accordingly. For example, Linda was asked whether or not she had engaged in sexual activity, and she immediately began to blush profusely, and did not respond immediately. The lead researcher responded to this non-verbal communication, by switching to asking if she had had sex education, which immediately changed her demeanor along with this less personal line of questioning. The significance of this is that even though Linda was struggling to verbalize her discomfort, she still communicated it in a way that could be understood by the lead researcher.

Each interview ended by asking what each adult with MID thought could be done to better support them in their relationships. Asking this question gave these participants the opportunity to provide explicit feedback to guide policy and practice for supporting socio-sexual well-being. Chantelle, like a number of these adults, took the opportunity to offer advice to those who support her, in regard to helping her talk about difficulties with her current romantic and sexual partner:

C: Um, maybe the staff should help me talk about it instead of saying—cause every time I ask for help, they don't wanna get involved. They would say, "Oh. I don't wanna hear about it."
I: Like talking about your relationship problems?
C: Yeah that's what they say, "I don't wanna hear about it, I don't wanna hear about it."

Tom used the opportunity to propose a "guy's night out" idea where he could meet with and hang out with other men to do things like shoot pool together. Having the adults with MID take part in identifying issues and proposing solutions is practical for guiding expert-informed policy and practice.

## Discussion

This chapter explores the methodological challenges of including adults with MID in qualitative research, particularly that which is of a sensitive nature. Our data support findings on research inclusion that adults with MID often require the support of caregivers, as well as researchers, to participate in studies (McDonald, 2012). This supports a relational view of autonomy whereby the decision (or not) to participate is embedded in the social context within which the participant resides (Sherwin and Winsby, 2010). The findings contribute new insights in regard to the vulnerability of adults with MID in research inclusion; that they are capable of negotiating their own participation, even when discussing sensitive topics. Researchers can support this by attending to relational autonomy, and being reflexive during the research process (Guillemin and Gillam, 2004; Phelan and Kinsella, 2013; Sherwin and Winsby, 2010).

One significant study finding was the integral role of caregivers in mediating the inclusion of adults with MID in social and sexual life. Most of the adults with MID in the study reported that they do the majority of their socializing within the context of segregated, structured activities; these spaces offer opportunities to meet and spend time with others for the purposes of friendship and dating. Unless, however, the adults with MID have the opportunity to meet outside of these activities in public or private, these adults must navigate their relationships within these supervised, structured contexts only. This does not allow much freedom to just "hang out" with friends, or go on dates; two activities that are typically afforded to adults without MID. Additionally, these spaces do not allow privacy for intimacy between partners; this is unfortunate for a couple of participants who were also restricted in terms of privacy in their homes. If these adults were considered to be sexual citizens, they would have the freedom to participate in sexual activity (Plummer, 1995; Weeks, 1998; Richardson, 2000), on an equitable basis as compared to their non-MID counterparts.

In the current study, community agencies and caregivers were capable of both facilitating and restricting opportunities for adults with MID to be included in the study. Gaining the interest and support of these entities was therefore necessary; however, this presented the most significant challenge to research inclusion. The reliance on caregiver schedules and ability to support the logistical aspects of participation reflects the important roles played by these supportive others in research inclusion (McDonald, 2012). There were, however, instances where this power was used in such a way as to undermine the autonomy of the adult with MID when the lead researcher was regarded with suspicion. This finding supports a relational view of autonomy, whereby an individual's capacity to be autonomous cannot be separated from the social context (Sherwin and Winsby, 2010); in this case the influence of caregivers who wish to protect the adult with MID from potential harm.

Adults with MID in the study demonstrated the ability to actively negotiate the limits of their own participation. This is contrary to the assumption of adults with MID being solely passive and vulnerable to the research process. Additionally, some participants did not want to answer certain questions that caused discomfort, and they communicated this to the lead researcher in order to protect their own interests. Even if the adult with MID was unable to express this verbally, the lead researcher was able to respond appropriately to the non-verbal communication that took its place, and did not probe further. Phelan and Kinsella (2013) contend that researchers can recognize and negotiate these moments of increased vulnerability by being reflexive. Reflexivity can be described as the process of the researcher being critically reflective of their interpretations of what is going on in the research process (Guillemin and Gillam, 2004). In this case, reflexivity involved the researcher's reflections on her interpretations of the participant's behavior as an expression of discomfort. Reflexivity requires a commitment on the part of the researcher to being attentive and prepared to respond to these "ethically-important moments" (Guillemin and Gillam, 2004, p.265) that arise during qualitative interviews (Guillemin and Gillam, 2004; Phelan and Kinsella, 2013). Adults with MID shared insights in regard to how they can be better supported to be included in social and sexual life—advice that will be shared with agencies and caregivers as an important part of dissemination. Adults with intellectual disability have stated that they want their participation in research to go towards educating others on their needs and desires in order to improve their lives (McDonald, 2012).

Researchers wishing to include adults with MID in qualitative research should consider the power of agencies and caregivers to both facilitate and restrict their inclusion. Efforts should be made to emphasize the importance of including adults with MID in research that will inform the very policies and practices that will shape their lives. A commitment to inclusion for adults with MID in all facets of life requires researchers, agency gatekeepers, and caregivers to challenge assumptions of vulnerability and autonomy by viewing these adults as experts in their own lives; capable of speaking and advocating for themselves. Researchers can also support the participation of adults with MID by attending to relational autonomy, working with ongoing consent processes, taking extra time to educate people with MID on their rights as research participants, within research, and engaging in ongoing reflexivity with respect to issues arising in the research process. The contributions to current knowledge of the first-hand experiences of these adults will go towards shaping supports to be more in line with what adults with MID want for themselves, rather than what others think is best.

## References


Abbot, D. and Horwath, J. (2007). "Still Off-limits? Staff Views on Supporting Gay, Lesbian and Bisexual People With Intellectual Disabilities to Develop Sexual and Intimate Relationships?" *Journal of Applied Research in Intellectual Disabilities*, 20: 116–126.

Beail, N. and Williams, K. (2014). "Using Qualitative Methods in Research With People Who Have Intellectual Disabilities." *Journal of Applied Research in Intellectual Disabilities*, 27: 85–96.

Bracken-Roche, D., Bell, E., Macdonald, M., and Racine, E. (2017). "The concept of 'vulnerability' in research ethics: an in-depth analysis of policies and guidelines." *Health Research Policy and Systems*, 15: 8.

Clarke, C. and Braun, B. (2006). "Using Thematic Analysis in Psychology." *Qualitative Research in Psychology*, 3: 77–101.

Foley, S. (2012). "The UN Convention on the Rights of Persons with Disabilities: A Paradigm Shift in the Sexual Empowerment of Adults with Down Syndrome or Sound and Fury Signifying Nothing?" *Sexuality and Disability*, 30:381-393.

Foucault, M. (1990). *The History of Sexuality: Volume 1: An Introduction*. London: Penguin.

Guillemin, M. and Gillam, L. (2004). "Ethics, Reflexivity, and 'Ethically Important Moments' in Research." *Qualitative Inquiry*, 10/2: 261–280.

Healy, E., McGuire, B. E., Evans, D. S., & Carley, S. N. (2009). "Sexuality and personal relationships for people with an intellectual disability. Part 1:service-user perspectives." *Journal of Intellectual Disability Research*, 5: 905-912.

Iacono, T. (2006). "Ethical Challenges of Including People With Intellectual Disability as Participants in Research." *Journal of Intellectual and Developmental Disability*, 31/3: 173–179.

Kelly, G., Crowley, H., and Hamilton, C. (2009). "Rights, Sexuality, and Relationships in Ireland: 'It'd be nice to be kind of trusted'. *British Journal of Learning Disabilities*, 37:308-315.

Kempton, W. and Kahn, E. (1991). "Sexuality and People With Intellectual Disabilities: A Historical Perspective." *Sexuality and Disability*, 9/2: 93–111.

Liamputtong, P. (2007). *Researching the Vulnerable*. London: SAGE.

McDonald, K. A. (2012). "We Want Respect: Adults with Intellectual and Developmental Disabilities Address Respect in Research." *American Journal on Intellectual and Developmental Disabilities*, 117/4: 263–274.

Phelan, K. and Kinsella, E. A. (2013). "Picture This ... Safety, Dignity, and Voice—Ethical Research With Children: Practical Considerations for the Reflexive Researcher." *Qualitative Inquiry*, 19/2: 81–90.

Plummer, K. (1995). *Telling Sexual Stories: Power, Change, and Social Worlds*. London: Routledge.

Richardson, D. (2000). "Constructing Sexual Citizenship: Theorizing Sexual Rights." *Critical Social Policy*, 20/1: 105–135.

Scotland, J. (2012). "Exploring the Philosophical Underpinnings of Research: Relating Ontology and Epistemology to the Methodology and Methods of the Scientific, Interpretive, and Critical Research Paradigms." *English Language Teaching*, 5/9: 9–16.

Siebers, T. (2008). *Disability Theory*. Ann Arbor, MI: The University of Michigan Press.

Shakespeare, T., Gillespie-Sells, K., and Davies, D. (1996). *The Sexual Politics of Disability: Untold Desires*. London: Cassell.

Sherwin, S. and Winsby, M. (2010). "A relational perspective on autonomy for older adults residing in nursing homes." *Health Expectations*, 14: 182–190.

Shildrick, M. (2012). Critical disability studies: rethinking the conventions for the age of postmodernity. In Watson, N., Roulstone, A., & Thomas, C. (Eds.), *Routledge Handbook of Disability Studies* (pp. 12–29). New York, NY: Routledge.

Siebers, T. (2008). *Disability theory*. Ann Arbor, MI: The University of Michigan Press.

Simmons, H. (1982). *From Asylum to Welfare*. Toronto, ON: Rocher Institute.

Snape, D. and Spencer, L. (2003). "The Foundations of Qualitative Research," in Ritchie, J. and Lewis, J., eds. *Qualitative Research Practice: A Guide for Social Science Students and Researchers*. Thousand Oaks, CA: SAGE, pp. 1–23.

Taylor, S. J., Bogdan, R., and Devault, M. (2016). *Introduction to Qualitative Research Methods: A Guidebook and Resource*. Hoboken, NJ: John Wiley & Sons.

Trent, J. W. (1994). *Inventing the Feeble Mind: A History of Mental Retardation in the United States*. Berkley, CA: University of California Press.

Walker-Hirsch, L. (2007). *The Facts of Life ... and More: Sexuality and Intimacy for People with Intellectual Disabilities. Baltimore:P.H Brookes.*

Weeks, J. (1998). "The Sexual Citizen." *Theory, Culture, & Society*, 15: 35–52.

Wellings, K., Branigan, P., and Mitchell, K. (2000). "Discomfort, Discord and Discontinuity as Data: Using Focus Groups to Research Sensitive Topics." *Culture, Health, and Sexuality*, 2/3: 255–267.

# 11

# Shifting Identities

## Research on Macro and Micro Aspects of Intellectual Disability College Programs

*Jack Trammell*

### Introduction

A significant long-term impact of the Americans with Disabilities Act (1990; 2008) and special education inclusion in the public schools in the United States has been a steadily increasing population of postsecondary students with disabilities attending colleges and universities. This trend has been similar in many other Western countries. To the extent that education beyond high school is often positioned culturally as the "road to success," and the trend in disability case law has steadily opened educational doors that had previously been closed (e.g., testing accommodations for entrance exams), students with disabilities of all types have increasingly transitioned into higher education in a series of waves. A recent wave has included many students with autism spectrum disorder (ASD), for example. Many institutions have developed specialized programs for students with ASD in response to, or in some cases to actively recruit, students who will utilize the new services.

A challenge, however, is that disability access has generally come about through disability activism, and not through an intentional framework designed by educators, with means for adequate assessment and consideration of ethical concerns. As this chapter will show, much of the research and accommodation has been reactive, rather than proactive.

Although it is easy to overgeneralize, the waves of students with disabilities over the past 50 years are recognizable and sometimes distinctive, as with ASD. Ed Roberts, US disability activist, was one of the first students in a wave of individuals with physical disabilities to attend university or college in the 1960s, and Roberts became part of the famous "rolling quads" at University of California, Berkeley (Fleischer and Zames, 2001). Students with learning disabilities and learning related disabilities constituted a wave in the 1980s and 1990s (Brinckerhoff, 2002). More recently, a wave of students with intellectual and developmental disabilities (ID/DD) are attending college and university in record numbers, some as degree-seeking students, and some in special programs.

The key difference with the current ID/DD wave is that elements of it challenge basic, long-standing educational paradigms and structures in ways that the other waves either did not, or that they affected to a much lesser degree. Many of the elements involve the cultural construction of intelligence and its educational interpretation, and the ethical concerns that accompany such interpretations Many students in the ID/DD wave cannot meet traditional academic curricular goals, even with significant accommodations. They often cannot meet traditional admission standards. Socially, they may not be able to live on campus comfortably within traditional student conduct policies. Whereas students with ASD, for example, may also struggle in the postsecondary environment with communication and "student conduct frameworks," which are based in normative codes, unlike students with ID/DD, many students with ASD can meet admissions and academic standards (sometimes with accommodations).

The ID/DD wave represents a unique development in the postsecondary landscape, and that is why some schools have built programs first, or simultaneously with bringing students with ID/DD to campus. The goals of such programs often fall outside of traditional academic curricula, and may instead involve more emphasis on cultivating independent living skills; improving basic job skills; fostering normalized community; and improving basic communication skills (McEathron et al., 2013). They typically have significantly different admission standards from degree-seeking programs, and sometimes involve special fees and additional costs to participants.

From a research standpoint, the analysis, evaluation, and development of an ethics for such programs has largely been sporadic, institution driven, and lacking a standardized set of terms, objectives, and measures. Although a few such programs date back to the 1970s, the majority of the several hundred that presently exist in the United States were created within the last decade or so. The newness and the uniqueness of these postsecondary education programs means that significant effort will be necessary to judge their success and impact, and perhaps some hindsight in years to come. There will also need to be an overt intentionality in finding the voices of these students and potential research subjects, who have valuable contributions to make about their own experiences (Fullana et al., 2017), as well as mediating the literature already in existence about employment preparation which has been a consistent emphasis in most programs (Walsh et al., 2018). In many medical studies related to ID/DD, for example, a greater emphasis is placed on caregiver voice (Shooshtari et al., 2017). In educational settings, where long-standing programs provide support for other types of disadvantaged students, no preparation or significant research has been completed looking at the impact of students with ID/DD coming to the university (Shetron, 2018, personal communication). New research will need to focus on participant voice, consent, and rethinking access, as well as concretizing the ethical framework that accompanies the research.

This chapter will briefly evaluate the success of one program at a small liberal arts school; examine the attempts recently made to research wider postsecondary effects and impacts of similar programs; and briefly suggest a series of ideas that will help position such programs in the wider educational narrative and provide a basis for ongoing research that includes the voice of participants.

## A brief case study

Postsecondary programs for students with ID/DD now exist at a wide variety of two- and four-year public and private institutions. An examination of a program at a small (1400 students), mid-Atlantic, private, liberal arts college will suggest many themes common to most of the current programs and also, perhaps, suggest some challenges in assessing and evaluating their true impact.

At this school, the program for ID/DD was an outgrowth of a first-year experience/colloquia collaboration with the local chapter of the ARC, the parent organization originally called the national Association for Retarded Citizens, but now renamed simply to its acronym to reduce stigmatization (Turney and Hughes, 2007). Full-time college students enrolled in the course received academic credit for psychology and philosophy. The other participants in the class were citizens from the ARC, who were not enrolled as full-time, degree-seeking students, but were treated as de facto members of the classes they attended. They were not registered as students in the college database. The first-year experience was grounded faced in objectives and pedagogy, which utilized elements of community-based learning and project-based learning. Some of the learning mimicked internships, including routine clerical work and other tasks associated with running a busy organization like the ARC.

Students and ARC citizens completed some assignments and activities together or in common, often organized around the philosophical theme of "minding" or "mindfulness"; other activities were aimed at just full-time students (e.g., regular academic exams). Mindfulness research has been shown to have anxiety-reducing effects and other positive outcomes for individuals with ID/DD (Idusohan-Moizer et al., 2015). A series of smaller and shorter assignments were usually linked to a much larger project that lasted throughout the semester, or even the entire academic year (Turney and Hughes, 2016).

At the end of the term, full-time students received a grade for their coursework, while ARC class members received an unofficial transcript/certificate documenting their completion of the course (this document was not technically produced by the college, but rather by the class). Perhaps uniquely, the parents of both students and citizens attended a final class event, sometimes termed a "graduation," an occurrence that would not typically occur in other standard classes on the campus.

Elements that made this program somewhat unique included the direct classroom learning and collaboration between students/citizens with ID/DD and full-time college students; the realization of the ideals of inclusion (shared classroom spaces, meals together, common physical activity, etc.); and the collaborative organizational partnership with the ARC that grew much closer over time. The professors, administrators, and students adjudged the program to be very effective in breaking down postsecondary and community barriers, as well as reducing community stigma. The program went on to expand to several other classes and larger contexts within the immediate college community (Turney and Hughes, 2005).

It is difficult to quantify from a research standpoint how successful this program was (or is, as it continues). There are some quantitative data to draw from, including classroom evaluations; retention statistics; ARC assessments and reports; and grant reports. But there are real concerns about generalizability given the unique nature of the school, the distinctiveness of the program (which when being limited to part of a single class does not formally comprise a college program), and its intended outcomes (which overlap in some cases but are not identical for college students and ARC citizens). ARC citizens and students also changed from semester to semester.

There are also unresolved ethical issues. For example, did ARC citizens ever mistakenly believe that they were actually college students in a sense that they really were not? Is that an acceptable misunderstanding? There are many such questions.

This is the research challenge when examining ID/DD programs. They often appear to be successful at the micro level, within limited objectives and within stated community goals, but are difficult as a genre to evaluate quantitatively and place into a larger context backed by empirical research. In contrast, medical conditions like stroke, which is the leading cause of disability in the United States, have been the subject of extensive and repeated study in terms of cause, effect, and outcomes, which also include ID/DD experiences (Hanel et al., 2018). Unlike more purely medical studies, postsecondary ID/DD programs lack such extensive research development, although efforts are now being made.

## Research on postsecondary education programs for ID/DD

Early research began on postsecondary education programs for ID/DD in the early part of the twenty-first century, concurrent with the growing popularity of offering them. In a 2011 review of the literature and research on postsecondary education programs for ID/DD, Thoma and colleagues found that postsecondary experiences for participants with ID/DD were primarily targeted at students between the ages of 18 and 21 years who were still receiving special education services (Thoma et al., 2011). As the anecdotal program discussed earlier, along with the existing research outlined in this chapter, suggests, the target audience and age range has diversified considerably since 2011. Thoma and colleagues also, at the time, lamented the lack of research on participant outcomes, and structural challenges, both of which remain research priorities into the present period (Thoma et al., 2011, p. 187).

McEathron and colleagues addressed these structural challenges in their 2013 creation of a taxonomy for postsecondary education programs targeting students with ID/DD (McEathron et al., 2013). Consistent with what has already been noted, their survey of the postsecondary programs for ID/DD landscape revealed a wide variety, size, and location of such programs in the United States, with little standardization or cross-pollination of methods and assessment. Many of the handful of studies that have been done on postsecondary education programs for ID/DD involve case studies or small sample sizes. Few of them examine ethical questions to the fullest extent. The creation of the taxonomy in this research was an attempt to bring more rigorous research structure to the examination of such programs for ID/DD (McEathron et al., 2013). The taxonomy itself consists of organizational, admissions, support, and pedagogical domains, and is reproduced with permission in Table 11.1.

Using the taxonomy as a guide, the researchers developed an online survey to collect data about postsecondary education programs for ID/DD programs and piloted it. Ultimately, 47 of the 119 invited programs participated in the study by completing the survey. The results indicated a number of noteworthy factors to consider.

In the organizational domain, a key finding involved sponsorship, which in the vast majority of cases was the home institution of higher learning, albeit with co-sponsors—when present—varying a great deal. Many co-affiliations were with offices on campus that historically have been associated with pedagogical differentiation: education departments, disability offices, or developmental education programs. The authors' findings suggest a degree of organic development to ID/DD programs driven by internal university forces, as well as external forces, which include organizations like the ARC.

In the admissions domain, the majority of programs were designed to serve students who were 18 years of age and older and had completed their secondary (high school) educational experience. The standards of admission varied, although many programs required at least a third-grade level of academic skill (McEathron et al., 2013, p. 312). Selectivity varied according to slots available, applicants, funding, and other factors. Costs varied widely, although the spread pattern was generally consistent with the types of schools and general costs associated with them for other degree-seeking students.

**Table 11.1** Postsecondary education taxonomy matrix

| | | | | | |
|---|---|---|---|---|---|
| **Organizational domain** | Type of Institution | Program administration or sponsor | Program length | Program funding sources | Program goals |
| **Admissions domain** | Student status | Student academic skills | Student functional and behavior skills | Selectivity | Tuition and fees |
| **Support domain** | School or program-based support | Agency-based support | Family support | Financial aid | |
| **Pedagogical domain** | Academic components<br>Integration<br>Credit<br>Certificate/degree | Vocational components<br>Coursework<br>Internships | Independent living components<br>Coursework<br>Housing | Social components<br>Coursework activities | |

Reproduced from McEathron, M. A., Beuhring, T., Maynard, A., and Mavis, A. "Understanding the Diversity: A Taxonomy for Postsecondary Education Programs and Services for Students with Intellectual and Developmental Disabilities." *Journal of Postsecondary Education & Disability*, 26/1: pp. 303–320 © 2013, The Associate on Higher Education and Disability.

The findings here suggest an ongoing dialogue about who can or should participate in college and who will pay for it that grows beyond the scope of just ID/DD.

In the support domain, there were myriad components and types of aid offered to students. These supports ran the gamut from residential support to specially trained counselors. Some programs reported working with external agencies. The findings in this area of the study suggest confirmation of a basic assumption, that postsecondary education programs for ID/DD programs require additional resources beyond what are typically offered to other students, and the funding must come from an internal commitment, or outside funding (e.g., grants), or most likely both.

In the pedagogical domain, most postsecondary education programs for ID/DD programs are not designed for students to earn a standard academic degree. There were widely varying degrees of course integration, often with auditing options, and some effort to focus on courses that were potentially transferable. Overall, the focus was more on developing social skills, communication skills, and job skills rather than on completing a traditional degree program. The results in this area directly connect to one of the biggest existential questions about ID/DD programs—what is their primary mission? If a degree-conferring institution is to educate non-degree-seeking students, is this not a fundamental shift in educational mission for many schools? It is also noteworthy that the ethical challenges attending such programs are really only hinted at in the domains, and not explicit in most cases.

There were program outcomes that were predictably measured, such as employment status, or growth of independent living skills. Ross and colleagues also examined those outcomes in the Taft College Transition to Independent Living program (Ross et al., 2013). But many studies do not adequately account for the barriers and unintended consequences of starting such programs.

Plotner and Marshall (2015) examined the facilitators and barriers to postsecondary education programs for ID/DD programs in a partial attempt to answer aspects of that question. Their general finding was that material conditions for the growth of ID/DD programs were improving and that an ongoing trend toward inclusion in postsecondary education continues. They are quick to point out, however, that such programs are funding dependent, limited in scope, and not accessible to all students with ID/DD. The authors also acknowledge the lack, at this point in time, of grounded empirical results of outcomes for such programs and suggest some general parameters for improvement in this area.

Although philosophical attitudes about increasing inclusion are generally reported as positive in the current literature, there are also indications that as postsecondary education programs for ID/DD programs grow, concerns about academic integrity and core school mission still remain at the forefront of conversation. Haney and Fisher (2017) interviewed liberal arts students about ID/DD programs and found that they were generally positive and inclusive in their reactions. But they also found concerns that "students with ID/DD would hold back other students in classes and that having students with ID/DD would negatively impact the college's prestige" (Haney and Fisher, 2017, p. 99).

There is also at this time a notable deficit in reporting on students' own perceptions of ID/DD postsecondary experiences. John Kubiak, reporting from Ireland where programs for ID/DD are also growing in higher education, suggests the students will ultimately have some of the most important things to say about program success and the long-term viability of such programs (Kubiak, 2017). Kubiak (2017, p. 42) argues that the issue of power, in the Foucauldian sense, remains at the heart of ID/DD initiatives and their position in academia. Power by its very nature demands an ethical framework to accompany it.

One issue related to power is disclosure. For a number of decades, student disclosure of disability at the postsecondary level was almost exclusively voluntary. In fact, the way disability law was crafted made it clear that institutions could not force or pressure student disclosure. Postsecondary education programs for ID/DD programs, like other disability-specific programs, require disclosure to the program in advance simply to participate, and therefore mostly remove that important element of decision-making from the process. While it may make eminent practical sense to do so, it runs contrary to the long trend of voluntary disclosure as a traditional structure in higher education. In effect, students with profound ID/DD are largely deprived of the ability to contemplate and decide about disclosure because their sole gateway to participation is through an action that presupposes disclosure; they are arguably denied an important act of self (Trammell, 2010).

Macro analysis of disability disclosure in higher education largely is silent on the matter of ID/DD, since students with profound ID/DD do not exist at the higher-education level (presumably) unless they have disclosed. In reality, many students at the higher end of the ID/DD spectrum do attend postsecondary and choose not to disclose for a wide variety of reasons. Studies of disclosure also presume that students have the ability to decide for themselves (Kerschbaum et al., 2017). In postsecondary education programs for ID/DD programs, students may not have that obvious ability or even a choice, and there has been little-to-no evaluation of what impact that has on their experience and outcomes, or the impact on the institution. By one line of logic, this again arguably is an indicator that these programs require a fundamental shift in institutional mission and thinking.

## Discussion

Research on programs for ID/DD at the postsecondary level has been limited for a number of reasons. A primary impact is that until recently there simply were not that many programs. But, in addition, a possible bias already mentioned that revolves around the concept of the norm, stigma, and flawed concepts of intelligence, has also limited research by constraining the vision of who really should be a college or university student. Finally, because there is no current ethical framework that significantly diverges from dominant postsecondary norms, this has served as an additional barrier to research.

There are a number of structural forces at the macro/cultural level that have affected ID/DD programs in postsecondary settings. One of the most important has been a general movement toward greater postsecondary access and inclusion, not just in the United States, but globally. The last 50 years have witnessed a mostly successful desegregation of higher education, the increase of women going to postsecondary schools, a learning support movement in the 1970s geared toward non-traditional and developmental students, the inclusion of students with disabilities and academic accommodations in the 1990s, and, more recently, the increase in English Second Language students and non-traditional adult students. The trend is unmistakable, and proponents of postsecondary education programs for ID/DD programs have strong evidence to support their own initiatives based on the actual historical curve.

Postsecondary education as a function for social justice or a pathway to a good life has become the new normal culturally in the United States, if not practically, as well. Since GIs returned from World War II and entered postsecondary institutions in record numbers, a college or university degree has increasingly become synonymous with better life opportunities, increased social capital, and greater income earned over time. The stigma of not going to college remains a negative stereotype in a variety of settings; the pressures to go to college are self-evident to almost every high-school senior. One application for a postsecondary education program for ID/DD even has as an admission requirement that applicants must “have an interest in going to college [to expand career opportunities]” (RRTC, 2013). This kind of anecdotal information reinforces the cultural norm which stigmatizes a number of groups of students, not just students with disabilities. Many non-disabled students go to college even then they don’t want to; why can’t students with disabilities go when they don’t want to?

This pressure or positive incentive to go to college is not necessarily a bad thing, and well within the traditions of a democratic education for citizenship for which John Dewey and others were early-twentieth-century proponents, and which is now a globalizing norm (Cogan and Derricott, 2012). It is also consistent with a late capitalist economy that seeks increasingly narrower markets as saturation occurs; or, to put it another way, as the percentage of college-bound students goes up, it becomes increasingly more difficult to include the smaller percentage that is left out, even as demand to include them goes up. Critics of late capitalism, like Chomsky, suggest that institutions like education imitate larger forces that become “natural” over time (2013, p. 143), and the trend with postsecondary education programs for ID/DD programs may just be vestigial “progress” toward a world where it is natural for everyone to go to college.

Postsecondary education programs for ID/DD programs are increasing and diversifying college participation, although that fact is possibly mitigated by two important a priori assumptions: first, the assumption that a college or university experience in a non-degree-seeking framework will serve vital functions in the global community analogous to those which higher education has typically served in degree programs for the last 50 or even 100 years or so; and second, the assumption that sending more students to college or university is a good thing for everyone, including the economy, and the students with ID/DD. Depending on whom one talks to, neither of these assumptions should be carelessly adopted as fact, and neither one has much empirical evidence to suggest what its true long-term effects might be if the postsecondary education programs for ID/DD movement is fulfilled. There is a popular cultural belief that "more is better" when it comes to students going to college typified by articles and reports that regularly appear in the media that does not necessarily mesh seamlessly with desired outcomes (Blumenstyk, 2018).

The functions of college and university experiences are of course myriad and complex. At a recent seminar discussion, undergraduate students studying college access identified a number of key functions that they believed were part of the societal integration with higher education. These included but were not limited to gateway to employment; growth in independence; sharpening and improvement of academic and empirical skills; learning and experiencing a life of the mind; development of a specific skillset in a major or program; enculturation into the adult world; a gateway to graduate level programs; strengthening sense of community; exposure to new people and new ideas; and the opportunity to play organized sports. On the darker side, students also believed that postsecondary education functions as a form of social control, and differentiates between people with varying talents, motivation, and ability, essentially serving a "sorting" function. In other words, it contributes to and even reifies stratification. But perhaps more importantly, students were adamant that they could think of no reasons why these objectives could not be met for non-traditional students with ID/DD in the postsecondary environment, as well (Trammell, 2018).

There can be little doubt that postsecondary education programs for ID/DD have already had an impact at the micro level. The program mentioned initially in this chapter is a good example—generally considered a great success based on student evaluations, qualitative evidence from participants, program completion rates, feedback from agencies, and so on.

However, there is an empirical link missing that should ideally connect theory to practice the way it does in other areas, like traditional learning assistance, and allow a more effective meta-analysis of where the ID/DD in postsecondary education program movement is headed, and why. One study in 2013, for example, suggested that less than 25% of students with ID/DD actually "succeeded" at the postsecondary level (diplomas, certifications, etc.) (Harrison and Holmes, 2013). That is arguably not a sustainable success rate. That type of more detailed analysis is missing in the present environment, although there are obviously those making efforts as have been reported here.

The research that should be done offers an important chance to revisit and reinterpret some of the most chimeric areas in the history of postsecondary education and educational research: the persistent existence of structural inequalities; the need to balance the practical side of education alongside character development; the uniqueness of the Western education system in a globalized world; and the social capital that education bestows upon and encultures within students, to name just a few. The research needed can also serve the greater dialogue ongoing about what postsecondary education intends to do and actually does accomplish.

## Conclusion

Many substantive questions are raised by an examination of postsecondary education programs for ID/DD programs: how much value and distinction does a *degree* have in comparison with an *experience*; what substantive objectives are realistic outcomes for postsecondary ID/DD programs; what is the long-term prognosis for ID/DD programs in the academy; and do ID/DD programs in the academy indicate a significant cultural shift in how people with disabilities are positioned in the mainstream? Many schools that have already piloted ID/DD programs continue to expand them. Some schools are including study abroad in their ID/DD programs (Kelley et al., 2016). Are there other avenues for ID/DD to enter or expand within the academy? Medical schools, for example, are not admitting students with ID/DD on a regular basis, but they are growing an academic focus for medical students on better awareness of ID/DD (Perkes, 2018).

The early pioneering research on ID/DD and postsecondary education generally demonstrates positive outcomes and the satisfaction of limited program and research-designed objectives. It does not, however, address the growing global issues that are important to resolve and the need for a much lengthier dialogue. These questions, as already outlined, include difficult ethical questions and conversations, as well as examination of the evolving nature of US (and global) postsecondary education itself.

The conclusion, based on the available evidence, is not perfectly clear. The available evidence suggests that researchers and educators are taking steps, and developing research frameworks, but will need to find answers to the bigger questions for ID/DD programs to have long-term viability as part of the academy. This is also a call for more rigorous research and assessment within such programs. Eventually meta-analysis will become more practical, and larger studies will expose more dramatic consequences and effects.

Perhaps of equal importance, the voices of students with ID/DD must be found and must be consistently heard. They will speak in part through employment rates and standard of living, but they ultimately must speak more directly for themselves in the wider narrative discourse of higher education. They are the co-beneficiaries of a more universal postsecondary experience that benefits all and should be treated as such.

There also is a need to keep sight of practical outcomes. Employment outcomes for individuals with ID/DD, while still abysmally low in the general economy compared with the overall numbers, do show signs of improving, specifically as a result of new postsecondary education programs for ID/DD (Magro, 2018). There is a need for global cooperation and sharing of data as postsecondary education continues to globalize. However, postsecondary education has been driven throughout the inclusive changes already mentioned by a performance-based framework that largely orbits around some measurement of intelligence and ability, whether it be GPA (grade point average), standardized test scores, or even perceived ability to communicate in traditional ways. The cultural power of IQ-based advancement remains problematic and entrenched. It might be realistic to question the long-term sustainability of postsecondary education programs for ID/DD programs if there is not a fundamental shift in this paradigm.

Nonetheless, the growth of postsecondary education programs for ID/DD likely signal an important shift in the wider culture, an increasingly globalized culture in which the challenge of access, and neurodiversity, demand a response from higher education

## References

Blumenstyk, G. (2018). "Fresh Ideas to Help Adult Learners Succeed," https://www.chronicle.com/article/Fresh-Ideas-to-Help-Adult/243834 (accessed March 5, 2019).

Brinckerhoff, L. (2002). *College Students With Learning Disabilities*. Boston, MA: AHEAD.

Chomsky, N. (2013). *Power Systems: Conversations on Global Democratic Uprisings and the New Challenges of U.S. Empire*. New York: Metropolitan Books.

Cogan, J. J. and Derricott, R. (eds.) (2012). *Citizenship for the 21st Century: An International Perspective on Education*. New York: Routledge.

Fleischer, D. Z. and Zames, F. (2001). *The Disability Rights Movement: From Charity to Confrontation*. Philadelphia, PA: Temple University Press.

Fullana, J., Pallisera, M., Catala, E., and Puyalto, C. (2017). "Evaluating a Research Training Programme for People With Intellectual Disabilities Participating in Inclusive Research: The Views of Participants." *Journal of Applied Research in Intellectual Disabilities*, 30: 684–695.

Hanel, R., Sauvageau, E. and Aghaebrahim, N. (2018). "Breakthroughs in Stroke Treatment," in *International Symposium on Cognitive Research & Disorders* ISCRD 2018, Feb 26–27, 2018, St. Augustine, FL.

Haney, M. R. and Fisher, K. (2017). "Student Attitudes and Perceptions About Postsecondary Education for People With Intellectual Disabilities (Practice Brief)." *Journal of Postsecondary Education & Disability*, 30: 97–104.

Harrison, A. G. and Holmes, A. (2013). "Mild Intellectual Disability at the Post-secondary Level: Results of a Survey of Disability Service Offices." *Exceptionality Education International*, 23: 22–29.

Idusohan-Moizer, H., Sawicka, A., Dendle, J., and Albany, M. (2015). "Mindfulness-based Cognitive Therapy for Adults With Intellectual Disabilities: An Evaluation of the Effectiveness of Mindfulness in Reducing Symptoms of Depression and Anxiety." *Journal of Intellectual Disability Research*, 59: 93–104.

Kelley, K. R., Prohn, S. M., and Westling, D. L. (2016). "Inclusive Study Abroad Course for College Students With and Without Intellectual Disabilities (Practice Brief)." *Journal of Postsecondary Education and Disability*, 29: 91–101.

Kerschbaum, S. L., Eisenman, L. T., and Jones, J. M. (eds.) (2017). *Negotiating Disability: Disclosure and Higher Education*. Ann Arbor, MI: University of Michigan Press.

Kubiak, J. (2017). "Using 'Voice' to Understand What College Students With Intellectual Disabilities Say About the Teaching and Learning Process." *Journal of Research in Special Educational Needs*, 17: 41–48.

McEathron, M. A., Beuhring, T., Maynard, A., and Mavis, A. (2013). "Understanding the Diversity: A Taxonomy for Postsecondary Education Programs and Services for Students With Intellectual and Developmental Disabilities." *Journal of Postsecondary Education & Disability*, 26: 303–320.

Magro, K. (2018). "Workforce 101: Disabilities in the Workplace and What You Need to Know," in *International Symposium on Cognitive Research & Disorders* ISCRD 2018, Feb 26–27, 2018, St. Augustine, FL.

Perkes, C. (2018). "Medical Schools Adding Focus on Developmental Disabilities," https://www.disabilityscoop.com/2018/03/12/medical-schools-focus-dd/24838/ (accessed March 5, 2019).

Plotner, A. J. and Marshall, K. J. (2015). "Postsecondary Education Programs for Students With an Intellectual Disability: Facilitators and Barriers to Implementation." *Intellectual and Developmental Disabilities*, 53: 58–69.

Ross, J., Marcell, J., Williams, P., and Carlson, D. (2013). "Postsecondary Education Employment and Independent Living Outcomes of Persons With Autism and Intellectual Disability." *Journal of Postsecondary Education & Disability*, 26: 337–351.

RRTC. (2013) "Ace-It Application," Richmond, VA: Virginia Commonwealth University, p. 22.

Shooshtari, S., Temple, B., Waldman, C., Abraham, S., Ouellette-Kuntz, H., and Lennox, N. (2017). "Stakeholders' Perspectives Towards the Use of the Comprehensive Health Assessment Program (CHAP) for Adults With Intellectual Disabilities in Manitoba." *Journal of Applied Research in Intellectual Disabilities*, 30: 672–683.

Thoma, C. A., Lakin, K. C., Carlson, D., Domzal, C., Austin, K., and Boyd, K. (2011). "Participation in Postsecondary Education for Students With Intellectual Disabilities: A Review of the Literature 2001–2010." *Journal of Postsecondary Education & Disability*, 24: 175–191.

Trammell, J. (2010). "Teach Students With Disabilities How to Become Better Information Managers." *Disability Compliance for Higher Education*, 15: 7.

Trammell, J. (2018). "What Are the Functions of 'Going Go College,'" in *Sociological Theory Seminar*. Ashland, VA: *Randolph-Macon College*.

Turney, D. and Hughes, A. (2005). "The Minding Class: Connecting the Academy and the Community," in *Virginia Transitions Conference*, Williamsburg, VA.

Turney, D. and Hughes, A. (2007). "Service Learning: Connecting the Academy and the Community," in *National Conference for the Humanities Education Conference*, San Francisco, CA.

Turney, D. and Hughes, A. (2016). "???", in Oxley, J. and Ilea, R., eds. *Experiential Learning in Philosophy*. New York and London: Routledge, pp. 189–197.

Walsh, E., Holloway, J., and Lydon, H. (2018). "An Evaluation of a Social Skills Intervention for Adults With Austism Spectrum Disorder and Intellectual Disabilities Preparing for Employment in Ireland: A Pilot Study." *Journal of Autism & Developmental Disorders*, 48: 1727–1741.

# SECTION 3
# SUCCESSES

# 12

# Recognizing the Voices of All Children, Including Those with "Cognitive Impairments," in Research

*Marjorie Montreuil, Gail Teachman, and Franco A. Carnevale*

## An introduction to child research ethics

A major research innovation of the mid-to-late twentieth century was the development of ethical standards for conducting research with human subjects. This development helped introduce norms and practices that should be used to protect research participants from harm, as well as respect any of their rights that the research might infringe upon. This includes the development of ethical standards for conducting research with children[1] and their families, which can entail some complex challenges. Additional challenges may arise in research with children with "cognitive impairments." We first present an overview of the current ethical standards for research with children, followed by a framework we propose for research with children, and share examples from our research.

## Ethical standards for conducting research with children and families

For the purposes of simplicity, Canadian standards will be used as a reference, which overlap significantly with other Western research ethics standards (e.g., United Kingdom, United States (Carnevale et al., 2008; CGP and MICYRN, 2012)). The dominant research ethics standards in Canada for research with children, as well as adults, require (1) balancing harms and benefits (e.g., promoting a favorable harms–benefits balance; the foreseeable harms should not outweigh anticipated benefits); (2) respect for free and informed consent (e.g., respecting the exercise of individual consent); (3) respect for privacy and confidentiality (e.g., regarding privacy and confidentiality as a form of respect for human dignity); (4) respect for justice and inclusiveness (e.g., ensuring a fair distribution of the benefits and burdens of research); and (5) respect

[1] We are using the term "children" to refer to people under 18 years old, as defined in the United Nations Convention on the Rights of the Child (1989).

for vulnerable persons (e.g., recognizing that having diminished competence and/or decision-making capacity can make people vulnerable) (TCPS2, 2014). In this section, we consider the implications of these standards for research with children.

Balancing research-related risks and benefits with children is difficult, in part because so little is known about children's experiences with research. It is important to guard against the exclusion of children from research when their participation is likely to contribute data different from what can be generated with adults. Such exclusion can unjustly compromise the advancement of knowledge regarding children's concerns and experiences. Although many studies with children may not directly benefit those who are participating in the study, the benefits to be considered should include the potential benefits for children in related contexts. Benefits should reasonably outweigh the risks that the research can imply for participating children and possible risks should be minimized. For non-therapeutic research, the projected risks should not exceed a *minimal risk* level. The Tri-Council Policy Statement (TCPS) defines *Minimal risk* as: the probability and magnitude of expected harm or discomfort are not greater than those ordinarily encountered in daily life (TCPS2, 2014).

Children's participation in a study also raises challenges related to free and informed consent. Consent to participation in research implies that the participant (or the person providing permission) is un-coerced. It also implies that participant has been given an explanation of the related purposes, expected duration, foreseeable risks and benefits, alternative procedures, confidentiality considerations, and who to contact for questions, as well as information about the voluntary nature of participation and that refusal to participate or subsequent withdrawal will not result in any loss of benefit that the participant is entitled to (TCPS2, 2014). Consent should be provided by a research participant who is considered legally capable, which is defined somewhat differently across legal jurisdictions. Chidren's capacity to consent to participation in research is narrowed in comparison with adults and commonly also requires permission of the children's parent(s) or guardian. Some minors may be considered capable to provide consent themselves to participate in research (e.g., mature minors). The applicable age and other related criteria can vary across jurisdictions. Moreover, the *assent* of children participating in a study should be sought where they are capable of doing so. Assent refers to a child's voluntary agreement (not only the absence of objection) to participate in a study (Carnevale et al., 2008). Relevant information should be provided and agreement to participate should be requested from children in a manner that is adapted to their individual capacities, understandings, and experiences. When children express an objection to participation in a study that provides no direct benefit for them individually, this objection should be respected as a refusal to participate (Carnevale et al., 2008).

Although respect for the privacy and confidentiality of research participants is a widely recognized standard, very little work has been published on how this should be operationalized for children (Noiseux et al., 2019). Aside from situations involving concerns regarding potential or actual maltreatment and additional concerns about risks and harms to self or others, there are significant uncertainties about the extent and the limits of privacy and confidentiality that should be accorded to children's disclosures. This is increasingly complex in light of the growing recognition of children's agential capacities and potential harms that can result from disregarding their wishes regarding privacy and confidentiality.

Respect for justice and inclusiveness requires a fair or equitable distribution of benefits, as well as the risks and burdens of participating in research. Children should not be unfairly burdened with the harms of research nor should they be systematically excluded or discriminated against as individuals and groups who may benefit from research-based innovations.

Given that children are frequently limited, by legal and ethical standards, in the scope of decisional autonomy granted to them; they are commonly dependent on others for the fulfillment of many of their needs, as well as protection of their rights. These dependencies, among other features of childhood deemed to make them "vulnerable," can disadvantage children. They are therefore generally considered entitled, on grounds of human dignity, caring, solidarity, and fairness, to special protection against abuse, exploitation, or discrimination (Canadian Pediatric Society, 2014). Whereas these protections can be necessary toward protecting children from risks and burdens, it is important to ensure that such practices are not applied in ways that limit the individual and collective benefits that can be derived from participating in research. This consideration becomes even more important for research with children identified as having "cognitive impairments."

## "Cognitive impairment" and participation in research

The construct of "cognitive impairment" is one that continues to shift and evolve over time; however, it is defined primarily through its binary relation to biomedical conceptualizations of "intact cognition." Across geographic and disciplinary boundaries and borders, children identified as having cognitive impairments are variously described as "intellectually disabled, "developmentally delayed," or "learning disabled" (McDonagh et al., 2018). In general, the term refers to "deficits" or "delays" in mental processes (thinking, learning, remembering, abstraction, judgment, problem solving, language, imagination, perception, planning, execution) (Suresh et al., 2015). Cognitive impairment is a potential feature of a wide range of pediatric diagnoses (including mental illness, degenerative conditions, autism spectrum disorder, cerebral palsy, and some chronic illnesses) and might occur as a transitory or relatively stable phenomenon. In this chapter, we use the term cautiously, acknowledging that understandings of human cognition continue to advance and are subject to cultural, historic, and political influences. We are mindful that it has been well established that children with cognitive impairments are subject to exclusionary and disabling social arrangements and conditions that restrict their life experiences and opportunities to acquire knowledge and self-awareness (Goodley and Runswick-Cole, 2015).

Children with cognitive impairments are often excluded from participation in research owing to (1) deficit approaches where vulnerability is conflated with an inability to provide free and informed consent; and (2) a paucity of well-prepared researchers and well-described inclusive methods for ensuring that children deemed highly vulnerable are able to share their experiences and perspectives on what matters to them (Carter, 2009). However, as we discuss later, the first of these rationales has been contested, and there is an emerging body of work to guide researchers in adopting more inclusive methodologies. Such methodologies acknowledge tensions between recognizing children's expertise and agency while acknowledging vulnerabilities and constraints that may be present in their lives (Baker and Plows, 2015).

Recent scholarship has pointed to the ways that vague conceptualizations of "vulnerability" act to perpetuate exclusion of entire groups of persons from participation in research, as a means of "protecting them" (Bracken-Roche et al., 2017; Peter and Friedland, 2017). Deficit approaches that equate cognitive impairment with prescribed incompetence and dependence risk restrict whole groups of children from participation in research. Such approaches fail to consider individual strengths and abilities, or the contextual factors that influence both children's intersecting "vulnerabilities" and their capabilities (Dowse, 2009) and, instead, reproduce stigmatizing social judgments and reinforce stereotypes about categories of individuals (Feudtner and Brosco, 2011). In short, vulnerability is too often simplified and conflated with an inability to provide free and informed consent. When vulnerability is envisioned as a relational construct that is context dependent rather than an individual trait, the way is opened to ask young participants directly about whether they think they are vulnerable and jointly plan for additional protections to be put in place (Bracken-Roche et al., 2017; Racine and Bracken-Roche, 2019).

In addition to challenging unexamined conceptualizations of vulnerability, researchers have reported on a range of alternative methods to generate data in research with people who have cognitive impairments (e.g., Hollomotz, 2017; Nind and Vanha, 2016; Stack and McDonald, 2014). With these advances, it has become clear that some of the challenges encountered in doing research with this group can be attributed as much to researchers' errors or lack of preparation as to participants' presumed limitations (Hollomotz, 2017). Still, with a few notable exceptions (e.g., Kelly, 2007; Robinson et al., 2018), much of what has been written discusses research with adults with cognitive impairment and there remains a relative lack of information to guide methodologies for doing research with children (especially those identified as cognitively impaired) in ways that balance recognition of children's agency with considerations of their best interests.

## A framework for research with children

Building on our interdisciplinary research in childhood ethics—a field that aims to identify, investigate, and develop strategies for addressing ethical concerns relating to young people—we argue for a shift in childhood research ethics norms toward more inclusive and participatory approaches anchored in the recognition of all children's voices and agential capacities. By participatory approaches, we refer to both participatory methods to generate and/or collect data with child participants, and participatory research approaches in which children are involved in the research process itself. This view challenges binary conceptions of children as either capable or incapable, and promotes a framework that integrates voice and agency with protection and best interests, highlighting their interrelation (Carnevale et al., 2015). We use the term "framework" to denote a set of underlying beliefs and values that can be used to guide approaches for doing research with children. Within this framework, children are viewed as active agents—in line with the field of childhood ethics—which we apply to the context of child-focused research (Carnevale et al., 2015; Montreuil and Carnevale, 2016, 2018). This framework contests taken-for-granted relations among "cognitive impairment" and agency, and highlights the intertwined nature of children's and parents' agency (Carnevale et al., 2017). We view "cognitive impairment" not as an impediment to participation in research, but as a catalyst for rethinking assumptions in research ethics more generally.

Children's agency is a key concept within this framework. It refers to "children's capacity to act, speak for oneself, actively reflect on their social worlds, shaping their lives and the lives of others" (Montreuil and Carnevale, 2016, p. 510). Children's agency differs from autonomy because it designates children's broader involvement in various processes affecting them. We apply this concept here to the context of research with children considered as having "cognitive impairments." In research projects involving or affecting children, recognizing children's agency would lead to the adoption of research approaches that include children in as many aspects of the projects as are relevant. However, recognition of children's agency does not override recognition of children's best interests. Children are disadvantaged in several important ways, for example being physically smaller than adults, having limited or no legal capacities, and being socially and economically dependent on adults, with some children additionally being identified as having a "cognitive impairment." This calls for a form of protection for children in their best interests, but should not prevent them from being recognized as full human beings with agential capacities (Lee, 2001).

For research, current protection mechanisms should still be employed but with deliberate actions on the part of researchers to involve children in research that affects them (Skelton, 2008). Different strategies can be used to involve children, ranging from conducting research directly with children, to engaging children in the research process or involving children as co-researchers (Bradbury-Jones and Taylor, 2015; Carnevale et al., 2008; James and Prout, 2015). This type of research is gaining increased recognition and more work is being conducted on children's participation in research, especially within childhood studies (e.g., Coyne and Carter, 2018; Groundwater-Smith et al., 2014; James and Prout, 2015; Montreuil and Carnevale, 2018; Teachman and Gibson, 2018). We review these approaches to contribute to the recognition of children as active agents.

## Strategies for recognizing children's agency in research

We now share concrete strategies for recognizing agency in research with children identified as "cognitively impaired" through examples from our own research. In the first study, one of us employed innovative participatory methods to collect data with children identified as disabled who communicate in ways other than speech. In the second study, some of us used a participatory research approach to involve children with mental health disorders in the research process itself.

## Doing research with children identified as disabled

One of this chapter's authors, Teachman, critically explored the notion of inclusion with 13 Canadian young people (aged 15–24 years, six young men, seven young women) who had little or no speech as a result of neurological impairments associated with cerebral palsy (Teachman, 2016). Research reports suggest that 50–60% of individuals with cerebral palsy have some degree of cognitive impairment, while up to 80% experience speech impairments (Odding et al., 2006; Aisen et al., 2011). Oriented by Bourdieu's (1990) theory of practice and Bakhtin's (1981) dialogism, the study design combined visual methods with interviews in order to optimize the data generated and to support analyses of participants' understandings of their social worlds alongside rich data that reflected the social, cultural, and material contexts that shaped their views (Teachman et al., 2018; Teachman and Gibson, 2018). The research demonstrated that some forms of so-called inclusion actually reproduced the exclusionary systems and structures they were intended to replace. Young people reported that their inability to communicate using speech was a key factor that contributed to stigmatization and negative social relations (Teachman, 2016).

Because young people in the study communicated primarily in ways other than speech—using augmentative and alternative communication (AAC)—it was necessary to interrogate normative assumptions in child-focused research about who makes a "good participant" (e.g., able to understand the research questions and procedures, able to articulate clearly their views, able to reflect on their experiences) and whose perspectives are recognized as "valid." Children with cognitive impairments often present with associated communication impairments and vice versa; however, because formal testing is so often reliant on oral expression, our experience, as well as empirical research, suggests that the actual and potential competencies and abilities of these young people is often underestimated (Nader et al., 2016; Racine et al., 2014). Until recently, children who use AAC were largely excluded from studies about disabled childhoods because researchers not only lacked well-described methods for eliciting their views, but also because they were judged as incapable of contributing "valid" accounts (Morris, 2003). Thus, to execute the research, and advance emergent methodologies for doing research with this population, Teachman and colleagues developed a critical dialogical methodology that explicitly reframes "voice" and communication generally, as always multiple and relational. A detailed discussion of the methodology has been described elsewhere (Teachman et al., 2018); here, we focus on the moral implications of the approach for designing and conducting research that recognizes the agency of all children, irrespective of their cognitive or communicative abilities.

The critical dialogical method forwarded through the study includes specific strategies and rationales for co-producing data with children attuned to their cognitive abilities and respect their multiple modes of communication. As noted by Barnes and Oliver, interviewers undertaking research with disabled persons should be mindful that the interview process becomes oppressive when it has the effect of "reinforcing into isolated individuals with impairments the idea that the problems they experience in everyday life are a direct outcome of subjective inadequacies or functional limitations and not the organization of society" (1993, p. 7). Accordingly, participants were encouraged to use all their preferred modes of communication, including mediation by a familiar communication partner (all but one participant elected to ask their mother to take on this role). By shifting away from expectations that young people in the study possessed an inner, wholly autonomous "voice" to be captured by a researcher, space was opened for participants to express themselves in a manner that more closely approximated their everyday communication modes. The following extract from the study field notes is an example of how interview relations unfolded:

> Peter, aged 17 [who with great effort could produce dysarthric, or slurred, speech that was understood only by familiar listeners], was relieved and pleased to have his mother join the interview as his communication partner. She took on the role in a somewhat formal way—initially asking permission to clarify Peter's speech with each utterance—but relaxed as the first interview progressed. There were a number of times when Peter's mother didn't know what he was saying, but the two of them worked through it in a practiced manner—neither seemed frustrated. During these moments, she rose from her chair to see Peter's face better, affectionately touching him and patiently working with him until she understood what he was trying to express.

Without a commitment to this methodology, the participants would not have been supported to express their views to the same extent. The combination of a number of methodological innovations in this work (direct video analysis of interviews, combining graphic and photo elicitation with interviews to align with existing visual communication strategies in AAC, and the development of a dialogical analytic framework) is unique and could be built on in other research with children generally. It could also be applied to help optimize data generation in research with a broad range of adult populations who experience cognitive and/or communication impairments.

The study contributed further ethical insights in relation to consent and assent processes, and the potential effects of participation in research for young people experiencing cognitive and communication challenges. One interaction illustrates the importance of approaching research with humility and attention to researcher/child participant/parent relations. The researchers made arrangements to meet and potentially enroll a participant whose mother had viewed a poster about the study and expressed a keen desire for her daughter to be included. At the visit, the young girl, who evidently had sensory, cognitive, and communication impairments, became extremely agitated by the prospect of talking with a stranger. Within a few minutes, she began to engage in destructive, potentially harmful behaviours and was unable to engage in conversations where she could ask questions and agree to participate in the study (or not). In consultation with the girl's mother, the researchers agreed that though the mother felt her daughter had wanted to participate, the potential benefits were outweighed by the likelihood that the types of interaction involved for participants were likely to produce undue stress. Still, this was a very disappointing outcome for the mother and a difficult decision for the researcher who was committed to optimizing the inclusivity of the research methodology.

This interaction exemplifies what Guillemin and Gillam (2004) termed "ethically important moments" that occur in the everyday practice of doing research. These "moments" relate less to procedural ethics or ethical dilemmas and more to the ethical responsibilities of researchers to interact with participants (and potential participants) in ways that are humane and non-exploitive, while reflexively attending to potential harms. Such approaches have been described as person-oriented research ethics (Cascio and Racine, 2018). In this case, the researcher's sense was that this single mother, who lived in barely furnished, dilapidated community housing, was desperate to access activities and supports for her daughter. However, the researcher's presence in their home had resulted in a distressing intrusion for the girl, and worse, the fact that she was not enrolled in the study might have been perceived as a rejection. For this mother, the interaction resulted in yet another professional informing her that her daughter was not a "fit." Although the researcher later followed-up to provide information about how to seek out other research studies and services which might be less stressful for her daughter, the interaction served as a reminder that all research (at all stages) has effects for participants and for researchers, and leaves each individual changed through the process. In this instance, participation in the research was judged to be not in the best interests of the child; however, the decision was not made based upon assumptions about her capacity to contribute valuable perspectives. If she had not demonstrated such significant anxiety, then she might well have contributed valuable insights to the research.

## Doing research with children in a child mental health setting

Mental illness does not imply cognitive impairment; however, links between the two have been made in the literature (Hawk Jr et al., 2018; Bora, 2015; Wagner et al., 2015). We address this topic here in the context of children with a mental illness diagnosis possibly being excluded from research based on the assumptions that it leads to cognitive impairment and a related incapacity to take part in research. Montreuil, Carnevale, and colleagues conducted a study in which children aged 7–12 years who had a mental illness diagnosis were involved in the research process. Within the study conducted, the institutional norms, structures, practices, and corresponding moral experiences of children, parents, and staff members around conflict and crisis management were examined. The study aimed to develop care approaches that promote an optimal reconciliation of ethical concerns in child mental health related to crisis management and the use of control measures (e.g., restraints and seclusion) with children in inpatient settings (in this case a day hospital) (Montreuil, 2017).[2] A methodological framework that recognized children as agents was developed to guide the conduct of the study, drawing on the hermeneutic philosophy of Charles Taylor (1971, 2004) and bridging it with ethnographic and participatory research approaches (Montreuil and Carnevale, 2018).

## Participatory research process

To involve children in the research process, the research team created an advisory committee to foster engagement of local partners in the study, which involved shared decision-making about different steps of the research process. Engagement with partners led to the co-creation of knowledge more anchored in the local context and more attuned to the experiences of the people in the setting, including children. The advisory committee was open to children who were receiving care at the study site and their parents, as well as staff members and managers from the day hospital program (children aged 7–12 years). Four children, two parents, and four staff members were partners to the study.

The members of the advisory committee were involved in key steps of the study process: refining the research question (e.g., the focus on crisis management changed to conflict and crisis management after the initial meeting); making decisions related to data collection (e.g., choosing when to do participant observation; identifying key informants; selecting the documents to review); interpreting the data and deciding who to disseminate the results with, following Green's definition of participatory research (Green et al., 1995). This process enhanced children's participation throughout the research process.

## Ethical considerations related to the participatory research process

One of the main ethical concerns in the participatory process was power differentials, particularly in relation to children. To recognize and try to decrease this power imbalance, children were asked for their preferences for the format and conduct of the meetings, which were conducted with children, parents, and staff members separately.

[2] This text is adapted and partially reproduced from an appendix present in the unpublished thesis on the participatory research process used in the study (Montreuil, 2017).

We preferred to ask children specifically for their preferences, not to assume children were incapable to take part in meetings with adults, while recognizing the power imbalance in place in the setting to their disadvantage due to their "vulnerable" status (Veale, 2005).

Since the different subcommittee members (i.e., children, parents, and staff members) did not discuss ideas together based on children's preferences, we shared the varied perspectives with one another to foster an exchange of ideas. This process led to rich discussions with the different members. For example, children and staff members shared whom they considered as potential key informants; we discussed the different perspectives, and the final decisions reflected the views of the different partners involved. During data interpretation, perspectives related, for example, to the punitive nature of the use of control measures differed: during the meeting with the staff, when researchers shared that many children perceived control measures as punitive, most staff members were surprised and explained it was not the case (though one staff member strongly argued it was punitive). Through discussion of the diverging perspectives, staff members agreed control measures were sometimes used as a punishment, which some preferred to call a consequence, in that the aim was to have something "not enjoyable" happen to the child in consequence for having done something wrong. If we had not sought or shared children's perspectives, the interpretive process would not have led to this depth and richness we accessed through the study, as we would only have reported the diverging perspectives as is, descriptively, and not contributed to better understand what led to both children and staff's perspectives. Also, for the staff members, this discussion triggered a team reflection on practices they are using and how they are labelled.

## Strengths and limitations of the participatory research process

Within a participatory research study, it is challenging to know the extent to which the partners will be involved and how the study will unfold since key decisions are taken collaboratively throughout the study process. Multiple opportunities for participation were offered throughout the project, and special attention was given to respecting partners' availability and interest in being part of the research process, as would be done for participation in the study itself. This led to different levels of involvements from partners, aiming for an equitable participation. Involvement of the partners led to a better fit of the research activities with the local context, more appropriate and relevant data collection procedures, an enriched interpretation of data, and enhanced recruitment as people were already aware of the study before the start of data collection. Meetings also contributed to the establishment of a rapport between children and the researcher, which is considered as particularly important with younger children in order for them to "get to know" the researcher and express their thoughts and opinions freely (Butler, 2012, p. 69). Involving children with mental illness diagnoses in the research process also contributed to defining children's best interests in ways that were more inclusive of their views, instead of pre-imposing what was considered as in their best interests by the researchers and/or clinicians.

Many children initially expressed being surprised to be asked directly for their perspectives. While most of them enthusiastically shared their views, one initially mentioned it was not worth sharing his perspective because it would not change anything. In this context, work still needs to be done to engage children meaningfully in research processes and recognize their capacity to be actively involved, and also follow-up with them about the changes resulting from their involvement. This was partially done in the project described here (through verbal exchanges with children) but could have been developed more significantly. The use of a participatory research approach in which children were involved contributed to the conduct of a study that was more attuned to the perspectives of children. It fostered the recognition of their agency, as well as best interests, with the aim of balancing these different concepts while involving them in a meaningful way.

## Conclusion

Rather than presenting a limitation for research with children, "cognitive impairment" affords opportunities to consider how to better recognize agency in research with *all* children. Conducting research that recognizes children's agency and best interests would allow for children's involvement in matters that affect them, while ensuring their involvement is performed in a way that is ethically sound and meaningful to them. As a child partner involved in a participatory research project related to public health in the United Kingdom stated: "People shouldn't assume that young people are not interested in research. We are. The key thing is making the research interesting and relatable to young people" (Skeels and Lewis, 2012, p. 48). It is up to researchers to find ways to make this possible, and ask children directly about how to enhance their engagement for each specific project.

## References

Aisen, M. L., Kerkovich, D., Mast, J., Mulroy, S., Wren, T. A., Kay, R. M., and Rethlefsen, S. A. (2011). "Cerebral Palsy: Clinical Care and Neurological Rehabilitation." *The Lancet Neurology*, 10/9: 844–852.

Baker A. and Plows V. (2015). "Re-Presenting or Representing Young Lives?" in Riele K. and Gorur R. (eds.) *Interrogating Conceptions of "Vulnerable Youth" in Theory, Policy and Practice. Innovations and Controversies: Interrogating Educational Change*. Rotterdam: SensePublishers, pp. 197–212.

Bakhtin, M. M. (1981). *The Dialogic Imagination: Four Essays*. Austin, TX: University of Texas Press.

Barnes, C. and Oliver, M. (1993). "Disability: A Sociological Phenomenon Ignored by Sociologists," https://disability-studies.leeds.ac.uk/wp-content/uploads/sites/40/library/Barnes-soc-phenomenon.pdf (accessed March 5, 2019).

Bora, E. (2015). "Developmental Trajectory of Cognitive Impairment in Bipolar Disorder: Comparison With Schizophrenia." *European Neuropsychopharmacology*, 25/2: 158–168.

Bourdieu, P. (1990). *The Logic of Practice*. Stanford, CA: Stanford University Press.

Bracken-Roche, D., Bell, E., Macdonald, M.E., and Racine, E. (2017). "The Concept of 'Vulnerability' in Research Ethics: An In-depth Analysis of Policies and Guidelines." *Health Research Policy and Systems*, 15/1: 8.

Bradbury-Jones, C. and Taylor, J. (2015). "Engaging With Children as Co-researchers: Challenges, Counter-challenges and Solutions." *International Journal of Social Research Methodology*, 18/2: 161–173.

Butler, V. (2012). "An Exploration of How Ethics Inform the Design of Social Research With Children Under 11 Years of Age," in Fleming, J. and Boeck, T. (eds.) *Involving Children and Young People in Health and Social Care Research*. New York: Routledge, pp. 63–72.

Canadian Pediatric Society. (2014). "Ethical Issues in Health Research in Children." *Paediatrics & Child Health*, 13/8: 707.

Carnevale, F. A., Macdonald, M. E., Bluebond-Langnerm, M. and McKeever, P. (2008). "Using Participant Observation in Pediatric Health Care Settings: Ethical Challenges and Solutions." *Journal of Child Health Care*, 12/1: 18–32.

Carnevale, F. A., Campbell, A., Collin-Vézina, D., and Macdonald, M.E. (2015). "Interdisciplinary Studies of Childhood Ethics: Developing a New Field of Inquiry." *Children & Society*, 29/6: 511–523.

Carnevale, F. A., Teachman, G., and Bogossian, A. (2017). "A Relational Ethics Framework for Advancing Practice with Children with Complex Health Care Needs and Their Parents." *Comprehensive Child and Adolescent Nursing*, 40/4: 268–284.

Carter, B. (2009). "Tick Box for Child? The Ethical Positioning of Children as Vulnerable, Researchers as Barbarians and Reviewers as Overly Cautious." *International Journal of Nursing Studies*, 46/6: 858–864.

Cascio, M. A., and Racine, E. (2018). "Person-oriented Research Ethics: Integrating Relational and Everyday Ethics in Research." *Accountability in Research*, 25/3: 170–197.

Centre of Genomics and Policy (CGP) and Maternal Infant Child and Youth Research Network (MICYRN). (2012). "Best Practices for Health Research Involving Children and Adolescents," http://www.genomicsandpolicy.org/en/best-practices-2012 (accessed March 5, 2019).

Coyne, I. and Carter, B. (2018). *Being Participatory: Researching with Children and Young People: Co-constructing Knowledge Using Creative* Techniques. New York: Springer.

Dowse, L. (2009). '"Some People are Never Going to be Able to do That". Challenges for People With Intellectual Disability in the 21st Century". *Disability & Society*, 24/5: 571–584.

Feudtner, C. and Brosco, J. P. (2011). "Do People With Intellectual Disability Require Special Human Subjects Research Protections? The Interplay of History, Ethics, and Policy." *Developmental Disabilities Research Reviews*, 17/1: 52–56.

Green, L. W., George, M. A., Daniel, M., Frankish, C. J., Herbert, C. J., Bowie, W., and O'Neill, M. (1995). "Participatory research in health promotion in Canada," http://lgreen.net/guidelines.html (accessed March 5, 2019).

Goodley, D. and Runswick Cole, K. (2015). "Critical Psychologies of Disability: Boundaries, Borders and Bodies in the Lives of Disabled Children." *Emotional and Behavioural Difficulties*, 20/1: 51–63.

Groundwater-Smith, S., Dockett, S., and Bottrell, D. (2014). *Participatory Research With Children and Young People*. London: Sage.

Guillemin, M. and Gillam, L. (2004). "Ethics, Reflexivity, and 'Ethically Important Moments' in Research." *Qualitative Inquiry*, 10: 261–280.

Hawk Jr, L. W., Fosco, W. D., Colder, C. R., Waxmonsky, J. G., Pelham Jr, W. E. and Rosch, K. S. (2018). "How do Stimulant Treatments for ADHD Work? Evidence for Mediation by Improved Cognition." *Journal of Child Psychology and Psychiatry* 59/12: 1271–1281.

Hollomotz, A. (2017). "Successful Interviews With People With Intellectual Disability." *Qualitative Research*, 18: 153–170.

James, A. and Prout, A. (2015). *Constructing and Reconstructing Childhood*: Contemporary Issues in the Sociological Study of Childhood. New York: Routledge.

Kelly, B. (2007). "Methodological Issues for Qualitative Research With Learning Disabled Children." *International Journal of Social Research Methodology*, 10/1: 21–35.

Lee, N. (2001). *Childhood and Society: Growing Up in an Age of Uncertainty*. London: McGraw-Hill Education (UK).

McDonagh, P., Goodey, C.F., and Stainton, T. (2018). *Intellectual Disability: A Conceptual History, 1200–1900*. Oxford: Oxford University Press.

Montreuil, M. (2017). "Moral Experiences of Crisis Management in a Child Mental Health Setting: A Participatory Hermeneutic Ethnographic Inquiry." Unpublished thesis, McGill University.

Montreuil, M. and Carnevale, F.A. (2016). "A Concept Analysis of Children's Agency Within the Health Literature." *Journal of Child Health Care*, 20/4: 503–511.

Montreuil, M. and Carnevale, F. A. (2018). "Participatory Hermeneutic Ethnography: A Methodological Framework for Health Ethics Research With Children." *Qualitative Health Research*, 28/7: 1135–1144.

Morris, J. (2003). "Including All Children: Finding Out About the Experiences of Children With Communication and/or Cognitive Impairments." *Children & Society*, 17.5: 337–348.

Nader, A. M., Courchesne, V., Dawson, M., and Soulières, I. (2016). "Does WISC-IV Underestimate the Intelligence of Autistic Children?" *Journal of Autism and Developmental Disorders*, 46/5: 1582–1589.

Nind, M. and Vinha, H. 2016. "Creative Interactions With Data: Using Visual and Metaphorical Devices in Repeated Focus Groups." *Qualitative Research*, 16/1: 9–26.

Noiseux, J., Rich, H., Bouchard, N., Noronha, C., and Carnevale, F.A. (2019). "Children Need Privacy Too: Respecting Confidentiality in Paediatric Practice." *Paediatrics & Child Health*, 24/1: e8–e12.

Odding, E., Roebroeck, M. E., & Stam, H. J. (2006). "The Epidemiology of Cerebral Palsy: Incidence, Impairments and Risk Factors". *Disability and Rehabilitation*, 28/4: 183–191.

Peter, E. and Friedland, J. (2017). "Recognizing Risk and Vulnerability in Research Ethics: Imagining the 'What Ifs?'" *Journal of Empirical Research on Human Research Ethics*, 12/2: 107–116.

Racine, E. and Bracken-Roche, D. (2019). "Enriching the Concept of Vulnerability in Research Ethics: An Integrative and Functional Account." *Bioethics*, 33/1: 19–34.

Racine, E., Bell, E., Yan, A., Andrew, G., Bell, L. E., Clarke, M., et al. (2014). "Ethics Challenges of Transition From Paediatric to Adult Health Care Services for Young Adults With Neurodevelopmental Disabilities." *Paediatrics & Child Health*, 19/2: 65–68.

Robinson, S., Hill, M., Fisher, K.R., and Graham, A. (2018). "Belonging and Exclusion in the Lives of Young People With Intellectual Disability in Small Town Communities." *Journal of Intellectual Disabilities*. DOI: 10.1177/1744629518765830.

Skeels, A. and Lewis, M. (2012). "Using National Standards for Children and Young People's Participation to Inform Health Research," in Fleming, J. and Boeck, T. (eds.) *Involving Children and Young People in Health and Social Care Research*. New York: Routledge, pp. 38–50.

Skelton, T. (2008). "Research With Children and Young People: Exploring the Tensions Between Ethics, Competence and Participation." *Children's Geographies*, 6/1: 21–36.

Stack, E. and McDonald, K.E. (2014). "Nothing About Us Without Us: Does Action Research in Developmental Disabilities Research Measure Up?" *Journal of Policy and practice in Intellectual Disabilities*, 11/2: 83–91.

Suresh, P., Ayyappan, A., Nandidn, J., and Ismail, T. (2015). "Cognitive Deficits and Behavioural Disorders in Children: A Comprehensive Multidisciplinary Approach to Management." *Annals of Behavioural Science*, http://behaviouralscience.imedpub.com/behavioural-science-psycology/cognitive-deficits-and-behavioral-disorders-in-children-a-comprehensive-multidisciplinary-approach-to-management.php?aid=7900 (accessed March 5, 2019).

Taylor, C. (2004). *Modern Social Imaginaries*. Durham, NC: Duke University Press.

Taylor, C. (1971). "Interpretation and the Sciences of Man." *The Review of Metaphysics*, 25/1: 3–51.

TCPS2 (Canadian Institutes of Health Research, Natural Sciences and Engineering Research Council of Canada, and Social Sciences and Humanities Research Council of Canada (CIHR, NSERC, SSHRC)) (2014). "Tri-Council Policy Statement: Ethical Conduct for Research Involving Humans," http://www.pre.ethics.gc.ca/pdf/eng/tcps2-2014/TCPS_2_FINAL_Web.pdf (accessed March 5, 2019).

Teachman, G. (2016). "Interrogating Inclusion: Critical Research With Disabled Youth Who Use Augmentative and Alternative Communication," https://tspace.library.utoronto.ca/handle/1807/73207 (accessed March 22, 2019).

Teachman, G. and Gibson, B.E. (2018). "Integrating Visual Methods With Dialogical Interviews in Research With Youth Who Use Augmentative and Alternative Communication." *International Journal of Qualitative Methods*, 17/1: 1609406917750945.

Teachman, G., McDonough, P., Macarthur, C., and Gibson, B.E. (2018). "A Critical Dialogical Methodology for Conducting Research With Disabled Youth Who Use Augmentative and Alternative Communication." *Qualitative Inquiry*, 24/1: 35–44.

Veale, A. (2005). "Creative Methodolgies in Participatory Research With Children," in Greene, S. and Hogan, D. (eds.) *Researching Children's Experience*. Thousand Oaks, CA: SAGE, pp. 253–272.

Wagner, S., Müller, C., Helmreich, I., Huss, M., and Tadić, A. (2015). "A META-Analysis of Cognitive Functions in Children and Adolescents With Major Depressive Disorder." *European Child & Adolescent Psychiatry*, 24/1: 5–19.

# 13

# Informed Consent for Next-Generation Deep Brain Stimulation Psychiatric Research

## Engaging End Users to Understand Risks and Improve Practice

*Eran Klein*

### Introduction

Research on innovative neurotechnology, such as deep brain stimulation (DBS), for treatment-resistant psychiatric illness, such as depression and obsessive–compulsive disorder, enroll potentially vulnerable research participants. Individuals with treatment-resistant depression are more likely to develop comorbid general medical or other psychiatric disorders and more likely to experience stressful live events, like relationship problems, financial difficulties, deaths of family members, and exposure to life-threatening situations (Amital et al., 2008). Neural devices that stimulate the brain, like DBS, are a promising new research direction in this population, but use of implantable devices to treat psychiatric illness raises important ethical issues (Fins et al., 2006; Rabins et al., 2009; Glannon, 2010; Dunn et al., 2011; Bell and Racine, 2012), including concerns related to patient selection criteria, clinical trial design, personal identity, enhancement, behavioral modification, and resource allocation (Grant, 2014). Informed consent is recognized as a particularly challenging area in psychiatric DBS (Bell et al., 2009, 2014; Glannon, 2009; Dunn et al., 2011; Synofzik and Schlaepfer, 2011; Lipsman et al., 2012).

Next-generation DBS devices in psychiatry will incorporate recording, as well as stimulating, capabilities. The move toward next-generation systems presents an opportunity to step back and consider research informed consent practices. Lipsman et al. (2012) identified three issues as particularly relevant to informed consent in psychiatric DBS research: Vulnerable research populations, decisional capacity in psychiatric illness, and scientific uncertainty in psychiatric DBS. Informed consent in next-generation DBS will need to not only address these issues, but also pay special attention to effects on agency, authenticity, and family relationships (Klein et al., 2016).

How should the challenges for informed consent in next-generation psychiatric DBS be approached? One promising avenue is user-centered design. User-centered design incorporates feedback given by targeted future users of devices early in the design process (e.g., which features are important to include and which are not). User-centered design can also be used to gather feedback on ethically salient aspects of research, including the informed consent process. This chapter provides a brief overview of user-centered design and its potential use in informed consent processes in next-generation neurostimulation systems in psychiatry. This is illustrated with results of a qualitative focus group and interview study recently conducted with individuals with first-generation DBS devices (Klein et al., 2016; Goering et al. 2017). By exploring issues of vulnerability, decisional capacity, scientific uncertainty, agency, authenticity, and family relationships with users of psychiatric neural devices, challenges of informed consent can be better understood, anticipated, and addressed.

## User-centered design

User-centered design prioritizes input of potential users into the design process to improve *usability*. The usability of devices reflects the extent to which the needs of targeted users are met. Originally focused on optimizing human–computer interaction (Norman and Draper, 1986), user-centered design now encompasses the design of assistive technology more generally. Six principles of user-centered design are codified in the ISO 9241-201: Understand the user, the task and environmental requirements; encourage early and active involvement of users; be driven and refined by user-centered evaluation; include iteration of design solutions; address the whole user experience; and encourage multi-disciplinary design. The rationale for user-centered design is that a design process that takes account of the perspectives of potential users of technology will be more likely to achieve a usable product. User-centered design overlaps with approaches to "participatory design" (Sanders, 2003) and "human centered design" (Gasson, 2003).

Users can offer input along the full spectrum of the design cycle from idea conception to testing of prototype. User-centered design can be used not only to improve usability of devices, but to address ethical concerns along the course of the research arc (Carmichael and Carmichael, 2014; Hariz et al., 2011; Sullivan et al., 2018). In part, this is because perspectives on ethical values, society norms, and worldviews are typically deemed outside the scope of science. By collecting this new form of "data," user-centered design allows for a broader range of device assessment. In addition, by gathering input from actual or potential end users, the user-centered design process demonstrates a kind of *respect* for users of devices, who can be members of disabled communities and whose voices and concerns are not always easily heard or appropriately valued (Goering and Klein, in press).

Implementation of user-centered design faces obstacles when applied to neural device development in psychiatry. Methods of gathering input from potential technology users—focus groups and interviews—can exclude participation based on cognitive or communicative capacities (for an exception to this, see Blain-Moraes et al., 2012). This can be a challenge if individuals with psychiatric illness have or are perceived to have cognitive or communicative disabilities. While specialized qualitative research methods have been developed for individuals with cognitive or communication disabilities (Gibson et al., 2004; Balandin and Goldbart, 2011), technology designers may not have the knowledge, expertise, or resources to implement specialized forms of end-user engagement. In addition, methods of user-centered design data gathering may require activities (e.g., focus groups, one-on-one interviews) that persons with psychiatric illness find particularly stressful or burdensome.

Thus, if the promise of user-centered design is to be realized in psychiatric device design, new approaches to gathering input from end users need to be explored. The next section provides an example of gathering input from users of psychiatric neural devices to improve research practice, specifically, informed consent.

## Informed consent challenges in psychiatric DBS

Informed consent is a bedrock principle in bioethics and an ethical and legal requirement for conduct of clinical research (National Commission, 1979 (45CFR46)). The basic elements of the informed consent process are: (1) disclosure of information, (2) decisional capacity, and (3) voluntariness (Beauchamp and Childress, 2012). At minimum, research participants must be provided with relevant information about their medical condition and therapeutic options, as well as potential risks and benefits of research participation. They must have the capacity to understand, appreciate, and make a reasoned decision specifically about study enrollment. Finally, though decisions about study participation may be influenced by others or by circumstance, the decision to enroll must be voluntary.

Klein et al. (2016) published a study exploring the phenomenology of psychiatric DBS, as well as views about next-generation psychiatric DBS. This study involved one focus group with eight individuals and separate interviews with seven individuals who could not participate in the focus group. Details about the methodology and ethics review of this study are described elsewhere (Klein et al., 2016). One of the themes evident in this study was a concern about informed consent. For instance, quotes from two individuals illustrate the complexity of informed consent in psychiatric DBS.

> Well, I do know, a lot of times, it really freaks me out that I had this done, and I have this... I've got this thing in my head. It *really*... I don't want to say I'm obsessed by it, because I'm not, but there are certain days I'm like, "Oh, my god, what on earth did I do?"... I just can't believe I did it! That's about all I can say. I, I do have to say I'm glad I did it. But I'm just saying, I just can't believe what state of mind that I would ever go get this...
>
> I think I made an informed... actually, I don't know if I made an informed decision, but, you have to question, "Can people make a truly informed decision about it?"

Here, published (and some previously unpublished) results from a recent study (Klein et al., 2016; Goering et al., 2017) are presented. These data illustrate three challenges for informed consent identified by Lipsman et al. (2012): vulnerability of psychiatric research populations, the effect of psychiatric illness on consent capacity, and scientific uncertainty related to DBS, as well as three challenges (i.e., agency, authenticity, and family relationships).

## Individual and group vulnerability

Individuals who enroll in psychiatric DBS can be vulnerable in various ways. Kenneth Kipnis (2003) describes seven types of vulnerability in biomedical research (capacitational, juridic, deferential, social, situational, medical, allocational). These types of vulnerability are present in psychiatric DBS research as well. Individuals can be *capacitationally* vulnerable in DBS psychiatric research owing to the effect of mental illness on decisional capacity. They can be *juridically* vulnerable if others (e.g., surrogates) exercise authority over their participation. They can exhibit *deferential* vulnerability if their participation comes about through patterns of deference to mental health professionals. Given the history of stigma experienced by those with mental illness, participants in DBS research can be *socially* vulnerable. They can experience *situational* vulnerability if medical exigency (e.g., suicide attempts) interferes with normal education and deliberation about study participation. The severity of mental illness can result in *medical* vulnerability, particularly if all effective treatment options have been exhausted. Finally, they can experience *allocational* vulnerability if participating in DBS research makes mental health expertise available that would otherwise be inaccessible because of cost or other barriers. DBS in psychiatry has been recognized as a particularly powerful example of the range of vulnerabilities in research practice (and the need for operationalization of constructive approaches) (Bracken-Roche and Racine, 2018).

In this study, social and medical vulnerabilities were particularly evident. The social vulnerability of severe depression took different forms. One individual expressed this in terms of isolation, noting that "We have a façade ... most people in our lives have no idea how sick we really are, and how much we struggle every minute of every day." Others experienced social vulnerability in terms of oversimplification of how DBS is used to treat mental illness and, in turn, how it leads to a reification of mental health stereotypes. Individuals in the study lamented that family and others came to view any depressive symptoms post-DBS as principally a technological problem, with family members stating that they should "go flip a switch" or "go get your settings adjusted." Depression was no longer seen as involving complex psychosocial influences, but as something to be fixed with a simple settings adjustment.

Moreover, participants experienced a kind of medical vulnerability related to feelings of desperation. The severity of symptoms and perceived lack of alternative therapies generated unrealistic expectations. One participant expressed that "[S]uffering from severe depression, you'll do anything to get out of it! Just excruciating! ... When you're at the end of the line, you're begging for DBS." This desperation was also associated with a willingness to take on high levels of risk. "I'm willing to try anything. I'm not ... like, I'm not even afraid if it's got a 50% chance of death, I'll still try it because I'm so desperate, and I'm ... I'm suffering so much."

An additional sense of medical vulnerability was experienced by participants who felt they would undergo a permanent change in the structure of their brains such that they might be precluded from future therapeutic options.

> I know that I won't qualify for other studies, because I've already had . . . essentially, damage done to my brain because it's been intruded. Um, any time you put anything in a brain, it's essentially, de facto, damaged . . . uh, material because it's not pure, for another study. Um, damaged in that sense because it, it's, you know, it's already had something else done to it.

## Decisional capacity

Decisional capacity is critical for informed consent in psychiatric DBS. Since DBS involves assessing surgical and other risks, the threshold for decisional capacity is higher than with most pharmacologic interventions (Glannon, 2010). Appelbaum and Grisso (2001) describe decisional capacity as involving understanding, reasoning, appreciation, and choice. They developed the MacArthur competency assessment tool for research (MacCat-CR) to measure decisional capacity in research contexts, including psychiatric research. Psychiatric illness can affect a range of cognitive processes—executive function (Snyder, 2013), attention and concentration (Kampf-Sherf et al., 2004), memory (Fossati et al., 1999)—but studies of individuals considering DBS for depression indicate that decision-making capacity can be maintained, despite severe depression (Rabins et al., 2009; Dunn et al., 2011).

In this study, individuals with psychiatric DBS retrospectively noted difficulty *understanding* and *appreciating* information provided to them during the initial informed consent process and attributed this difficulty to their underlying psychiatric symptoms. For some, difficulty understanding manifested as impairment in reading and comprehending informed consent documents ("I could not read [the forms] to save my life."), or even just "pay attention" to information provided. Others commented on their difficulty *appreciating* the risks involved in research. One participant noted "I could have cared less about the risks," while another stated "I was so depressed I didn't even care. I, 'Whatever.' You know?"

## Scientific (and other) uncertainty

Meaningful informed consent relies on research participants having a reasonable approximation of risks and benefits. Some of the risks of DBS are well known. Risks of surgical implantation of electrodes and batteries have become clearer over time as DBS therapy for movement disorders has become standard of care. This information can help inform psychiatric DBS research. Other risks of psychiatric DBS research are hard to estimate, in part because of a lack of understanding of how DBS works. Even in

DBS used successfully to treat movement disorders, there is a lack of consensus on its mechanism of action (Wichmann and DeLong, 2011). The mechanism gap is wider in psychiatric DBS where the appropriate target of stimulation is still a matter of debate (Graat et al,. 2017). Uncertainty affects not just whether psychiatric DBS will have its intended immediate effect (e.g., enhance mood), but how long this effect will last and whether induced changes to mood will have unanticipated effects (e.g., to cognition, personality, etc.). Anticipating the risks of psychiatric DBS is challenging.

In this study, respondents acknowledged the uncertainty attending research in this area. One individual summarized this uncertainty as "there's just so many unknowns." Another respondent expressed similar sentiment, noting:

> I don't think a whole lot of [subjects and researchers] had a whole lot of information. We had some real good ideas, we had some real good possibilities and some real good hypotheses, but until you stick something like this into somebody's body, and you watch them change over time, then, you don't know.

In addition to unscientific unknowns, uncertainties relate to conduct and funding of research, including what will happen to participants and their devices at study conclusion. One respondent expressed frustration about the impact of economic forces on the conduct of research and the difficulty posed for the informed consent process:

> [I]t would be nice if you could tell people, "There's no way this study can work, um, because we're not getting enough people, we're not . . . we're not funding to enroll . . . enroll enough people, to show that this can work or not. So, you know, don't be surprised, um, if the funding gets pulled." Um, I mean, I was specifically told several times, that the funding could NEVER get pulled, "It's not gonna happen, not gonna happen." I was even stopped in the hallway by one of the PI's [principal investigators] who was impressed with how well I was looking, and he said, "Well, you know, it's not gonna happen. You look so great. They're never gonna pull the funding on this." Um . . . I don't think you can do that in informed consent if you want to get any patients!

## Additional informed consent challenges

The use of neural devices to treat psychiatric illness also raises questions about authenticity, agency, and familial relationships (Klein et al., 2016). The incorporation of next-generation control schemes for psychiatric DBS devices requires giving attention to these underappreciated challenges.

### Authenticity

Treatment of psychiatric illness can have effects on individuals' sense of authenticity. Carl Elliott (1998) has written about psychopharmacologic treatment and the "ethics of authenticity". He argues that some psychiatric treatments, like the antidepressant Prozac, have adverse effects on authenticity, which can lead to a sense of alienation. Interventions can "work"—lead to changes in personality and subsequent improvements in financial or social standing—but leave a sense of emptiness if how one feels or acts is at some level out of sync with who one takes oneself to be. To illustrate, Elliott offers the example of Percy, an accountant who uses Prozac to more "successfully" navigate an unfulfilling suburban middle class life. Conversely, David DeGrazia (2000, 2005) argues for the positive effect of psychopharmacology on authenticity. When chosen autonomously and honestly, medications allow an individual with psychiatric illness to live a *more* authentic life. An analogous debate about authenticity is found in discussions about psychiatric DBS (Schöne-Seifert and Talbot 2010).

Eric Parens (2005, 2014) describes the appeal to authenticity as generally conforming to one of two frames: self-creation or self-discovery. That is, interventions promote a sense of authenticity by allowing for self-creation, becoming the person one wants to be, or by allowing an uncovering (or discovering) of one's hidden or deeper self. DBS study participants expressed views implicating both kinds of authenticity. With respect to self-discovery, some expressed that they were able to get "back to sort of a baseline" or be "more like yourself." Others described effects on authenticity that were more in line with self-creation. One respondent noted that after receiving DBS she became "entirely different" and "aware of having feelings that I never knew existed before."

## Agency

Agency can be broadly understood as the capacity or exercise of the ability to perform (or hold back from performing) an action (Schlosser, 2015). An individual exercises agency when she intends to act and, consequently, does perform an action. A sense of agency helps people distinguish between things they do (as an actor) and things that happen to them (as a recipient).

Psychiatric interventions, including DBS, can raise questions about agency when they blur the line between actor and recipient. In this study, one person with DBS described acting in socially insensitive or inappropriate ways and wondering whether this behavior was due to depression, the effect of the device, or to neither. "There are three things—there's me, as I was, or think I was; and there's the depression, and then there's depression AND the device and, it, it blurs to the point where I'm not sure, frankly, who I am" (Goering et al., 2017). Another person described questioning whether an inability to cry at a loved one's funeral was a DBS effect or due to some other factor (e.g., depression, medications, or circumstances) (Goering et al., 2017). Such experiences lend credence to the idea that psychiatric DBS can lead some individuals to question whether changes in their emotional states are due to the device or to their agency.

A focus on agency in the informed consent process will help research participants recognize when their agency is affected by a neural device and how to deal with it. It may be inevitable that certain neural devices, particularly if they include features of machine learning, will generate experiences at odds with how participants understand their agency. This may require developing a kind of trust in devices (Goering et al., 2017). This need not (and usually should not) be a blind trust, but a kind of relational trust in which participants "entrust" some of their agency to neural devices. So long as devices are constructed in such a way as to be trustworthy, researchers and participants can explore ahead of time in the informed consent process what effects on agency are anticipated and acceptable.

## Impact on family

Discussions about informed consent paradigmatically center on the *individual*. The decision to get an implanted device, however, often involves families as well. Families are affected by what transpires after DBS implantation. In the case of DBS for Parkinson disease, Schüpbach et al. (2006) and Agid et al. (2006) describe family members whose lives were upended by "successful" DBS surgery, owing to personality or other changes in their loved ones after DBS. Taking account of effects on family is particularly important in the case of psychiatric DBS due to the effect that severe mental illness has on not just the individual, but on family members as well (Glannon, 2010; Lipsman et al., 2012).

Treatment with DBS can potentially improve the lives of caregivers and enhance relationships between treated individuals and families, but it can also exacerbate problematic familial relationships. One member of the focus group expressed that having a device in some ways fed into established and undesirable relationship dynamics with her family member:

> [T]he problem's [always] with me. It's like, "Oh, you're just too sensitive." And I'm like, "Well, you're not sensitive enough." And, um, but if... things are bad, and I'm feeling bad about what's going on at home, his solution is always to get it turned up, "Why can't you get turned up?"... Yeah, just because there's like a little candyman in your head, [he thinks] "I don't have to be nice to you, I just have to turn it up and you'll be OK with me yelling at you." And, that's kind of how it was when it was first turned up, I was like... I, I mean, I didn't like it, but I just didn't react, and it was like... "Well, I'm feeling good." And so it gave him an excuse to just... he's actually been worse since I've had it. He... it's funny—I'm better, he's worse!

Varied and complex effects of devices on relationships need to be explored in the informed consent process. This involves discussing with family members—not just DBS recipients—expectations for life post-DBS. Do family members think that there will be less need for caregiving post-DBS? As such, do family members expect their quality of life (or even health) to improve after their loved one gets DBS, perhaps due to reductions in caregiving responsibilities? Or do family members worry that they won't be "needed" as much or in as meaningful a way as before? Exploring these kinds of questions with both device recipient and family *before DBS* is preferable to confronting a mismatch of expectations and reality post-DBS.

## Conclusion

Research on implantable neurotechnology may open new avenues for treatment of psychiatric illness. Such research involves risks that need to be carefully considered in the informed consent process. The vulnerabilities of research participants need to be considered, as do impairments of decisional capacity and scientific uncertainty. Attention also needs to be paid to effects of devices on agency, authenticity, and familial relationships. Understanding *how* to attend to these concerns in the informed consent process requires learning from individuals who have lived experience with psychiatric neural devices. Adopting a user-centered design approach to research on new neural devices provides a promising path forward.

## Acknowledgements

I would like to thank Sara Goering and Alik Widge, who were collaborators on the interview and focus group study out of which this paper originated. This work was supported by the National Science Foundation through EEC#1028725.

## References

Agid, Y., Schupbach, M., Gargiulo, M., Mallet, L., Houeto, J. L., Behar, C., et al. (2006). "Neurosurgery in Parkinson's Disease: The Doctor is Happy, the Patient Less So?" *Journal of Neural Transmission, Supplement*, 70: 409–414.

Amital, D., Fostick, L., Silberman, A., Beckman, M., and Spivak, B. (2008). "Serious Life Events Among Resistant and Non-Resistant MDD Patients." *Journal of Affective Disorders*, 110/3: 260–264.

Appelbaum, P. and Grisso, T. (2001). *MacCAT-CR: MacArthur Competence Assessment Tool for Clinical Research*. Sarasota, FL: Professional Resource Press.

Balandin, S. and Goldbart, J. (2011). "Qualitative Research and AAC: Strong Methods and New Topics." *Augmentative and Alternative Communication*, 27: 227–228.

Beauchamp, T. L. and Childress, J. F. (2012). *Principles of Biomedical Ethics*, 7th ed. New York: Oxford University Press.

Bell, E., Mathieu, G., and Racine, E. (2009). "Preparing the Ethical Future of Deep Brain Stimulation." *Surgical Neurology*, 72/6: 577–586.

Bell, E. and Racine, E. (2012). "Ethical Guidance for the Use of Deep Brain Stimulation in Psychiatric Trials and Emerging Uses: Review and Reflections," in Denys, D., Feenstra, M., and Schuurman, R. (eds.) *Deep Brain Stimulation: A New Frontier in Psychiatry*. New York: Springer, pp. 273–288.

Bell, E., Racine, E., Chiasson, P., Dufourcq-Brana, M., Dunn, L.B., Fins, J.J., Ford, P.J., Glannon, W., Lipsman, N., Macdonald, M.E., and Mathews, D. J. (2014). "Beyond Consent in Research." *Cambridge Quarterly of Healthcare Ethics*, 23/03: 361–368.

Blain-Moraes, S., Schaff, R., Gruis, K.L., Huggins, J.E., and Wren, P.A. (2012). "Barriers to and Mediators of Brain-Computer Interface User Acceptance: Focus Group Findings." *Ergonomics* 55: 516–525.

Bracken-Roche, D. and Racine, E. (2018). "Enriching the Concept of Vulnerability in Research Ethics: An Integrative and Functional Account." *Bioethics* 2018, https://rdcu.be/48zY.

Carmichael, C. and Carmichael, P. (2014). "BNCI Systems as a Potential Assistive Technology: Ethical Issues and Participatory Research in the BrainAble Project." *Disability and Rehabilitation: Assistive Technology*, 9/1: 41–47.

DeGrazia, D. (2000). "Prozac, Enhancement, and Self-creation." *Hastings Center Report*, 30/2: 34–40.

DeGrazia, D. (2005). "Enhancement Technologies and Human Identity." *Journal of Medicine and Philosophy*, 30/3: 261–283.

Dunn, L.B., Holtzheimer, P.E., Hoop, J.G., Mayberg, H.S., Weiss Roberts, L., and Appelbaum, P. (2011). "Ethical Issues in Deep Brain Stimulation Research for Treatment-Resistant Depression: Focus on Risk and Consent." *American Journal of Bioethics*, 2/1: 29–36.

Elliott, C. (1998). "The Tyranny of Happiness: Ethics and Cosmetic Psychopharmacology," in Parens, E. (ed.) *Enhancing Human Traits: Ethical and Social Implications*. Washington, DC: Georgetown University Press, pp. 177–188.

Fins, J.J., Rezai, A.R., and Greenberg, B. D. (2006). "Psychosurgery: Avoiding an Ethical Redux While Advancing a Therapeutic Future." *Neurosurgery*, 59/4: 713–716.

Fossati, P., Amar, G., Raoux, N., Ergis, A.M., and Allilaire, J. F. (1999). "Executive Functioning and Verbal Memory in Young Patients With Unipolar Depression and Schizophrenia." *Psychiatry Research*, 89/3: 171–187.

Gasson, S. (2003). "Human-Centered vs. User-Centered Approaches to Information System Design." *Journal of Information Technology Theory and Application*, 5/2: 29–46.

Gibson, G., Timlin, A., Curran, S., and Wattis, J. (2004). "The Scope for Qualitative Methods in Research and Clinical Trials in Dementia." *Age and Ageing*, 33: 422–426.

Glannon, W. (2009). "Stimulating Brains, Altering Minds." *Journal of Medical Ethics*, 35/5: 289–292.

Glannon, W., (2010). "Consent to Deep Brain Stimulation for Neurological and Psychiatric Disorders." *Journal of Clinical Ethics*, 21/2: 104–111.

Goering, S., Klein, E., Dougherty, D.D., and Widge, A. S. (2017). "Staying in the Loop: Relational Agency and Identity in Next-generation DBS for Psychiatry." *AJOB Neuroscience*, 8/2: 59–70.

Goering, S. and Klein, E. (in press). "Neurotechnologies and Justice By, With and For Disabled People," In Wasserman, D. and Cureton, A. (eds.) *Oxford Handbook of Philosophy and Disability*. Oxford: Oxford University Press.

Graat, I., Figee, M., and Denys, D. (2017). "The Application of Deep Brain Stimulation in the Treatment of Psychiatric Disorders." *International Review of Psychiatry*, 29/2: 178–190.

Grant, R.A., Halpern, C.H., Baltuch, G.H., O'Reardon, J.P., and Caplan, A. (2014). "Ethical Considerations in Deep Brain Stimulation for Psychiatric Illness." *Journal of Clinical Neuroscience*, 21/1: 1–5.

Hariz, G.M., Limousin, P., Tisch, S., Jahanshahi, M., and Fjellman-Wiklund, A. (2011). "Patients' Perceptions of Life Shift After Deep Brain Stimulation for Primary Dystonia—A Qualitative Study." *Movement Disorders*, 26/11: 2101–2106.

ISO 9241-210 (2008). "Ergonomics of Human System Interaction—Part 210: Human-Centred Design for Interactive Systems (Formerly Known as 13407)." Geneva: International Organization for Standardization (ISO).

Kampf-Sherf, O., Zlotogorski, Z., Gilboa, A., Speedie, L., Lereya, J., Rosca, P., and Shavit, Y. (2004). "Neuropsychological Functioning in Major Depression and Responsiveness to Selective Serotonin Reuptake Inhibitors Antidepressants." *Journal of Affective Disorders*, 82/3: 453–459.

Kipnis, K. (2003). "Seven Vulnerabilities in the Pediatric Research Subject." *Theoretical Medicine and Bioethics*, 24/2: 107–120.

Klein, E., Goering, S., Gagne, J., Shea, C.V., Franklin, R., Zorowitz, S., Dougherty, D.D., and Widge, A. S. (2016). "Brain–Computer Interface-Based Control of Closed-Loop Brain Stimulation: Attitudes and Ethical Considerations." *Brain-Computer Interfaces*, 3/3: 140–148.

Lipsman, N., Giacobbe, P., Bernstein, M., and Lozano, A. M. (2012). "Informed Consent for Clinical Trials of Deep Brain Stimulation in Psychiatric Disease: Challenges and Implications for Trial Design." *Journal of Medical Ethics*, 38/2: 107–111.

National Commission for the Protection of Human Subjects of Biomedical and Behavioral Research (1979). *The Belmont Report: Ethical Principles and Guidelines for the Protection of Human Subjects of Biomedical and Behavioral Research*. Washington, DC: US Department of Health and Human Services.

Norman, D.A. and Draper, S. W. (1986). *User-Centered System Design: New Perspectives on Human–Computer Interaction*. Hillsdale, NJ: CRC Press.

Parens, E., (2005). "Authenticity and Ambivalence: Toward Understanding the Enhancement Debate." *Hastings Center Report*, 35/3: 34–41.

Parens, E. (2014). *Shaping Ourselves: On Technology, Flourishing, and a Habit of Thinking*. Oxford: Oxford University Press.

Rabins, P., Appleby, B.S., Brandt, J., DeLong, M.R., Dunn, L.B., Gabriëls, L., Greenberg, B.D., Haber, S.N., Holtzheimer, P.E., Mari, Z., and Mayberg, H. S. (2009). "Scientific and Ethical Issues Related to Deep Brain Stimulation for Disorders of Mood, Behavior, and Thought." *Archives of General Psychiatry*, 66/9: 931–937.

Racine, E. and Bracken-Roche, D. (2018). "Enriching the Concept of Vulnerability in Research Ethics: An Integrative and Functional Account." *Bioethics*, https://doi.org/10.1111/bioe.12471.

Sanders, E.B.N. (2002). "From User-Centered to Participatory Design Approaches," in Frascara, J. (ed.) *Design and the Social Sciences*. London: Taylor & Francis Books, pp. 1–8.

Schöne-Seifert, B. and Talbot, D. (2010). "(Neuro-) Enhancement," in Helmchen, H. and Sartorius, N. (eds.) *Ethics in Psychiatry*. Dordrecht: Springer, pp. 509–530.

Schlosser, M. (2015). "Agency," in Zalta, E. N. (ed.) *The Stanford Encyclopedia of Philosophy*, https://plato.stanford.edu/archives/fall2015/entries/agency (accessed May 22, 2018).

Schüpbach, M., Gargiulo, M., Welter, M. L., Mallet, L., Behar, C., Houeto, J. L., Maltete, D., Mesnage, V., and Agid, Y. (2006). "Neurosurgery in Parkinson Disease. A Distressed Mind in a Repaired Body?" *Neurology*, 66: 1811–1816.

Snyder, H.R. (2013). "Major Depressive Disorder is Associated With Broad Impairments on Neuropsychological Measures of Executive Function: A Meta-Analysis and Review." *Psychological Bulletin*, 139/1: 81–132.

Sullivan, L.S., Klein, E., Brown, T., Sample, M., Pham, M., Tubig, P., Folland, R., Truitt, A., and Goering, S. (2018). "Keeping Disability in Mind: A Case Study in Implantable Brain–Computer Interface Research." *Science and Engineering Ethics*, 24/2: 479–504.

Synofzik, M. and Schlaepfer, T. E. (2011). "Electrodes in the Brain—Ethical Criteria for Research and Treatment With Deep Brain Stimulation for Neuropsychiatric Disorders." *Brain Stimulation: Basic, Translational, and Clinical Research in Neuromodulation*, 4/1: 7–16.

Wichmann, T. and DeLong, M. R. (2011). "Deep-Brain Stimulation for Basal Ganglia Disorders." *Basal Ganglia*, 1/2: 65–77.

# 14

# Using Ethnographic Methods to Determine Capacity to Consent in Individuals Diagnosed with Chronic Mental Illnesses

*Saira A. Mehmood*

## Introduction

This chapter reports on an ethnographic research project conducted with people diagnosed with chronic mental illnesses and often economic and educational vulnerabilities as well. It focuses particularly on strategies for assessing capacity to consent—both formal assessment instruments and informal assessments over time through a process of participant observation. Through ethnographic methods, I discuss how successful participation of individuals diagnosed with chronic mental illnesses with impaired cognition can be included in non-clinical research to ensure the principle of autonomy, which requires respect for the decision-making capacities of autonomous persons, while also following the bioethical principle of justice (Beauchamp, 2007), as a way to include individuals with chronic mental illnesses and empower them.

## Research objectives

My dissertation research, conducted primarily from January 2015 to December 2017, examined how mental health discourse and government policies affected the lived experiences of individuals with chronic mental illnesses in New Orleans, Louisiana. How do these polices affect how individuals navigate the mental health care system? To explicate the main research objective, the following questions drove my research: (1) How do individuals diagnosed with chronic mental illnesses perceive mental illness and stigma? (2) What services do individuals use to address their mental health needs and what barriers do they face in this process? (3) How do individuals diagnosed with mental illness and their family members understand and embody recovery?

## Research site

Given my research questions, one of the primary research populations for my ethnographic study included individuals diagnosed with chronic mental illnesses who lived in a community setting. The decrease in both hospital-based and community-based psychiatric services led to an increasing number of individuals diagnosed with chronic mental illnesses living a nomadic life in New Orleans post-Hurricane Katrina. They moved between supported housing, jail, hospitals, homeless shelters, and the street, otherwise called "the institutional circuit" (Hopper et al., 1997; Luhrmann, 2008). Thus, I utilized a site-based approach (Arcury and Quandt, 1999) to recruit participants from community-based programs that provided mental health resources. The primary site where I recruited individuals to participate in my research was Vista,[1] a non-profit organization where the mission is to provide help to people living with mental illness and family members through family support, education, advocacy, and psychosocial programs.

Vista provided numerous programs, including peer-to-peer classes about mental illnesses, support groups for family members, housing programs, a psychosocial rehabilitation day program, case management, and a low-barrier access "Drop-In" where anyone with a mental illness could come in and utilize the space. I spent much of my time in the psychosocial rehabilitation day program, which I will refer to as "the day program" and Drop-In, which convened in the same space as the day program, but during later hours in the afternoon for two to three times a week. The day program convened during the morning hours in the workweek.

Some of the same members[2] who were in the day program often stayed for Drop-In later in the day. I was more familiar with members in the day program as I saw them more often; some members came in two or three times a week, while others came in every day of the week. Drop-In attracted not only members from the day program, but also homeless individuals or anyone who just wanted to see what Vista offered. Because Drop-In offered free coffee and a light meal or snack, this attracted a lot of homeless or low-income individuals since they could get food and benefit from an air-conditioned space during the hot summer months, as well as access computers with Internet, and clean restrooms. These were often the reasons members would tell me why they came to Vista during Drop-In hours. As a low-barrier service for individuals with mental illness, members just had to sign in when they came to Drop-In. Some of the members at Drop-In came for years, but others were in transition coming from one city and on their way to another. These included homeless individuals and military veterans.

[1] Vista is a pseudonym.

[2] I use participants and interlocutors for individuals that actually participated in my research. In this chapter, I also use the term "members" when describing individuals at Vista in general, as it was the most commonly used phrase used by staff. Although the staff used various terminologies to describe members (e.g., clients, consumers, users, etc.), the language within social work shifts regarding what to call members. Unless I use the phrase participants or interlocutors explicitly, members did not participate in my research.

Another major difference between the day program and Drop-In is that mental health professionals ran the day program, but during Drop-In hours, the staff primarily kept to their offices; peers who were diagnosed with a mental illness were employed by Vista and ran Drop-In.

## Methods

To answer my research questions, I had a three-phase design project. In phase one, I collected demographic data and employed the use of stigma scales to determine how stigma affected individuals with mental illness (Ritsher et al., 2003; Link, 1987). During phase two, I conducted life histories and illness narratives (Kleinman, 1988). Lastly, during phase three, I utilized the McGill Illness Narrative Interview (Groleau et al., 2006), with modifications for my study, as I found this worked better than the eight-question illness narrative (Kleinman, 1988). I also gave research participants a composition journal for time diaries, where they wrote what they did outside of Vista for two weeks. When I told one staff member about the time diaries, she remarked, "They just sit at home all day and watch TV." Since many ethnographies on mental health tend to focus on staff–client relationships or on mental health programs, I wanted to know what research participants were doing when they were not at Vista instead of making the assumption the staff member had.

### Participant observation

In addition to the tools and interviews I used during the three-phase design, an essential method to anthropology and ethnography that I utilized included participant observation (Spradley, 1980). During the time I conducted research, I spent, on average, between 15 and 20 hours a week at the day program and Drop-In. I participated in many of the activities the members did during the day program, including journaling, arts and crafts, reading about mental illness, simple exercise units, and chores after lunch. During Drop-In, I often played various board and card games with members.

Throughout my research, I made it clear that I was not a mental health professional, and that I was an anthropology student working on my dissertation project. While I did talk to staff and also interviewed them for my research, I usually spoke to them when members had gone home. I also ate lunch with members instead of joining staff in one of the larger offices, to emphasize that I was not a staff member. While there are anthropologists who also identify as clinicians (Kleinman, 1988; Lester, 2013), I do not consider myself a mental health professional and did not want to be viewed as one, given the complexities of this role.

## Research population

One key population in my research were participants diagnosed with a mental illness. The most common diagnoses were schizophrenia, schizoaffective, and bipolar disorder, though many of my interlocutors had more than one diagnosis with post-traumatic stress disorder, obsessive–compulsive disorder, and anxiety as additional diagnoses. Another commonality with my interlocutors was that most received income either from Social Security Disability Income (SSDI) or Supplemental Security Income (SSI). If they did not receive SSDI or SSI, many were in the process of applying for income from these sources.

Given the various diagnoses my interlocutors had, I use the phrase chronic mental illness amongst my interlocuters. Because the severity of the same mental illness and diagnosis can vary for different individuals, the cognitive impairment amongst members with the same diagnoses could be drastically different. Most members in the day program at Vista had some symptoms of psychosis, impacting their cognition. Depending on the severity of the psychosis, they may or may not have had the capacity to understand my research. Psychosis does impair cognition for many individuals with mental illness, but psychosis alone did not necessarily mean members lacked cognition to participate in my research project, since many learned coping skills over the years on how to deal with their symptoms. In the next sections, I discuss the ethical concerns of studying my research population, traditional tools I used to determine capacity to consent and the problems with those, and I suggest alternative methods to determine capacity to consent for individuals with impaired cognition in non-clinical research studies.

## Determining capacity to consent

One of the challenges in recruiting participants for my research was determining if they had the capacity to consent to participate in my research project. According to The Belmont Report (National Commission for the Protection of Human Subjects of Biomedical and Behavioral Research, 1978), "special revision may need to be made when comprehension is severely limited—for example, by conditions of immaturity or mental disability." In addition, The Belmont Report suggests adapting the presentation of the information to the subject's capacities because the "subject's ability to understand is a function of intelligence, rationality, maturity and language".

The United States Department of Health and Human Services' (HHS) criteria for Institutional Review Board (IRB) approval of research includes that "selection of subjects is equitable" (Office for Human Research Protections, 2009a). This includes considering the purpose of the research, the setting where the research will be conducted, and being mindful of research which involves vulnerable populations, including children, prisoners, pregnant women, mentally disabled persons, and economically or educationally disadvantaged persons (Office for Human Research Protections, 2009a).

"The HHS regulations are silent on the consent procedures specific to subjects with impaired decision-making capacity, for example, as a result of trauma, mental retardation, some forms of mental illness, or dementia, whether temporary, progressive, or permanent" (Office for Human Research Protections, 2009b). The HHS regulations do require that the IRB ensure "additional safeguards have been included in the study to protect the rights and welfare" of subjects that are "likely to be vulnerable to coercion or undue influence." The HHS regulations include "mentally disabled persons" in this category (Office for Human Research Protections, 2009a).

## Vulnerability

Because the population I was trying to recruit was appropriate for my research questions, I did not have trouble explaining to my IRB why individuals with chronic mental illnesses were recruited for my study. However, assessing the vulnerability of individuals was a different matter. Vulnerability is not a term clearly defined in HHS regulations, but the Collaborative Institutional Training Initiative (CITI)[3] I completed before fieldwork states critically ill individuals "may have limitations in their ability to process information, make complex decisions, and communicate their wishes. This may lead to them being in a state of diminished capacity to make autonomous decisions and protect their own interests" (Block and Gordon, 2017).

## **Informed consent**

Because most members of Vista received income from SSDI or SSI, they were economically disadvantaged. Many, but not all, were educationally disadvantaged with a high-school degree or lesser education, and all the members at Vista had a mental illness diagnosis. The economic disadvantages, educational disadvantages, and mental illness diagnoses placed Vista members in the "vulnerable" category. To address the first two disadvantages, following IRB protocol, I acknowledged that informed consent "includes both the process of sharing information and documenting that the process took place" (Hicks, 2014). Thus, the fliers I used to share information about my research project and the scripts I used from the beginning of fieldwork to explain who I was to members at Vista were pre-approved by my IRB.

Addressing the third possible disadvantage, just because persons are diagnosed with a chronic mental illness does not necessarily mean that they are "critically ill" or have

[3] The Collaborative Institutional Training Initiative (CITI Program) was founded by Paul Braunschweiger, Ph.D., and Karen Hansen in March 2000. The CITI Program provides web-based educational courses in research, ethics, regulatory oversight, responsible conduct of research, and other topics relevant to member organizations and researchers. Many universities, including my IRB, now require training through the CITI Program to promote ethical research and to enhance "the knowledge and professionalism of investigators, staff, and students conducting research in the United States and internationally" (CITI Program Mission and History, 2018).

impaired cognition. However, some members at Vista were in psychosis, which is a symptom, not a diagnosis, and that affected their cognition and status as being "vulnerable." During the three years I conducted research at Vista, someone who participated in phase 1 may have gotten too sick to participate in later phases. The opposite also occurred. Someone who was too sick in my first year of research to participate may have improved considerably, enough to participate at a later time. Since this was my first project that dealt directly with individuals diagnosed with chronic mental illnesses, it was important to me to ensure members at Vista who wanted to participate had the capacity to consent to participate in my research. Furthermore, I had a different consent form for each phase of my project, to ensure members knew what the purpose of each part of my research project concerned and to reconsent.

## Traditional instruments

Decision tree and sample quiz instruments have been traditionally used to determine capacity to consent. I was required to have these for my IRB. While the decision tree I had in my IRB protocol was helpful conceptually to determine who could participate, it was less useful in helping determine *how* to conduct explicit assessments to determine if members could participate in my research (see Figure 14.1). One of the assessments I did use in my IRB was a quiz to evaluate decisional capacity (see Figure 14.2).[4] The challenge with the quiz was it made members anxious because it was a quiz, making potential participants nervous because it evoked an examination or test-taking situation with an implication of judgment on correct or incorrect answers. Potential participants had to answer all questions correctly on the quiz in order to participate in my research, and they could take the quiz up to three times on different days. In addition, the information on my consent forms could be relayed through different methods because of literacy issues. I used other methods to enhance understanding of what my research consisted of including PowerPoint as a visual aid and teach-back (VoICE, 2018), where I asked prospective participants to explain my research project in their own words. These alternative methods were more useful because the primary challenge with the quiz was individuals who did not have a mental illness or impaired cognition might not even answer all the questions correctly (Kass et al., 2015).

## Ethnographic methods

As an anthropologist, participant observation was an essential method in determining if members at Vista had the capacity to consent to participate in my research

[4] The sample instrument for evaluating decisional capacity in Figure 14.2 was the form I used in my research and is modified from the UCSD Human Research Protections Program (2012) Decisional Capacity Assessment Instrument Samples.

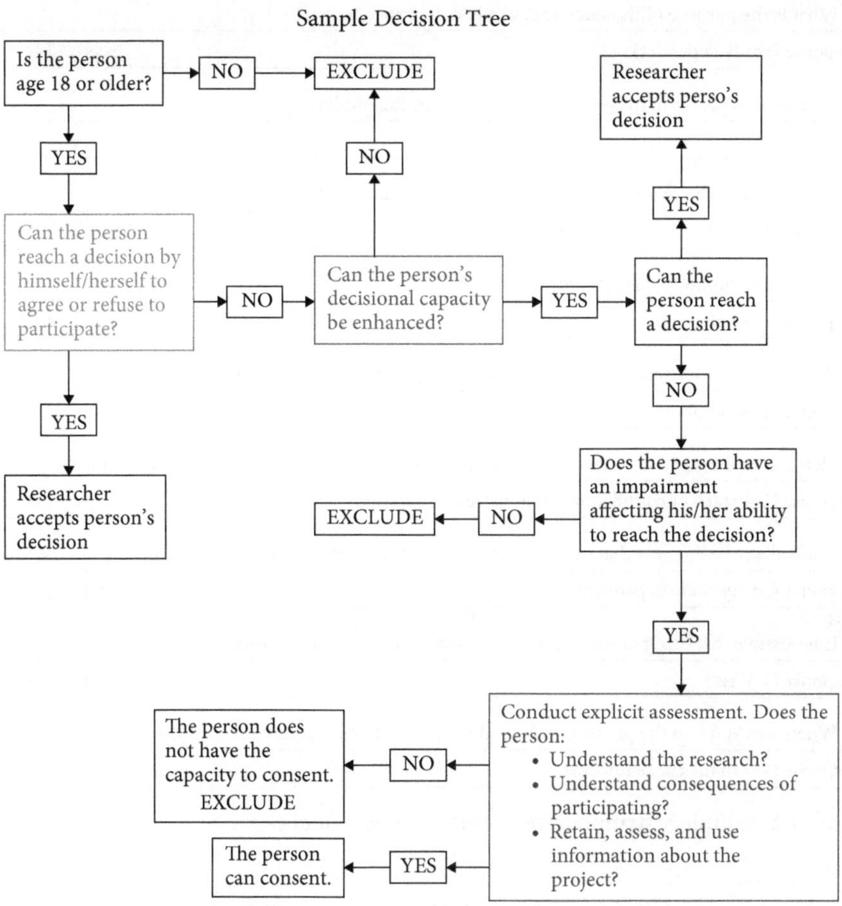


**Figure 14.1** Sample decision tree.

and also allowed opportunities to enhance capacity to participate. Before even conducting any interviews from the three-phase design of my project, I spent several months just observing members in the day program and Drop-In. Watching the members interact with staff allowed me to understand which members were actually vulnerable, educationally or economically, since I provided a gift card in return for participation in my research, or too sick to be able to consent to participate in my project. This initial period of observation also allowed me to understand a member's "baseline," a term the staff used. For instance, some members continuously showed signs of nervousness, and the staff would not worry since that was the person's baseline. However, if an individual behaved extremely differently from their baseline (e.g., showing signs of psychosis or crisis), then that was a cause for concern. Participant observation helped me determine who had the capacity to consent for day program members at Vista, but it was less helpful for Drop-In members because many of these individuals were transitional, came from other cities, especially during the summer months, and the staff did not know too much about these members either.

1. What is the purpose of the sutdy that was just described to you?

| | | | |
|---|---|---|---|
| Response (Study dependet) | Score: | 0 | 1 |

2. What makes you want to consider participating in this study?

| | | | |
|---|---|---|---|
| Response (Study dependet) | Score: | 0 | 1 |

3. Do you have to be in this study if you don't want to participate?

| | | | |
|---|---|---|---|
| Response (1 = No) | Score: | 0 | 1 |

4. Can you withdraw from this study at any time?

| | | | |
|---|---|---|---|
| Response (1 = Yes) | Score: | 0 | 1 |

5. Please describe one thing that will happen to people who decide to be in this study.

| | | | |
|---|---|---|---|
| Response (1=interviewed) | Score: | 0 | 1 |

6. Please describe one risk or discomfort you may experience if you participate in this study

| | | | |
|---|---|---|---|
| Response (1=breach of confidentiality or distress questions) | Score: | 0 | 1 |

7. Please describe one way that people might benefit if they participate in this study.

| | | | |
|---|---|---|---|
| Response (partly study dependent) | Score: | 0 | 1 |

8. Is it possible that being in this study won't have any direct benefit to you?

| | | | |
|---|---|---|---|
| Response (1 = Yes) | Score: | 0 | 1 |

9. Where can you find the phone numbers of the people to contact if you have questions?

| | | | |
|---|---|---|---|
| Response (1 = In the consent form) | Score: | 0 | 1 |

**Figure 14.2** Sample instrument for evaluating decisional capacity.

The unstructured nature of Drop-In had its advantages. Because Drop-In was a low-barrier mental health program, members were free to choose from using the computers, playing board games, chatting with others, or just keeping to themselves. Many members enjoyed playing board games during Drop-In, and I joined the games when I could. Some of the most popular games were UNO, Scrabble, and Monopoly.

Playing these games alongside Drop-In members was extremely useful for my research. Similar to the day program, whenever a new member came to Drop-In, I explained who I was so members knew I was present as a student anthropologist and not staff. During many of these games, members opened up about themselves, but the games allowed me to determine a member's ability to focus and helped me evaluate a member's reading level. In addition, returning members did not always have the capacity to consent even if they did previously, especially if their health status changed after a recent hospitalization.

Because my research design consisted of three phases, I found that some members went through periods of psychosis during the time of my research. While they may not have struggled playing any games in the first phase, it was possible that they were too sick to even play the same game later on or they tried to play but could not focus or remember when it was their turn. For games such as Monopoly, the "Chance" and "Community Chest" cards also gave away when a member did not know how to read or had limited reading capacity. Members who had trouble reading often just handed me these cards when they landed on those spots, since I was often the banker anyway, and I did not mind reading these cards or explaining them. Gauging the reading level of members allowed me to determine how to relay information about my project. At the other end of the spectrum, some members taught me how to play more difficult games such as Rummikub, a tile game based on colors and numbers.

The ability for more than two people to participate in these games at one time gave me a sense of how well several members could focus at the same time and also helped me sense if there were any substantial changes within a person's diagnosis. For example, even some of the people who showed me how to play Rummikub became sicker at one point and eventually were hospitalized. When members showed lack of interest in a game they previously wanted to play frequently, I realized there was something more to the "lack of interest," and they were potentially getting sicker.

The games helped me evaluate the decisional capacity for new clients at Drop-In and also for returning clients who participated in the initial phase of my research. I used the quiz for evaluating decisional capacity (Figure 14.2) when I thought there was a gray area between a member who was in psychosis at a previous point but seemed better later on and expressed interest to participate in my research.

## Research success

While the ethnographic methods I employed for my research project are time consuming and work best in non-clinical research projects such as mine, the benefits of using these methods were worth it. For members who were able to participate in all three phases of my project, including writing the time diary, I learned about aspects of their lives, beyond Vista, which I would not have known if they had not completed the time diaries (see Figure 14.3). For example, many participants had transportation issues and difficulty getting to places using public transportation, including Vista, and trouble paying rent. Since my project was at the intersections of medical and urban anthropology, this was essential data illustrating the complexities of living in New Orleans. Furthermore, I had a chance to talk to participants after they had completed the time diaries and ask questions about the information they wrote. I sought clarification, and this aspect of the research project gave my interlocutors some agency in what they wanted to share in their own narratives. I could have not completed the time diaries without conducting participant observation and playing games during the earlier phases of my research project to determine individuals' capacity to consent to participate in my research.

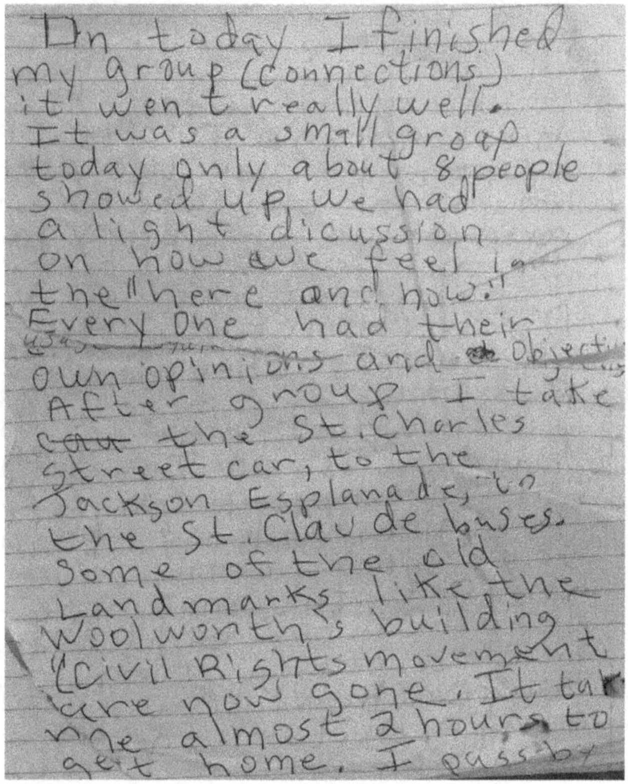
On today I finished
my group (connections)
it went really well.
It was a small group
today only about 8 people
showed up, we had
a light dicussion
on how we feel in
the "here and now."
Every One had their
own opinions and Objecti
After group I take
the St. Charles
street car, to the
Jackson Esplanade, to
the St. Claude buses.
Some of the old
Landmarks like the
Woolworth's building
(civil Rights movement
are now gone. It tak
me almost 2 hours to
get home. I pass by

**Figure 14.3** Sample of a time diary from a participant.

## Future directions

I found games such as Monopoly and UNO to be helpful before administering a sample instrument (Figure 14.2) to evaluate a client's decisional capacity. In a future research design, redoing such sample instruments from a quiz into an actual game may help enhance a person's decisional capacity (red text in Figure 14.1) or be used as an explicit assessment itself (blue text in Figure 14.1) for a more beneficial and time-efficient method to determine an individual's ability to consent to participate in research. In addition, the time diaries gave individuals control over their own narratives and provided a form of empowerment.

While ethical concerns based on the bioethical principle of autonomy need to be considered for vulnerable populations with impaired cognition, the principle of justice also needs to be considered to give the same populations agency, empowerment, and the ability to be included in the Disability Rights Movement's call for "Nothing About Us Without Us" and to acknowledge that individuals with disabilities, including those with mental illness, know what is best for them (Charlton, 2000).

## References


Arcury, T. and Quandt, S. (1999). "Participant Recruitment for Qualitative Research: A Site-Based Approach to Community Research in Complex Societies." *Human Organization*, 58/2: 128–133.

Beauchamp, T. L. (2007). "The '4 Principles' Approach to Health Care Ethics," in Ashcroft, R., Dawson, A., Draper, H., and McMillan, J. (eds.) *Principles of Health Care Ethics*. 2nd ed. Chichester: John Wiley & Sons, Chapter 1.

Block, J. and Gordon, B. (2017). "Populations in Research Requiring Additional Considerations and/or Protections," CITI Program, https://www.citiprogram.org (accessed April 23, 2018).

Charlton, J. I. (2000). *Nothing About Us Without Us: Disability Oppression and Empowerment*. Berkeley, CA: University of California Press.

CITI Program Mission and History (2018). CITI Program Mission Statement, https://about.citiprogram.org/en/mission-and-history/ (accessed October 14, 2008)

Groleau, D., Young, A., and Kirmayer, L. J. (2006). "The McGill Illness Narrative Interview (MINI): An Interview Schedule to Elicit Meanings and Modes of Reasoning Related to Illness Experience." *Transcultural Psychiatry*, 43/4: 671–691.

Hicks, L. (2014). "Informed Consent-SBE," CITI Program, https://www.citiprogram.org (accessed April 23, 2018).

Hopper, K., Jost, J., Hay, T., Welber, S., and Haugland, G. (1997). "Homelessness, Severe Mental Illness, and the Institutional Circuit." *Psychiatric Services*, 48/5: 659–665.

Kass, N. E., Taylor, H. A., Ali, J., Hallez, K., and Chaisson, L. (2015). "A Pilot Study of Simple Interventions to Improve Informed Consent in Clinical Research: Feasibility, Approach and Results." *Clinical Trials*, 12/1: 54–66.

Kleinman, A. (1988). *The Illness Narratives: Suffering, Healing, and the Human Condition*. New York: Basic Books.

Lester, R. J. (2013). "Lessons from the Borderline: Anthropology, Psychiatry, and the Risks of Being Human." *Feminism & Psychology*, 23/1: 70–77.

Link, B. G. (1987). "Understanding Labeling Effects in the Area of Mental Disorders: An Assessment of the Effects of Expectations of Rejection." *American Sociological Review*, 52/1: 96–112.

Luhrmann, T. M. (2008). "'The Street Will Drive You Crazy': Why Homeless Psychotic Women in the Institutional Circuit in the United States Often Say No to Offers of Help." *American Journal of Psychiatry*, 165/1: 15–20.

National Commission for the Protection of Human Subjects of Biomedical and Behavioral Research (1978). "The Belmont Report: Ethical Principles and Guidelines for the Protection of Human Subjects of Research," https://www.hhs.gov/ohrp/regulations-and-policy/belmont-report/read-the-belmont-report/index.html#xinform (accessed April 23, 2018).

Office for Human Research Protections (2009). "Code of Federal Regulations. Part 46: Protection of Human Subjects," https://www.hhs.gov/ohrp/regulations-and-policy/regulations/45-cfr-46/index.html (accessed April 23, 2018).

Office for Human Research Protections (2009). "Informed Consent FAQs," https://www.hhs.gov/ohrp/regulations-and-policy/guidance/faq/informed-consent/index.html (accessed April 23, 2018).

Ritsher, J. B., Otilingam, P. G., and Grajales, M. (2003). "Internalized Stigma of Mental Illness: Psychometric Properties of a New Measure." *Psychiatry Research*, 121/1: 31–49.

Spradley, J. P. (1980). *Participant Observation*. New York: Holt, Rinehart and Winston.

UCSD Human Research Protections Program (2012). "Decision Making Capacity Guidelines," http://irb.ucsd.edu/decisional.shtml (accessed June 6, 2012).

Valid Informed Consent Education Program (VoICE) (2018). "Giving Research Participants a Voice," https://www.dartmouth.edu/~cphs/tosubmit/teachback/index.html (accessed October 14, 2018).

# 15

# Making Research More Ethical for Adults with Fetal Alcohol Spectrum Disorder

## A Story of Stakeholder Engagement, Accommodation, and Inclusion

*John Aspler*

### Introduction

The first time I spoke with stakeholders about my thesis project, I received complimentary critiques. My supervisor and I sought feedback from researchers, clinicians, and parents of people with fetal alcohol spectrum disorder (FASD)—a complex neurodevelopmental disability caused by prenatal alcohol exposure. We listened to their concerns, took them seriously, and made the necessary adjustments. I felt good about being inclusive and open to criticism. Which is why, months later, I worried and stressed after a difficult phone call with other key stakeholders. The call had been both instructive and upsetting; the people I spoke with had taken great pains to review my focus group study materials, concluding that they needed to be reworked. This feedback came from several adults with FASD, a group we had not—but should have—included in the design stage. As a student new to qualitative research, I now worried about the inclusiveness and emotional safety of my study. I also stressed about my personal goals and timelines. I thought I had been doing a good job, but negative feedback, especially from people you hope your work will help, can be difficult—though necessary—to sit with and work through.

Their criticism included three points:

(1) Given that we were conducting focus groups, they felt that our script and interview questions were too abstract for some individuals with FASD to understand—including our consent form.
(2) They suggested that some of the media content was too negative and potentially triggering.
(3) Most importantly, since our ability to support participants post-study was both limited and geographically restricted, we could not provide adequate mental health services to those who experienced emotional distress later on. They also described our list of resources as not geographically specific enough, and as too focused on children rather than adults.

These were all problems we had anticipated, and thought we had already addressed.

In this chapter, I reflect on some of the challenges I experienced in designing and executing a safe and inclusive group interview study for people with cognitive disability or difference. First, I describe what FASD entails, and then explain our research project and its goals. Second, I outline anticipated sources of participant vulnerability and how we initially planned to mitigate them. Third, I explore the above stakeholder feedback, as well as the adjustments we made in response. Fourth, I discuss several key research ethics and methodological tensions that arose in the process of resolving previous challenges. Finally, I reflect on the experience of seeking stakeholder feedback, exploring the necessity of such input, as well as the difficulty and importance of remaining open and vulnerable to critique as a researcher. While other chapters in this book defend or justify the importance of inclusive research practices, here, I will take their importance as a given and explore their practical realities.

## What is FASD?

FASD results from exposure to alcohol in the womb (Chudley et al., 2005; Cook et al., 2016). Individuals with FASD can experience difficulties across a broad range of "brain domains"—including executive function, intellectual disability, motor control, and language, among others. In a small portion of cases (roughly 10%), people with FASD also present with characteristic facial features (Andrew, 2011). In the 1970s, these visible cases were first described as a "fetal alcohol syndrome" (FAS), affecting the children of "chronic alcoholic mothers" (Jones and Smith, 1973)—which soon expanded, controversially, to include a broader spectrum of both children without observable physical features and mothers who were not chronic alcoholics (Armstrong, 1998; Chudley et al., 2005). FASD eventually emerged as an umbrella term for a number of other diagnoses, including FAS, partial FAS, and alcohol-related neurodevelopmental disability (ARND) (Chudley et al., 2005). In most cases, diagnosis requires confirmation that the mother consumed alcohol while pregnant.

In qualitative studies about their lives, people with FASD discuss feelings of difference, social exclusion, difficulty in school, and problems in employment (Salmon and Buetow, 2012; Stade et al., 2011). Given the cause of FASD, women who consume alcohol during pregnancy can also experience stigmatization, blame, and shame (Salmon, 2008).

Owing to the wide range of areas that can be affected by prenatal alcohol exposure, it can be difficult to describe a "typical case" of FASD. This, in turn, makes it hard to develop a uniform set of accommodations for people with FASD, which is a helpful reminder that, no matter the project, participants should be recruited and accommodated based on their individual and diverse support needs, strengths, and weaknesses.

## Our research projects

The research team conducted two main studies related to FASD. First, we undertook a media content analysis (Macnamara, 2005) using ten top English-language Canadian newspapers to better understand the landscape of information presented to Canadians about FASD, alcohol, and pregnancy (Aspler et al., 2018). Second, we used the results of that media analysis to fuel the design of a focus group study in which we interviewed three key FASD stakeholder groups: (1) adults with FASD; (2) their parents or caregivers (mostly adoptive); and (3) healthcare and allied professionals with relevant experience (mostly social workers) (Racine and Aspler, 2018). In this second study, our objectives were to understand the perspectives and lived experiences of people affected by FASD, and to solicit their views about the media content we analyzed. It was in this second study that concerns about participant support arose.

Our group interviews focused on four key areas of discussion: (1) participant experiences with FASD; (2) experience with a potential diagnosis; (3) stereotypes about people with FASD and about women who consume alcohol while pregnant; and (4) participant reactions to specific media examples from our previous media analysis (Aspler et al., 2018). The interviews were two hours long, audio recorded, and semi-structured (Morgan and Krueger, 1998). We conducted 12 focus groups of 4–8 participants, four with each category, for a total of 65 participants (19 of whom had FASD). A few had identities across participant categories (e.g., a social worker who was a parent of someone with FASD, a person with FASD who had a child with FASD), so they chose which group to join based on their personal preferences.

Our project was motivated by the importance of centring the voices of marginalized persons in discussions about their own lives (i.e., instead of leaving "solutions" to professionals) (Racine et al., 2013), as well as an interest in fostering deliberation around troubling ethical tensions in FASD communication from a multitude of key stakeholder perspectives (Racine, 2016). We aimed for real-world relevant outcomes, aiming to destigmatize and demystify the lives of people with FASD and their birth mothers. Most previous qualitative research about FASD had focused on the experiences of adoptive or foster caregivers, with very few studies taking the time to talk to people with FASD themselves (Domeij et al., 2018). Consequently, we wanted to turn our attention to those missing central voices.

## Anticipated challenges for participant inclusion

We knew that some people with FASD may struggle to understand complex informed consent documents, interview questions, and study instructions. Consequently, our original protocol called for the recruitment of people with ARND—at the time, a supposedly milder version of FASD. We would still screen participants individually (e.g., by email, by phone, by recruitment survey) and discuss the consent document in detail (both one-on-one and as a group before the interview), but we could also sidestep more serious questions of competence to consent by removing people in other categories of FASD from consideration (like those with the most severe version, FAS).[1] This very quickly proved to be an untenable recruitment strategy for several practical reasons, as well as a clearly troubling approach to certain responsibilities surrounding the principle of justice in research ethics (Canadian Institutes of Health Research et al., 2014; Lai et al., 2006).[2]

First, around the time we finished designing the focus group study, updated Canadian diagnostic guidelines changed existing diagnostic categories from FAS and ARND to FASD with or without sentinel facial features (Cook et al., 2016). In this way, the spectrum became a key part of the diagnostic label, instead of a broad umbrella term encompassing other diagnoses; the idea of a spectrum of alcohol effects had been radically reimagined. This aligns with reconfigurations in the way we think about other spectrum disorders, like autism—i.e., what does it mean to be "high functioning" versus "low-functioning," to use outdated terminology, when individuals have strengths and weaknesses across multiple axes (Happe and Ronald, 2008). For example, when trying to position someone who can cook and clean independently on the spectrum, but who has a low IQ, where would they fall in comparison to someone with the exact opposite strengths and weaknesses? A linear, one-dimensional understanding of a spectrum of possible challenges hardly seems helpful here.

Second, many potential participants did not have a diagnosis of any FASD (never mind ARND). This kind of participant typically did not have confirmed prenatal alcohol exposure, but otherwise met diagnostic criteria—or else were still on their diagnostic journeys. We concluded that it did not matter much for our study; what mattered most was understanding how people who identified with the diagnostic label (formally or informally) felt about it and about FASD media coverage. And so we dropped the specific category of ARND and the need for a mandatory diagnosis from our inclusion criteria, relying more heavily on participant self-identification and our team's research expertise and judgment.

We also knew that some of our questions and media content were negative and possibly emotionally distressing. Consequently, we mentioned this negative content and the risk of emotional distress in the informed consent document. We also talked to participants ahead of time about this kind of possibly-distressing content in more depth, to explore with them how they felt, to ensure they could comfortably participate.

[1] Given FASD's expansion from observable physical difference with brain effects (i.e., FAS) to subtle cognitive symptoms alone (i.e., ARND), FAS is often positioned at the "severe" end of a linear spectrum. This can be true, but given the heterogeneity of the diagnosis, reality is more complex.

[2] The principle of justice includes the notion of equity, which means ensuring that the benefits and burdens of research are distributed among appropriate segments of the population. Sometimes, in protecting potentially vulnerable groups from undue burdens, researchers and research ethics board members neglect to distribute benefits of knowledge equitably; they exclude difficult-to-include groups for both practical and ethical reasons. This makes sense when concerned with participant welfare and protection, but can mean leaning too far away from inclusion (Martino and Schormans, 2018). Since our project focused on the voices of often-excluded groups with cognitive disability or difference, we had to include them effectively and appropriately. As is clearly articulated in the Tri-Council Policy Statement (TCPS2): "... individuals who lack capacity to decide whether or not to participate in research shall not be inappropriately excluded" (Canadian Institutes of Health Research et al., 2014).

Importantly, a social worker (who was part of the research team) was always present—ready to assist any participant who found the questions, media quotes, or discussion topics difficult to handle.[3] A weakness that we recognized in our plan was that, as a Montreal-based research team talking to people about English-language news media, we were conducting the study in different cities around the country, meaning we could not provide in-person assistance several days post-interview. To mitigate this problem, we provided both a list of Canadian resources and the social worker's contact information for any who wished to contact us later—something we emphasized to participants. Ultimately, only one parent reached out, but to ask for more specific local resources and programs (a gap later identified by the adults with FASD who provided feedback).

Finally, as discussed, we presented our questions, media coverage, study documents, and plans for accommodating and mitigating vulnerabilities to several clinical and research professionals with expertise in FASD, as well as several parents of people with FASD and other developmental disabilities. We acted on most of their suggestions (e.g., changing complicated language, the addition of a cool-down question about positive experiences or coverage), but recognized that we had not received feedback from any adults with FASD. In not including one of our three key stakeholder groups in early discussions, we missed some potential major problems.

## Responding to feedback about inclusion

The three aforementioned critiques from adults with FASD included (1) a lack of local support systems once we left a city; (2) concerns about participant resilience in the face of negative media content; and (3) a lack of linguistic clarity related to linguistic abstraction for adults with potential cognitive disability or difference. Although we thought that having access to our social worker post-study (by email, by Skype, etc.) would be sufficient, we were informed that participants might not reach out due to (1) a lack of familiarity with this social worker; and (2) only processing emotional reactions to negative content several weeks after the study had taken place. Based on these concerns, we formalized several informal practices (e.g., a break halfway through the interview—something we did not provide to parents or professionals) and added new support protocols.

### Local support

We wanted our participants to have access to strong local support once we left, since stakeholders had identified this lack of support as the biggest barrier to research

[3] The social worker was also present for interviews with parents for the same reason. Although we did not think parents overall would have the same support needs for comprehension, the topics being discussed could still have been very emotionally draining for anyone with personal stakes in discussions about FASD.

inclusion. We decided to recruit through programs that already had readily available support staff with expertise in—and knowledge of—FASD, who would also be familiar to participants. We would provide all of the study tools to these workers beforehand (i.e., the consent form, the questions, the script, and the media quotes), and they would be present during the interviews.

Furthermore, they could assist us with parts of the consent process, by identifying comprehension gaps for specific participants. Some stakeholders suggested that some participants might pretend to understand, nodding in agreement so as not to appear confused in front of their peers, even if they did struggle to understand. Consequently, support staff who knew them well could provide more precise insight into these kinds of concerns prior to and during the interviews. They could also help respond to questions (and communicate with me) after the study. In this way, when we left a city, if participants decided not to reach out to us with further questions or about any potential emotional distress, they could instead turn to a familiar face who knew them well, and who knew what could have troubled them during or after the interview.

## Negative content

We also worked with local programs and support workers to recruit adults with FASD who the staff felt could best handle more negative content, given concerns about the potential risks and emotional harm to participants. In this way, the support workers who assisted us acted as gatekeepers, to improve protections for potential participants. Prior to the interview, we would still interact with participants one-on-one as part of our own assessment of capacity to consent (again, by phone, by email, and through the recruitment survey), but we now had an extra layer of protection.

We also began to conduct these interviews with groups who largely knew each other, to enhance their initial comfort levels and to provide peer support throughout and after the interview. Although the staff were absolutely essential (i.e., one participant had to leave the room during an interview, so a support worker followed them out and spoke with them until they felt comfortable enough to return), this peer support was perhaps even more essential. Through very respectful discussions of similar experiences and different emotional reactions, plus a clear sense of solidarity, it became apparent that many of these participants already relied on each other for emotional support. They encouraged each other to share upsetting experiences with the group, and then provided support (e.g., hugs, verbal validation, paper for colouring, stress balls) if the discussion grew too difficult.

## Understanding

To enhance understanding, we took two key actions. First, we simplified some of the questions and explanations from our original script. For example, one suggestion was to remove abstract or metaphor-based language—i.e., "And don't worry, we'll have plenty of time later in the interview to *dive into the ideas you bring up in more depth*" [emphasis added]. In this example, the notion of "diving into" the conversation was seen as confusing, since we were not diving into a body of water. Second, we worked with local centres to take the time to go through the consent document with participants. This translated into a number of strategies for enhancing comprehension, including asking local centres to print copies of the form for potential participants weeks before our arrival, answering any grammar questions they may have as they go through the form, and facilitating some of the communication we would have from afar as I discussed the study with them. In these ways, we were able to reduce the language level of the interview script and questions (which, despite having been reviewed and approved by several experts and parents, was still seen as too complex by some adults with FASD), and provide stronger local support for understanding before our arrival. Notably, we could not reduce the complexity of the media quotes, as these were taken verbatim from various newspapers around Canada. Instead, we took extra time during the discussion of these quotes to explain words and phrases as needed. For example, after reading each quote, I would ask participants if anything seemed unfamiliar. In an early interview, the first time someone asked for clarification about the word "scourge," another participant defined it using pirates (i.e., "the scourge of the sea"). I then used a similar definition in other interviews (and not just for people with FASD).

With these three key suggestions, we were able to enhance both the process of recruitment and participant protections in order to create successfully more comfortable, more ethical, and more inclusive research.

## New challenges

In changing our practices, new research ethics and methodological problems arose. First, in working closely with local services, we gave up some control over participant recruitment. This raised important questions about the voluntary character of consent, our capacity to assess risks to individual participants, and the informed consent process itself. Second, in conducting interviews with support workers or parents in the room, or in finding participants who largely knew each other, we may have affected or inadvertently shaped participant involvement in the discussion (i.e., the kinds of things they felt comfortable talking about)—since group dynamic is central to understanding and analyzing the results of focus group data (Lunt and Livingstone, 1996).

### Research ethics challenges

#### Voluntary and informed consent

Our previous process of recruitment, which included all three stakeholder groups, involved one-on-one communication with prospective participants who themselves got in touch with us based on purposive and snowball recruitment strategies—so it was their choice to reach out to us. Now, we were asking local social service groups across the country to identify and recruit participants in our place by approaching them—making it a more top-down kind of recruitment. We would still, of course, have control over participation; however, it was a control mediated through a gatekeeper, which could at times become complicated. For example, one participant (in filling out our recruitment screening survey online) provided the email address of one of the local social workers with whom we were working, instead of a way for me to reach out to them directly.[4] Consequently, it became more difficult to speak with participants (both alone and at all), in order to more independently assess their capacity and volition to take part in the study.

The same concerns also applied to risk–benefit assessments—i.e., in working through gatekeepers, we gave up some control over individual risk–benefit analyses (since workers would be choosing clients to approach based on their clinical judgment about participant resilience in our place). At the same time, these workers were in a much better position to make those judgments, knowing their clients far better than we ever could after only a few one-on-one discussions.

Finally, asking local support staff to identify and approach potential research participants raised questions about the impact of trusted authority figures on the voluntary component of consent. Since previous participants (none of whom we knew) had to reach out to us themselves, the researcher–participant power dynamic was less problematic. Ultimately, we were satisfied that everyone taking part in our study wanted to be there (e.g., by talking one-on-one beforehand, following non-verbal cues, reminding participants they could take a break or even stop entirely), but these ethical concerns were specifically introduced by our solutions to making our project more comfortable, more ethical, and more inclusive. In short, by involving local staff in other cities to ensure a more supportive space, different concerns about participant voluntariness arose.

## Methodological challenges

### The presence of support workers or parents during the interviews

Prior to the phone call described at the beginning of this chapter, we had already conducted one focus group with adults with FASD. Even at that time, we knew we would have to make participant accommodations; however, these accommodations were spontaneous. They were absolutely vital to the success of this particular interview, but were not part of a formal process or deeply thought through. On the day of this focus group, a few participants were anxious about the study. They each reacted in their own ways: some asked to speak with me alone about what to expect, and so I shared study questions with them prior to their participation—something I had not done for parents

[4] To resolve this case, I contacted the worker and asked them to pass along my phone number. In the end, the participant called me and we were able to chat for about 15 minutes regarding their worries and concerns.

or for health and allied professionals. Others had brought items to fidget with.[5] One participant felt anxious enough to request that a parent stay with us throughout the interview. Although the parent did not sit at the table with us, they remained in the room, behind their child, which could have influenced the kinds of stories and experiences members of the focus group were willing to share with me.

At the same time, had I not shared the questions prior to the interview, or allowed the parent to stay, I would have affected what participants felt comfortable sharing with me anyway. If they did not feel secure throughout the interview, then their discomfort would have influenced the direction of the discussion. In addition, unlike later groups, these participants started as strangers. And yet, through their positive, constructive, and supportive engagement with each other, a sense of community seemed to grow. After the interview, I watched as all the participants exchanged contact information, promising to keep in touch, to keep discussing their traumas and successes, and to maintain a circle of support. I do not know if, in the end, they maintained that contact, but I did come away from that particular focus group feeling like we had built exactly the kind of safe and inclusive space we wanted. Still, I recognized that this interview was the best-case scenario, with the later formalization of accommodations helping us prevent the worst. Thankfully, we were able to accommodate this group's particular needs, so that they could comfortably share their deeply personal challenges (e.g., experience in jail, a struggle to forgive a birth mother), as well as their joys and successes (e.g., graduation, parenthood).

Ultimately, the key piece of feedback from that phone call—that our participant support system was insufficient—had already been somewhat addressed early on (if informally, without explicit articulation in our study protocol). We were already working with a local service provider—though again, without the formal structures in place for later interviews. We had already found ways to help participants feel comfortable, like including a parent in the room (though not support workers). However, I had not yet realized the necessity of always including each of these options, and formalizing them in the protocol.

## Conclusion

In this chapter, I have explored the importance of including robust accommodations for participants with cognitive disability or difference—in this case, for people with FASD. The final form of our accommodations was borne out of some difficult-to-hear but ultimately necessary input from adults with FASD. It was hard for me as a researcher to receive negative feedback—both in terms of my hopes for success and regarding the well-being of my participants. As a researcher in training, my advice to others is to

[5] This was not something we formalized in the protocol; however, all of the centres we later worked with independently provided participants with amazing accommodations we had not considered—not just fidgets (e.g., stress balls, colouring pencils and paper), but also lifts to and from the interviews and even free childcare services.

proactively seek out stakeholder feedback even if it takes extra time, take their criticism seriously, build positively on any feedback you receive, and know that it is okay to feel upset—this kind of work can be emotional, intense, and difficult as we foster spaces for participant dialogue and the expression of sensitive experiences and feelings. Their feedback and those feelings, yours and theirs both, can help you push toward inclusion at every stage of research, whatever form that takes based on your particular project and the population(s) involved.

The research process and the experiences shared in this chapter speak, in my opinion, to the need for greater inclusion of marginalized voices throughout the development of a research project about them, as well as the need for strong local support in the form of familiar faces and support staff. Even if new challenges arise in the process of accommodation (either ethical or methodological), justice in research requires us to create safer environments for purposes of inclusion. Environments where richer dialogue can unfold—dialogue that could not have happened without the kinds of changes we had to make. Although we ran into a number of issues, our research was made better for the support structures we built into the study—both in terms of ensuring participant emotional safety and with regard to the generation of rich and meaningful discussion data. Most importantly, the voices of a group of people who are often excluded from research became central to the way the study unfolded, not just the study findings.

## References


Andrew, G. (2011). "Diagnosis of FASD: An Overview," in Riley, E., Clarren, S., Weinberg, J., and Jansson, E. (eds.) *Fetal Alcohol Spectrum Disorders: Management and Policy Perspectives of FASD.* Weinheim: Wiley-Blackwell, pp. 127–148.

Armstrong, E. (1998). "Diagnosing Moral Disorder: The Discovery and Evolution of Fetal Alcohol Syndrome." *Social Science & Medicine*, 47/12: 2025–2042.

Aspler, J., Zizzo, N., Di Pietro, N., and Racine, E. (2018). "Stereotyping and Stigmatising Disability: A Content Analysis of Canadian Print News Media About Fetal Alcohol Spectrum Disorder." *Canadian Journal of Disability Studies*, 7/3: 89–121.

Canadian Institutes of Health Research, Natural Sciences and Engineering Research Council of Canada and Social Sciences and Humanities Research Council of Canada (2014). "Tri-Council Policy Statement: Ethical Conduct for Research Involving Humans (TCPS-2)," http://www.pre.ethics.gc.ca/eng/policy-politique/initiatives/tcps2-eptc2/Default/ (accessed March 7, 2019).

Chudley, A., Conry, J., Cook, J., Loock, C., Rosales, T., and LeBlanc, N. (2005). "Fetal Alcohol Spectrum Disorder: Canadian Guidelines for Diagnosis." *CMAJ* 172/5 Suppl.: S1–21.

Cook, J., Green, C., Lilley, C., Anderson, S., Baldwin, M.E., Chudley, A., Conry, J., LeBlanc, N., Loock, C.A., Lutke, J., Mallon, B.F., McFarlane, A.A., Temple, V.K., and Rosales, T. (2016). "Fetal Alcohol Spectrum Disorder: A Guideline for Diagnosis Across the Lifespan." *CMAJ*, 188/3: 191–197.

Domeij, H., Fahlstrom, G., Bertilsson, G., Hultcrantz, M., Munthe-Kaas, H., Gordh, C.N., and Helgesson, G. (2018). "Experiences of Living With Fetal Alcohol Spectrum Disorders: A Systematic Review and Synthesis of Qualitative Data." *Developmental Medicine & Child Neurology*, 60/8: 741–752.

Happe, F. and Ronald, A. (2008). "The 'Fractionable Autism Triad': A Review of Evidence From Behavioural, Genetic, Cognitive and Neural Research." *Neuropsychology Review*, 18/4: 287–304.

Jones, K.L. and Smith, D.W. (1973). "Recognition of the Fetal Alcohol Syndrome in Early Infancy." *Lancet* 302/7836: 999–1001.

Lai, R., Elliott, D., and Ouellette-Kuntz, H. (2006). "Attitudes of Research Ethics Committee Members Toward Individuals With Intellectual Disabilities: The Need for More Research." *Journal of Policy Practice in Intellectual Disabilities*, 3/2: 114–118.

Lunt, P. and Livingstone, S. (1996). "Rethinking the Focus Group in Media and Communications Research." *Journal of Communication* 46/2: 79–98.

Macnamara, J. (2005). "Media Content Analysis: Its Uses, Benefits and Best Practice Methodology." *Asia Pacific Public Relations Journal* 6/1: 1–34.

Martino, A.S. and Schormans, A.F. (2018). "When Good Intentions Backfire: University Research Ethics Review and the Intimate Lives of People Labeled With Intellectual Disabilities." *The Forum: Qualitative Social Research* 19/3.

Morgan, D.L. and Krueger, R.A. (1998). *The Focus Group Guidebook.* Thousand Oaks, CA: Sage Publications.

Racine, E. (2016). "Can Moral Problems of Everyday Clinical Practice Ever Be Resolved? A Proposal for Integrative Pragmatist Approaches," in Rosenbaum, P., Ronen, G. M., Racine, E., and Johannesen, J. (eds.) *Ethics in Child Health: Principles and Cases in Neurodisability.* London: Mac Keith Press, pp. 33–48.

Racine, E. and Aspler, J. (2018). "Keynote: Neuroéthique, pragmatisme, et la stigmatisation envers les parties prenantes touchées par les troubles du spectre de l'alcoolisation fœtale." The 29th Annual Canadian Bioethics Society Conference. Halifax, NS.

Racine, E., Bell, E., and Shevell, M. (2013). "Chapter 21 – Ethics in Neurodevelopmental Disability." *Handbook of Clinical Neurology*, 118: 243–263.

Salmon, J. (2008). "Fetal Alcohol Spectrum Disorder: New Zealand Birth Mothers' Experiences." *Canadian Journal of Clinical Pharmacology*, 15/2: e191–213.

Salmon, J. and Buetow, S. (2012). "An Exploration of the Experiences and Perspectives of New Zealanders With Fetal Alcohol Spectrum Disorder." *Journal of Population Therapeutics and Clinical Pharmacology* 19/1: e41–50.

Stade, B., Beyene, J., Buller, K., Ross, S., Patterson, K., Stevens, B., Sgro, M., Ungar, W., Watson, W., and Koren, G. (2011). "Feeling Different: The Experience of Living With Fetal Alcohol Spectrum Disorder." *Journal of Population Therapeutics and Clinical Pharmacology* 18(3): e475–85.

# 16

# A Conversation with Research Ethics Boards About Inclusive Research with Persons with Intellectual and Developmental Disabilities

*Virginie Cobigo, Lynne A. Potvin, Casey Fulford, Hajer Chalghoumi, Mariam Hanna, Natasha Plourde, and Whitney D. Taylor*

## Introduction

As we were writing this chapter, a medical historian published an article about the troublesome contributions of Hans Asperger to the Nazi regime and the extermination of children with intellectual and developmental disabilities (IDD) during the Second World War (Czech, 2018). Asperger is, however, still considered a pioneer in autism research. Unfortunately, this is not a unique example of human rights violations during the conduct of research with persons with IDD. Indeed, a survivor of the Canadian institutionalization era recounted how he was unethically and severely punished for refusing to participate in research (Park and Hutton, 2018). When Mr. Park refused to ingest unknown medications, he was labelled as non-compliant and confined. In other words, his participation in clinical drug trials was coerced.

The history of our field renders researchers accountable to persons with IDD. The Nuremberg Code (see Office for Human Research Protections, 1949), Declaration of Helsinki (World Medical Association, 1964), and The Belmont Report (Office for Human Research Protections, 1979) are influential documents that encompass ethical principles to guide research. Moreover, most countries have signed and ratified the United Nations' (2006) *Convention on the Rights of Persons with Disabilities*, urging respect, protection, and promotion of persons with disabilities' rights. Upholding these rights when conducting research with persons with IDD is, however, challenged by limited formal procedures (Carey and Griffiths, 2017). The application of ethical guidelines and regulations in IDD research requires further study, as translation from theory to practice is inconsistent (Hamilton et al., 2017; Lai, et al., 2006). Ethical principles frequently come into conflict, requiring researchers and members of research ethics boards (REBs) to make personal judgments (Truscott and Crook, 2013); decisions are inevitably influenced by their personal experiences with and attitudes toward persons with IDD (Lai et al., 2006).

## Context

We conduct research to inform evidence-based practices and policies for persons with IDD. We strive to adopt an inclusive approach, as the perspectives of individuals with IDD are critical to inform practices and policies relevant to them. Qualitative methods are considered an effective way to involve persons with IDD in research (Ottmann and Crosbie, 2013). Interviews and focus groups are our primary methods of data collection. Our recent research topics include ethical development of information and communication technology (e.g., Chalghoumi et al., 2017), knowledge mobilization in community service agencies, strategies to support reciprocal relationships and a fulfilling sexuality, experiences during physical health exams (e.g., Potvin et al., in press), and perinatal social support (e.g., Potvin et al., 2016). These studies were conducted in Ontario, Canada, between 2013 and 2019.

We illustrate concerns raised by REBs, or our team in response to feedback from REBs, during reviews of ethics' applications for the aforementioned projects. These projects were approved by various academic and hospital REBs, depending on team members' affiliations and recruitment locations (none of these projects consisted of clinical intervention research). We propose solutions to ethical dilemmas that emerged from our exchanges with these REBs. We also discuss situations encountered during our projects that were not raised by REBs but could pose a potential risk to persons with IDD during research.

## Challenges and recommendations for ethical research conduct

Accessible information and communication, free and informed consent, confidentiality, and risks associated with research participation were themes that often emerged as challenging in our conversations with REBs.

### Accessible information and communication

Processing complex information and understanding abstract ideas are common challenges for persons with IDD (Schalock et al., 2010). Persons with IDD report that information complexity is frequently a barrier to research participation (Lennox et al., 2005). For example, recruitment templates (i.e., information letters and consent forms) provided by REBs are typically inaccessible to persons with IDD due to complex language (Scott et al., 2006; Truman, 2003). Therefore, IDD researchers and REBs should consult accessibility guidelines to provide only necessary information using simple words, short sentences, and simple fonts and layouts (Financial Consumer Agency of Canada, 2017; Your Health Matters, 2018). Additionally, using illustrations and demonstrations can facilitate comprehension (Dalton and McVilly, 2004).

In collaboration with REBs, we developed accessible recruitment materials and consent forms (see Box 16.1 for an excerpt of the information provided for Chalghoumi et al., 2017b). Determining essential information to include was challenging. For example, one REB requested that we provide the names and contact information of all researchers. We judged this information unnecessary and confusing for some individuals with IDD. Consequently, we agreed on including only the coordinates of the principal investigator and the REB with which he or she is most closely affiliated. In addition, most institutional telephone numbers are not direct lines, and some participants have difficulty navigating systems using voice recognition or extension numbers. We now only provide direct toll-free telephone numbers to facilitate participation.

Most researchers rely on written means to convey information, which may exclude individuals who have difficulty reading (Hamilton et al., 2017). Participants should have the option to have recruitment materials read and explained to them verbally (Dalton and McVilly, 2004; McDonald et al., 2015). Although participants should be encouraged to call the researchers if they require further explanation, literacy is assumed in recruitment materials that provide this instruction. We find that collaborating with service providers and caregivers facilitates recruitment of participants with IDD (Becker et al., 2004) and increases information accessibility (McDonald et al., 2015). For example, collaboration provides persons with IDD the opportunity to have research materials explained to them by a trusted individual who is familiar with their needs. Adults with IDD have reported that this collaboration is reassuring; many have expressed concerns associated with disrespectful treatment from researchers

## Box 16.1 Example of accessible recruitment material

**What is the study about?**

We want to develop an app. It is a program that can be put in tablets and cell phones. It will help people to take their medications.

At the end of our project, people can buy this application if they want to use it.

Your opinion will help us make the application better.

If you want to participate in our study, we will invite you to try this application. You will talk with other participants about it.

We will ask you questions like these ones:

- Do you use technology such as cell phones or tablets?
- Why do you use technology? Or why do you not use technology?
- Why is it difficult to use technology? Or why is it easy to use technology?

You do **not** have to answer all of our questions.

(McDonald et al., 2015). However, in these instances, researchers should carefully consider the impact of support persons' influence on potential participants' freedom of choice.

## Free and informed consent

### Considering the influence of third parties in participant recruitment

The disadvantage of collaborating with third parties is that these individuals may play a gatekeeper role that affects potential participants' self-determination and introduces biases into research samples (Gerrish and Lacey, 2007). For example, third parties might deny participation because of their personal opinions about research or about the relevance of the project. Moreover, they might want to protect individuals with IDD from harm, especially when the topic is sensitive (e.g., sexuality) or they might think individuals will not be interested or able to participate (McDonald et al., 2015). Some of these concerns might be well intentioned, but they raise ethical questions. These practices might be overprotective and prevent persons with IDD from having their voices heard in research (McDonald and Kidney, 2012; Walker and Read, 2011). Moreover, because of their caregiving role, service providers or family members might coerce individuals to participate, intentionally or unintentionally. It is also possible that third parties may not adequately or accurately explain the study to potential participants. For example, during a focus group on sexuality, we realized that some participants did not know they were attending a discussion for research purposes. The risks and benefits of including third parties, or caregivers, must therefore be carefully weighed.

We recommend that researchers clarify caregivers' roles during the research process and emphasize the freedom of choice of the persons whom they support. Researchers are encouraged to meet with caregivers to develop partnerships (Taylor et al., 2016) and to provide instructions to explain research using accessible language (Carey, 2010). Also, it is crucial researchers review research materials with participants and answer their questions preceding data collection, even if consent forms were previously signed (Carey and Griffiths, 2017). Additionally, researchers are urged to directly address persons with IDD, even in the presence of third parties (McDonald et al., 2015).

Working with caregivers is not always feasible or desirable, and alternative recruitment strategies may need to be considered. Contacting individuals with IDD directly may sometimes be the preferred strategy because it might increase response rates versus recruitment relying on third parties (Cleaver et al., 2010). During a study on the experiences of persons with IDD undergoing a physical health exam, we recruited using a mass mailing list of persons with IDD receiving social assistance (Potvin et al., in press). Letters were sent to 39,868 individuals with IDD throughout the province of Ontario, Canada. We therefore had no opportunity to work collaboratively with caregivers to potentially increase the accessibility of our recruitment letters. A link to a video of the researcher explaining the project in accessible language with closed captioning was included in the recruitment package with the intent of increasing accessibility. Unfortunately, very few individuals visited the web page.

### Assessing capacity to consent

Although information can be conveyed in a variety of ways to meet the communication needs of persons with IDD, clear guidelines for assessing their comprehension of research participation are essential. Disagreements remain regarding best practices for assessing (1) capacity to consent, (2) comprehension of the study, (3) understanding of rights as research participants, and (4) understanding of risks and benefits associated with research participation (McDonald et al., 2015). REB members have requested that we disclose the level of impairment and the communication skills of the participants to appraise their capacity to consent:

> The REB's main concern with this study is the obtained assent of the individuals with intellectual deficits. [ . . . ] What will be done to determine that the participants truly understand the research, and their role in this research? Will only highly functional individuals be invited to participate? [ . . . ] If some participants may need to be accompanied for the group discussion, does it mean that some may not be able to fully consent for themselves?

In our experience, REB members frequently question the capacity to consent of individuals with IDD. They may also have limited knowledge about assessing capacity to consent in this context (e.g., they used the word assent instead of consent, despite the application form only mentioning consent). It is also concerning that some REBs questioned participants' capacity to consent when they require support to communicate (e.g., sign language, communication technology). Communication abilities are not representative of individuals' overall cognitive functioning and capacity to consent (Jepson, 2015). To address REB members' concerns, we suggest that researchers clarify support persons' roles during the consent process. The following is an example of our response to a REB's concerns:

> The purpose of having a support person accompany persons with IDD to the focus group is to support communication with the moderator and other participants, and not to answer questions for them. [ . . . ] The individual accompanying the participant serves therefore as an interpreter and facilitates informed consent.

Another challenge is obtaining consent from individuals who are not able to sign consent forms, but have the capacity to verbally or non-verbally provide consent. Restricting consent to written formats impedes the participation of many individuals, such as those with limited literacy or upper-body mobility (Hamilton et al., 2017).

Finding alternative ways of recording consent is needed to make research accessible to all.

### Consent is a process

Consent should be approached as an ongoing process (Dalton and McVilly, 2004). For many, participating in research is a novel situation that often entails discussion of abstract or hypothetical concepts. Assessment of individual needs can be facilitated by meeting with participants prior to obtaining consent (McDonald and Kidney, 2012; Carey and Griffiths, 2017). Individuals with IDD have indicated that it is important for them to feel safe and respected by researchers (McDonald et al., 2015); therefore, this meeting may also provide an opportunity to foster participants' comfort and trust (Carey and Griffiths, 2017). Moreover, it also provides an occasion for researchers to ask participants what supports they require, if any.

As recommended by other researchers (Kidney and McDonald, 2014), we suggest conducting an interview to assess participants' comprehension of the study and the implications of participation (see Box 16.2). If participants provide responses demonstrating comprehension, we assume that their consent is valid. If not, we explain the study again and repeat the comprehension test. If they still do not understand, we investigate whether a caregiver can support their decision-making and participation. Researchers should also be sensitive to verbal and non-verbal signs of withdrawal or dissent throughout the project (Carey and Griffiths, 2017). For example, clear questions about if they want to continue participating should be asked to those presenting signs of dissent or disengagement. However, observing these signs remains the responsibility of the researchers who rely on their personal judgment.

**Box 16.2 Example of an interview for determining participants' comprehension**

Participants' capacity to consent will be determined according to the following steps in the consent protocol.

1. The researcher will explain the study details to participants.
2. To check for comprehension and evaluate capacity to consent, the researcher will ask participants a series of questions:
   a. Do you have to answer every question that I ask you?
   b. What will I ask you about?
   c. Who gets to choose if you answer these questions?
   d. Can you stop answering the questions at any time?
3. If the potential participants give an incorrect response, the correct response will be explained. If they still do not understand after a second explanation, they will be asked if they know someone (e.g., caregiver) who can help facilitate communication between them and the researcher.

## Confidentiality

### Communicating about confidentiality with persons with IDD

Many persons with IDD understand the concept of confidentiality in their daily lives; however, data collection and result dissemination are abstract and unfamiliar contexts. For example, participants with IDD might have difficulty understanding that some researchers who are not physically present will have access to the data and report findings to different audiences (Chalghoumi et al., 2017a).

Persons with IDD have expressed concerns regarding disclosed information being shared with their caregivers, who may be key knowledge users, and about information sharing that may affect their support receipt (McDonald et al., 2015). Therefore, researchers should be diligent when explaining confidentiality to individuals with IDD. We find it useful to address these concerns during member-checking. Member-checking is an opportunity to ask participants if they agree with the way we represent the information they provided and to explain how and with whom this information will be shared.

### Communicating about confidentiality with third parties

Participants with IDD have the right to choose if they desire the presence of a support person during data collection, and, if so, to determine this person. Benefits of including a support person include comfort, safety, and facilitated communication (McDonald et al., 2015). However, involving a third party during data collection can lead to confidentiality concerns. For example, the support person may gain access to new information about the individual because of the questions asked, which may go beyond what the support person would learn about the individual in daily interactions. We recommend having confidentiality agreements for third parties who are present during research activities (see Box 16.3).

Confidentiality may also be jeopardized when multiple respondents from the same system are interviewed separately (Margolin et al., 2005). For example, when doing research with families navigating transitions, we collected the voices of persons with IDD, their parents and siblings, and other support persons. In these circumstances, it is crucial that researchers remember who disclosed what information to prevent accidental confidentiality breaches amongst participants. We have never received feedback

**Box 16.3 Third-party confidentiality agreement**

I, ________________, am present with ________________ for an interview conducted for the purpose of research. I am present to help with communication and offer support. I understand that everything said during this interview is to be kept strictly confidential and shall remain between me (named above), the participant (named above), and the researcher.

from REBs about these risks, however. Researchers should nevertheless convey the added risk of having multiple members of a system involved in a research project and diligently protect privileged information.

### Re-identification risks

Protecting participants' confidentiality is often naïvely understood as not disclosing information that would directly identify participants, such as their name, date of birth, and place of residence. However, in qualitative research, aggregated details presented in participants' quotes may result in re-identification, such that participants become indirectly identifiable, especially when using small samples recruited by community or health service providers (Damianakis and Woodford, 2012; Kaiser, 2009). Balancing the need to present sufficient methodological details and meaningful findings, while not disclosing information that can breach confidentiality, is a challenging task.

### Managing confidentiality threats

Many REBs, research funding agencies, and academic institutions are moving towards mandatory data-management plans. Typically, these plans outline procedures for collecting, storing, and securely protecting data, as well as the resources required to fulfill the data-management plan (Czechowski et al., 2018; Czechowski and Sylvestre, 2018). We suggest that data-management plans should include a section on re-identification risks and provide specific measures to protect the confidentiality of participants recruited from small populations, especially those vulnerable to stigma (Damianakis and Woodford, 2012; Kaiser, 2009). When involving persons with IDD in research, data-management plans should also include procedures for protecting confidentiality when participants require or desire the involvement of a support person.

## Risks associated with research participation

Researchers must be sensitive to stigma that participants may experience due to their research participation. Moreover, researchers and REBs should be careful not to perpetuate stereotypes about persons with IDD. We recommend the use of person-first language and awareness of stigmatizing comments and behaviors. It is not uncommon to find recruitment materials that include stigmatizing language or highlight disabilities. For example, one REB recommended that we develop a recruitment poster that advertised, "Do you have a cognitive impairment?" This recruitment headline may be viewed as stigmatizing. Even experienced researchers struggle with finding proper or inoffensive wording. In one of our studies, a participant expressed that she was insulted that we had mentioned "disability" during recruitment. Adults with IDD have emphasized that they should be treated respectfully, and their competence and decision-making abilities should be recognized (McDonald et al., 2015). Using respectful language and focusing on abilities, rather than disabilities, diminishes the risks of discomfort or distress that participants may experience during research. There is a need for guidance, for both researchers and REB members, on how to communicate with participants in a respectful way while also adhering to the scientific requirements of research.

REBs have raised concerns that participants may incur significant burden or distress due to their participation in research. Some concerns were due to the topics of our studies (e.g., sexuality and childbearing), while others were specific to the characteristics of the participants. For example, risks related to traveling to data-collection sites were queried: "The REB would like also to know which mechanisms will be put in place to ensure that participants do not take on unsupervised travel if they do not do so in ordinary life." Although this is a valid concern, REBs should avoid proposing mechanisms that are potentially paternalistic and stigmatizing. Rather, researchers should strive to remove unnecessary barriers to participation, as when we responded:

> Mechanisms are in place to ensure that participants can travel to the meeting location: 1) Participants who so desire or who are not able to travel unsupervised may be accompanied by the person of their choice; 2) the location of [data collection] will be a familiar place for most participants. Directions to the location will be provided to participants by mail or email prior to [data collection].

However, these mechanisms may add demands on persons with IDD and their support persons. Often, paid or unpaid caregivers arrange transportation, leading them to incur expenses or take time to support persons with IDD to participate in research. Despite efforts to increase accessibility, some persons with IDD may remain unable to participate, despite their desire to do so, because of barriers associated with transportation to data collection sites. The REBs that reviewed our projects have never raised this issue, and we do not claim that we have found a way around this challenge. However, we have attempted to alleviate transportation-related burdens by providing a financial incentive to participants, reimbursing their travel expenses, or, when possible, conducting interviews over the telephone or at the residences of the participants.

### Protecting participants from harm

All researchers who include participants with IDD should be sensitive to the history of IDD research and associated human rights violations. Protecting research participants with IDD from unfair, cruel, and degrading treatment also means not exposing them to persons who might harm them. One recruitment site asked for a police record check for vulnerable sector verifications for each of the researchers interacting with participants. In our projects, we have worked collaboratively with several organizations, and only one requested vulnerable sector verifications; none of the academic REBs requested these verifications for conducting research. Under the Canadian Criminal Record Act (Criminal Records Act, c.47, 1985) those who are vulnerable are "in a position of dependency on others; or is otherwise at a greater risk than the general population of being harmed by a person in a position of trust or authority towards them." Persons with IDD and other cognitive disabilities are, therefore, considered vulnerable.

Researchers and REBs should explore the necessity of police record checks in their field of work.

## Conclusion

Research involving persons with IDD has generated important ethical issues; movements toward inclusive and participatory action research methods are a response to historical shortcomings. That said, significant challenges related to the ethical conduct of research with persons with IDD remain. Some of these are routinely discussed in the IDD literature, such as capacity to consent (e.g., Carey and Griffiths, 2017; Jepson, 2015; McDonald and Kidney, 2012) and gatekeeping by third parties (e.g., Carey and Griffiths, 2017; Lennox et al., 2005; McDonald et al., 2015); however, practical recommendations have yet to be formalized, translated to practice, and enforced by researchers and REBs. Other challenges, such as potentially offensive recruitment materials and confidentiality in the presence of support persons, have received insufficient attention in the IDD literature and REB application reviews.

Those who conduct or review the ethics of research concerning persons with IDD should obtain training in ethical issues pertinent to this population, accessibility guidelines, and respectful interactions with persons with IDD and their support networks. Persons with IDD comprise a heterogeneous population with varying levels of autonomy and needs; therefore, a person-centred approach is highly recommended to facilitate their participation in research (Hamilton et al., 2017). Moreover, research designs are enhanced when researchers consult and collaborate with persons with IDD (McDonald et al., 2015).

Persons with IDD have the right to participate in research. A knowledge-mobilization plan is required to ensure researchers, REB members, and funding agencies become aware of the ethical considerations and guidelines in this research context. Our research team is currently developing online training resources to inform inclusive research practices with persons with IDD. We hope the experiences and recommendations provided in this chapter also accomplish this aim.

## References

Becker, H., Roberts, G., Morrison, J., and Silver, J. (2004) "Recruiting People With Disabilities as Research Participants: Challenges and Strategies to Address Them," *Mental Retardation*, 42/6: pp. 471–475.

Carey, E. (2010). "Navigating the Process of Ethical Approval: A Methodological Note." *The Grounded Theory Review*, 9/3: 14.

Carey, E. and Griffiths, C. (2017). "Recruitment and Consent of Adults With Intellectual Disabilities in a Classic Grounded Theory Research Study: Ethical and Methodological Considerations." *Disability & Society*, 32/2: 193–212.

Chalghoumi, H., Cobigo, V., Dignard, C., Gauthier-Beaupre, A., Jutai, J. W., Lachapelle, Y., Mcheimech, R., and Perrin, M. (2017a) "Information Privacy for Technology Users With Intellectual and Developmental Disabilities: Why Does It Matter?" *Ethics & Behavior*, 29/3: 201–207.

Chalghoumi, H., Cobigo, V., and Jutai, J. (2017b) "Ethical Issues Related to IT Adoption by Elderly Persons With Cognitive Impairments." *Studies in Health Technology and Informatics*, 242: 59–63.

Cleaver, S., Ouellette-Kuntz, H., and Sakar, A. (2010) "Participation in Intellectual Disability Research: A Review of 20 Years of Studies." *Journal of Intellectual Disability Research*, 54/3: 187–193.

Criminal Records Act, c.47 (1985). "Procedure (continued)," https://laws-lois.justice.gc.ca/eng/acts/C-47/page-2.html (accessed November 5, 2018).

Czech, H. (2018). "Hans Asperger, National Socialism, and 'Race Hygiene' in Nazi-Era Vienna." *Molecular Autism*, 9: 29.

Czechowski, K. and Sylvestre, J. (2018) "Best Practices for Secure Handling and Storage of Confidential Research Data," http://hdl.handle.net/10393/37559 (accessed May 6, 2018).

Czechowski, K., Sylvestre, J., and Morneau, K. (2019). "Secure Data Handling: An Essential Competence for Evaluators." *Canadian Journal of Program Evaluation*, DOI: 10.3138/cjpe.43319 (Epub ahead of print).

Dalton, A. J. and McVilly, K. R. (2004) "Ethics Guidelines for International, Multicenter Research Involving People with Intellectual Disabilities1,2,3,4," *Journal of Policy and Practice in Intellectual Disabilities*, 1/2: 57–70.

Damianakis, T. and Woodford, M. R. (2012) "Qualitative Research With Small Connected Communities: Generating New Knowledge While Upholding Research Ethics." *Qualitative Health Research*, 22/5: 708–718.

Financial Consumer Agency of Canada (2017). "CG-3 Clear Language and Presentation Principles and Guidelines for the Industry," https://www.canada.ca/en/financial-consumer-agency/services/industry/commissioner-guidance/guidance-3.html (accessed May 6, 2018).

Gerrish, K. and Lacey, A. (2007) *The Research Process in Nursing*. 5th edn. Oxford: Blackwell.

Hamilton, J., Ingham, B., McKinnon, I., Parr, J. R., Tam, L. Y.-C., and Le Couteur, A. (2017) "Mental Capacity to Consent to Research? Experiences of Consenting Adults With Intellectual Disabilities and/or Autism to Research." *British Journal of Learning Disabilities*, 45/4: 230–237.

Jepson, M. (2015) "Applying the Mental Capacity Act to Research With People With Learning Disabilities." *British Journal of Learning Disabilities*, 43/2: 128–134.

Kaiser, K. (2009) "Protecting Respondent Confidentiality in Qualitative Research." *Qualitative Health Research*, 19/11: 1632–1641.

Kidney, C. A. and McDonald, K. E. (2014). "A Toolkit for Accessible and Respectful Engagement in Research." *Disability & Society*, 29/7: 1013–1030.

Lai, R., Elliott, D., and Ouellette-Kuntz, H. (2006) "Attitudes of Research Ethics Committee Members Toward Individuals with Intellectual Disabilities: The Need for More Research." *Journal of Policy and Practice in Intellectual Disabilities*, 3/2: pp. 114–118.

Lennox, N., Taylor, M., Rey-Conde, T., Bain, C., Purdie, D. M., and Boyle, F. (2005). "Beating the Barriers: Recruitment of People With Intellectual Disability to Participate in Research." *Journal of Intellectual Disability Research*, 49/4: 296–305.

Margolin G., Chien, D., Duman, S. E., Fauchier, A., Gordis, E. B., Oliver, P. H., Ramos, M. C., and Vickerman, K. A. (2005). "Ethical Issues in Couple and Family Research." *Journal of Family Psychology*, 19/1: 157–167.

McDonald, K. E. and Kidney, C. A. (2012) "What Is Right? Ethics in Intellectual Disabilities Research: Research Ethics." *Journal of Policy and Practice in Intellectual Disabilities*, 9/1: pp. 27–39.

McDonald, K. E., Schwartz, N. M., Gibbons, C. M., and Olick, R. S. (2015). "'You Can't be Cold and Scientific': Community Views on Ethical Issues in Intellectual Disability Research," *Journal of Empirical Research on Human Research Ethics*, 10/2: 196–208.

Ottmann, G. and Crosbie, J. (2013). "Mixed Method Approaches in Open-Ended, Qualitative, Exploratory Research Involving People With Intellectual Disabilities: A Comparative Methods Study." *Journal of Intellectual Disabilities*, 17/3: 182–197.

Park, P. and Hutton, S. (2018). "Nothing About Us Without Us! That Includes Research." Keynote Address Presented at the Ontario Association of Developmental Disabilities. Research Special Interest Group, Kingston, Ontario.

Potvin, L. A., Brown, H. K., and Cobigo, V. (2016). "Social Support Received by Women With Intellectual and Developmental Disabilities During Pregnancy and Childbirth: An Exploratory Qualitative Study." *Midwifery*, 37: 57–64.

Potvin, L., Fulford, C., Ouellette-Kuntz, H., and Cobigo, V. (in press) 'What Adults With Developmental Disabilities Say They Need to Access the Annual Health Exam: System Navigation Support and Person-Centered Care." *Canadian Family Physician.*

Schalock, R. L., Borthwick-Duffy, S. A., Bradley, V. J., Buntinx, W. H. E., Coulter, D. L., Craig, et al. (2010). *Intellectual Disability: Definition, Classification, and Systems of Supports. 11th edn.* Silver Spring, MD: American Association on Intellectual and Developmental Disabilities.

Scott, J., Wishart, J., and Bowyer, D. (2006). "Do Current Consent and Confidentiality Requirements Impede or Enhance Research With Children With Learning Disabilities?" *Disability & Society*, 21/3: 273–287.

Taylor, S. J., Bogdan, R., and DeVault, M. L. (2016). *Introduction to Qualitative Research Methods: A Guidebook and Resource.* 4th edn. Hoboken, NJ: John Wiley & Sons.

Office for Human Research Protections (1949). "Trials of War Criminals Before the Nuremberg Military Tribunals Under Control Council Law No. 10," http://www.hhs.gov/ohrp/references/nurcode.htm (accessed May 6, 2018).

Office for Human Research Protections (1979) "The Belmont Report: Ethical Principles and Guidelines for the Protection of Human Subjects of Research," http://ohsr.od.nih.gov.proxy.library.carleton.ca/guidelines/belmont.html (accessed May 6, 2018).

Truman, C. (2003). "Ethics and the Ruling Relations of Research Production." *Sociological Research Online* 8/1: 1–11.

Truscott, D. and Crook, K. H. (2013). "Ethics for the Practice of Psychology in Canada," http://www.deslibris.ca/ID/446511 (accessed May 6, 2018).

United Nations. (2006). Convention on the rights of persons with disabilities. Retrieved May 28, 2017, from United Nations website: http://www.un.org/disabilities/documents/convention/convoptprot-e.pdf

Walker, S. and Read, S. (2011) "Accessing Vulnerable Research Populations: An Experience With Gatekeepers of Ethical Approval." *International Journal of Palliative Nursing*, 17/1: 14–18.

World Medical Association (1964). "World Medical Association Declaration of Helsinki: Ethical Principles for Medical Research Involving Human Subjects." *JAMA*, 310/20: 2191–2194.

Your Health Matters (2018). "Easy Read is Just One Way of Making Information More Accessible (2018) What is easy read?" http://www.easyonthei.nhs.uk/accessible-information-standard-what-is-easy-read (accessed May 6, 2018).

# 17

# Assuming Capacity

## Ethical Participatory Research with Adolescents and Adults with Down Syndrome

*Anne Kohler*

### Introduction: Using theory to account for method

When I began planning a long-term research project with the central aim of understanding how individuals with Down syndrome, their parents, and their clinicians navigate healthcare decision-making and care relationships, there was limited literature to guide the development of a methodologically robust study that assured full and rich participation on the part of participants with intellectual disabilities. Ethnography, a hallmark of anthropological research, is characterized by the systematic study of people's perspectives and social relationships within a given sociocultural and structural milieu. The tools of ethnography are varied and include participant observation, structured and unstructured interviews, and surveys. Although such methods are flexible and work across multiple social worlds, they are designed and taught in methods seminars with the underlying supposition that research participants meet the culturally constructed baseline for cognitive "normality." My hunch was that participants would struggle to conform to a set of methods ill-equipped to elicit information from people who think, process, and express themselves in a manner diverging from expected social norms. My intuition, however, was that all participants with Down syndrome had rich and varied perspectives on their lives, social situations, healthcare encounters, social and sexual relationships, and futures. Indeed, many held passionate opinions on the current US president Donald Trump, the Black Lives Matter movement, and the #MeToo Campaign. The most illustrative examples confirming that my hunch was correct were those responses that passionately conveyed opinions on the disability rights movement, anti-institutionalization, and healthcare policy. One participant, a 30-year-old man with Down syndrome who lives in a group home and works at a well-known local restaurant, was adamant that healthcare encounters must not invoke fear, and that healthcare and other social benefits provided by the state must be maintained:

> Whenever it's about healthcare [ … ] you don't want the individual, or individuals, to always fear it. Because when you have fear, it's going to take away the purpose out of your life [ … ] It's not just about benefits, it's about healthcare, it's about raising the bar, money, the Affordable Care Act, the ABLE [Achieving a Better Life Experience]

> account, certain things that elude you your whole life, that you need. And part of me is that I'm outspoken. [ . . . ] I [can] be wacky, or smacky, or funny, or whatever. But when it comes to huge things like this? I need to focus on, to champion, people with disabilities. Make sure they have success, strive for the future, and [that lawmakers] *don't do cuts.*

Here, David highlights a clear political position on not only his own quality of healthcare access, but also that of others utilizing the current healthcare system

Eliciting this answer was not a straightforward matter. David, although eager to talk when we had met a few months earlier at a local self-advocacy meeting, seemed shy and anxious during our interview. It took a great deal of encouragement to help him feel comfortable, and I found myself making the mistake of measuring whether he was "high functioning" in certain moments and "low functioning" in others. Despite my continued commitment to interrogating intellectual disability as a way of being-in-the-world (Jackson, 2012), I fell back on questions of function, cognition, memory, and the potential (or not) to narrativize one's life.

I offer this moment to spark discussion about how adapting and creating whole-cloth methods for participants with intellectual disabilities ought never to be disconnected from a theoretical account of personhood, as well as how we configure capacity and "competence" both as social scientists and as a society. This is not to suggest that personhood or cognitive difference must be configured similarly across the board, but rather that we as researchers ought to get a clear view of how our research methods might rely on such exclusionary notions of personhood—a trap easy enough to fall into, as detailed earlier. Further, in adapting or creating new methods, I believe it is worth rooting such changes in a thorough accounting of how we, as researchers, theorize the personhood of people with intellectual disabilities.

In the United States, those with disabilities have often been excluded from political and social life based on their "failure" to live up to a Western, liberal-democratic view of personhood (Carlson, 2009; Simplican, 2015). Intellectual disability—as a diagnosis, an experience, and a theoretical bogeyman—seeps into a variety of political, social, and legal spaces, including immigration policy (Baynton, 2013), feminist political movements (Kafer, 2013), reproductive rights (Cohen, 2017), and conversations regarding the distribution of healthcare resources (Ervin and Merrick, 2014). As anthropologists, we have acknowledged that our own, and our field's, positionality is never disconnected from our social context (Closser and Finley, 2016). Following this logic, it is possible to see how certain research methods, particularly eliciting an illness narrative (Kleinman, 1989), can exclude those who think and process their experiences differently. I argue that many anthropological research methods rely on a specific imagined person: one who conceives of their life as a narrative with a start and an end, one who will be concrete or abstract at the "right" times, one who will make the expected connections between question and answer. Some imagine an agentive, individual subject, and feel especially uneasy if someone is helped by a parent, friend, or support person to answer questions. It goes to the heart of what we consider "good data": was this sentence uttered or that pile sort completed alone, without influence from other persons?

In response I offer three methodological adaptations for including people with varied cognitive strengths in social science research. The first is *assisted interviewing*, which entails undertaking interviews with participants with intellectual disabilities with a generous openness to informal assistance from parents, siblings, and others who know the participant well. Assisted interviewing acknowledges the interrelatedness of individuals and their families and caregivers without adopting a confirmatory bias. *Adapted photovoice* is the second methodological adaptation useful for robust inclusion of individuals with intellectual differences in research. Third, I urge researchers, when possible, *to hire a research assistant with an intellectual disability*. My research assistant, Ben, a young man with Down syndrome, has been invaluable as both a key informant and a research partner. Ben and I have collected, coded, and analyzed data together. He also assists in ensuring that all research materials are in plain language and provides emic insight into researcher quandaries or questions about data. Further, given anthropologists' strong ethical obligations to research communities, as well as the long history of research abuse among people with intellectual disabilities, hiring a research assistant with intellectual disability can serve as an important step towards more inclusive research design.

If sociocultural values regarding personhood, cognition, and independence undergird established research methods, then any methodological innovation is also necessarily underwritten by a particular set of values. In this particular case, I draw on the feminist care ethics of Eva Feder Kittay in which assistance and interdependence are central to all human experiences (2011)—not just of those with cognitive disabilities—and in which rationality and autonomy are philosophical fictions used to justify entrenched systems of social inequality (2005). Therefore, the success of any of these methodological interventions ought to be judged by their ability to partner with those with cognitive differences in dismantling the fiction of cognitive difference as pathology across multiple social contexts.

Readers might well be asking themselves an important question at this point: how does this seemingly eclectic approach result in the collection of the kind of data required for (1) generalizing findings in order to build on existing social science theory and (2) translating ethnographic findings for policy audiences? In the conclusion I will offer one possible answer, arguing that recent critiques of metrics and reliance on "objectivive statistics" in global health (Adams, 2016) open up a space for re-thinking what data "count," and how ethnographic findings on intellectual disability and health can be translated into new kinds of "data that count" for multiple audiences.

## Assisted interviewing

Assisted interviewing is a process in which the interjections of parents and caregivers are acknowledged and taken as additional data rather than as simply confirming or denying the opinions of those with intellectual disabilities. Assisted interviewing draws inspiration from dyadic interviewing. Used here (Caldwell, 2014), dyadic interviewing contextualizes the answer given by participants with intellectual disabilities. Attention to interdependence as an important factor in designing a research study is admirable, but it may also serve to reproduce the notion that the words and thoughts of participants with intellectual disabilities only become legible when partnered with those of typically developed parents, friends, or support persons. Assisted interviewing provides researchers with a way to acknowledge the interjections of such individuals while avoiding a confirmatory lens that, I suggest, rests on the notion that those with intellectual disabilities live in a radically different (and perhaps not entirely legible) world.

There are two key modes for utilizing assisted interviewing. The first is *formal assisted interviewing*, in which interlocutors who struggle with vocal communication use a parent or support person to help them answer questions and engage with the researcher. The second is *informal assisted interviewing*, in which the researcher takes (sometimes unwelcome) interjections by parents or support people as a useful tool to better understand how the participant with intellectual disability feels constrained within their social world. I offer two illustrative examples of each format.

Alice is a 22-year-old woman with Down syndrome who lives with her parents in an upper-middle-class neighborhood. She is short, with fine brown hair and a palpable shyness. When we first met, I struggled to connect with her. Alice has severe anxiety, chronic depression, and a possible post-traumatic stress disorder diagnosis related to severe and previously untreated nerve pain. Her diagnostic journey, which included dismissal and several incorrect diagnoses, is beyond the scope of this chapter. However, when I met her on a muggy July afternoon, it was clear that a traditional semi-structured ethnographic interview was too constraining a format. When we began, Alice gave short answers, taking a long time to think about each one:

ANNE: So, what's your name?
ALICE: . . . Alice. [Her voice is whispery, breathless, and tentative.]
ANNE: Alice. And how old are you?
ALICE: . . . 22
ANNE: That's a good age! And let's see, do you live at home?
ALICE: [Silence.]
ANNE: With your parents?
ALICE: Yeah.

Alice was uncomfortable. Taking a break, I wrote down some of the questions on paper—switching media can be another good way to draw out interviewees who may not be comfortable in the verbal mode. When I did this, Alice's mother Gayle—sitting on a stool on the other side of Alice—started helping her to read the question.

ANNE: How about this question?
GAYLE: What do you like to do during the day? Jumping jacks?
ALICE: Yes.
GAYLE: No, you don't, I was teasing you! [Alice cracks a smile, the first one I've seen.]

Gayle's intervention helped to put Alice at ease, and also signaled to me that humor would be a good way to help Alice feel more comfortable. For the rest of the interview we took turns joking with her, using humor to elicit her opinions on eating healthy (sandwiches, watermelon, and no junk food), her goals (getting a job, visiting Miami), and her pop-culture idols (musical artist Michael Jackson). Given Alice's anxiety around strangers, Gayle's assistance helped me to better understand her life and opinions in a way that recognized her relationship with her mother without cross-checking her answers or turning to Gayle to "fill in" any gaps. During the back-and-forth between the three of us, Alice grew visibly more at ease and indicated that she would like to provide written answers to some of the questions—something that she had rejected when I first offered. While Gayle and I chatted quietly about her qualms regarding the politics of one of the local advocacy organizations, Alice bent her head to the paper and wrote. When she was done, we read her answers together. One, shown in Figure 17.1, stood out immediately:

Grief, and the way in which those with intellectual disabilities experience it, is something that unexpectedly peppered data collection from the very beginning. Clinicians and other care workers often spoke of "delayed grief," and suggested grief might manifest as "behavioral" issues—assuming the capacity to name or understand one's grief would be lacking in those with Down syndrome. However, I found participants often spoke of both grief and death. Alice, it seemed, was no different—although in the medical world she was often described as "low-functioning" and, goes the suggestion, perhaps less inclined to focus on such abstract concepts as grief and death. Our conversation ensued:

ALICE: My grandma died.
GAYLE: Three years ago.
ALICE: Heart attack.
ANNE: Yeah, when we get older sometimes our family members pass away. It's sad, isn't it? It does happen to everyone though.

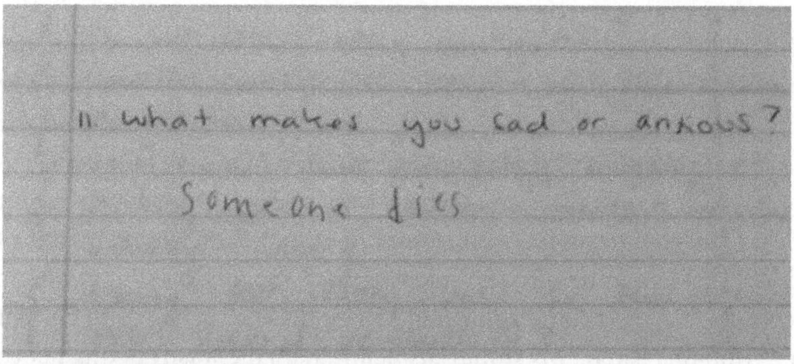


**Figure 17.1** Alice's written answer to a photovoice prompt.

Alice is preoccupied with the death of those close to her, a hypothesis supported by the fact that her mental health problems began almost immediately after her grandmother's passing. In being open to Gayle's participation, an interview that started out with Alice having difficulty stating her name and place of residence opened into a discussion of her grief, illustrating that clinical expectations on the part of mental health professionals regarding mental and behavioral health were incomplete in Alice's case: she is well aware of death, and can convey how it makes her feel. Given that my data also show that a significant barrier to mental health care for those with intellectual disability has been the assumption that individuals cannot adequately narrativize their feelings in a therapeutic environment, the use of *formal assisted interviewing* illustrates that such barriers can be overcome if one assumes capacity rather than inability.

The second mode of assisted interviewing, *informal assisted interviewing*, takes the interruptions of parents or other support people as ultimately valuable, despite the fact that they are often an unwanted disruption. While interviewing Grace, a woman in her early thirties with Down syndrome, her mother Jane sat nearby and prompted Grace much more than was necessary. Grace has indicated to me several times that she would like to see a therapist—in fact, the first time we met I introduced myself as being a researcher, and she immediately asked if I would help her find a therapist. When she mentioned this again, Jane interjected: "Is that something you still want to do?" When Grace answered yes, her mother asked again, seeming surprised: "Do you?" When her daughter again answered in the affirmative, Jane explained to both of us that she has a lead on an appropriate therapist but simply hasn't called due to her busy schedule. Further, she explained her perception of barriers to accessing mental health care for someone with an intellectual disability:

JANE: The trick is, you can't just go get any therapist. You've got to get someone who is used to working with people with developmental disabilities [ . . . ] they may not know what to say, you know? They may not have the best advice [ . . . ]. And some can cause damage, I think. So, [you've] got to get the right person, and that's a trick, and that's why I haven't jumped and just grabbed someone Grace, because I want to make sure to get someone who knows what they're doing. Right?

GRACE: I wasn't sure.

Although at the time I was sympathetic to Jane's position, given the documented lack of mental health services for people with intellectual disabilities, I eventually grew frustrated with the interview dynamic after spending more one-on-one time with Grace. One day, a few weeks after our initial interview, Grace and I met for coffee. When she sat down, I asked her how things had been going, and she immediately responded she needed help managing her alcohol consumption. Would I be willing to find a therapist or an Alcoholics Anonymous group? We also spoke several times about how lonely she felt and how she did not feel that she could share these struggles with her parents because they "wouldn't listen." My initial suspicion that Jane wasn't taking her daughter's desire for therapy seriously was confirmed, and the experience of re-framing her interjections as informal assisted interviewing gave me a better sense of the social and familial barriers Grace was facing in her support for mental health care.

Formal and informal assisted interviewing provide researchers a chance to better understand social networks and modes of interdependence without seeking confirmation from parents and other support persons. In the two examples, participants shared valuable information in the ways they felt comfortable, and I left each interaction with a better understanding of how and why both continued to struggle with mental health and access to treatment. By better considering interdependence—even the kind that can appear detrimental, such as Jane's interjections—researchers can develop a more complete picture of participants' lives and how social networks can facilitate or constrain their experiences of being in the world.

## Adapted photovoice

The method of photovoice, designed as a way for researchers unfamiliar with the local language(s) to engage participants, was originally developed by public health researchers (Wang and Burris, 1997). During a photovoice project research participants are provided with a camera and asked to take photographs that respond to prompts related to the research topic. In this particular study, prompts included "your favorite things," "going to the doctor," "things that are healthy," and "things that are unhealthy." Generally, participants share and discuss their photographs in a focus-group setting. The photovoice method has also been used among research participants with physical disabilities (Newman et al., 2010), but for participants with intellectual disability it has been slower to catch on in ethnographic settings (but see Poveea et al., 2014). Although promising for intellectual disability research, the often-rigid guidelines for photovoice—particularly the process of participating in focus groups—requires the ability for sustained concentration. Participation in focus groups constituted a significant barrier for many in my study. The men and women I got to know cited reasons such as transportation issues and anxiety induced by group settings. Instead of abandoning this method I carried out individually adapted projects with a number of participants. This perceived limitation turned out to be an ethnographic boon: pursuing individual projects increased the number of research visits by necessity, resulting in stronger relationships and rapport with participants.

For participants like Alice, whose first interview is detailed in the previous section, photography proved an especially helpful medium for gaining more insight into her life. It was initially very difficult to establish a relationship with her, as detailed above. Getting a deeper sense of "who Alice is" and what was important to her was difficult. When she started sending me the photographs she took, or the ones of herself that she staged, I saw an entirely different Alice: an artist, dancer, and a basketball, and tennis player, as well as a yoga enthusiast. Figures 17.2 and 17.3, respectively, show her kayaking in a local river, an open and happy look on her face, and standing proudly in front of her paintings, which are striking in their use of color and composition.

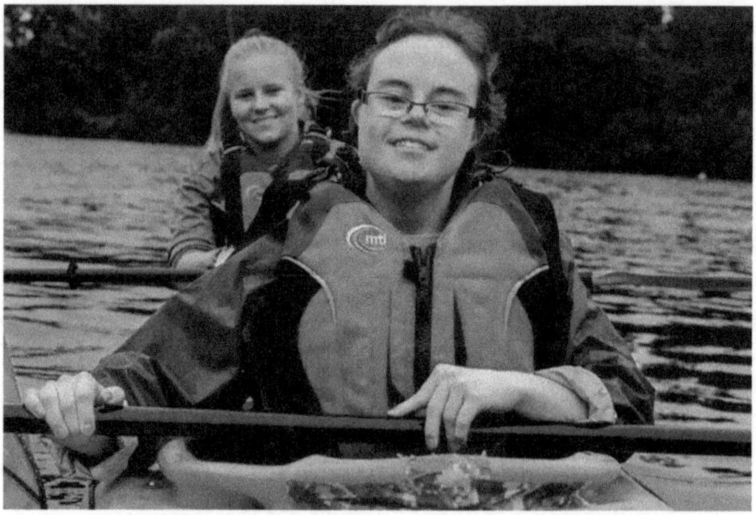

**Figure 17.2** Alice kayaking on a local river.

Alice's mother also mentioned that she planned to use the photographs to help motivate Alice during the worst of her anxious and depressed moments: "I like giving her positive reinforcement that she can do [things] again." This was a key moment in which I saw the promise of an adapted, flexible photovoice. The visual medium of photography allowed Alice to present herself and her world in the way she most felt comfortable, and

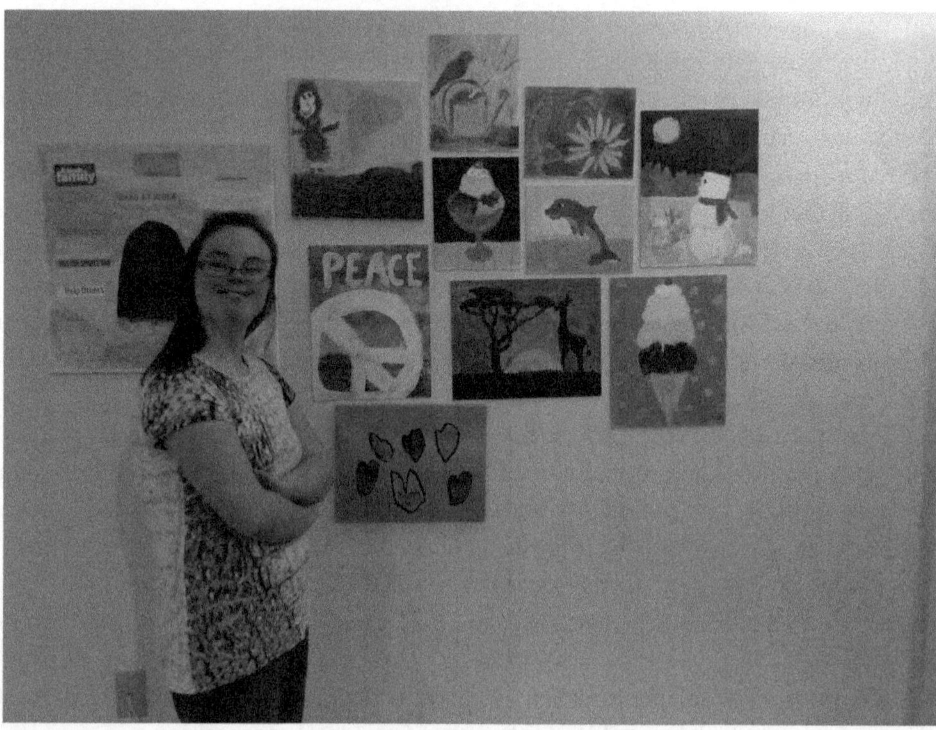


**Figure 17.3** Alice showing off her artwork.

the figures above provide a better sense of what is important to her. Further, Gayle's plan to use the project as a therapeutic tool illustrates how mental health status became a matter of familial care and concern.

Another participant chose to use the photovoice directions as a writing prompt. Although at first concerned about the "correctness" of her participation, I soon realized that Ana's way of interacting with the project was no less valuable as a source of data. Ana's written answers gave a *very* clear picture of her position on the role health plays in her life, as well as her rejection of a paternalistic model of care. For the prompt "what are your least favorite things?" Ana wrote: "People [ ... ] tell me what to do or not," "people don't tell me the rules," "tell me what healthy or not." In discussing these answers with her, Ana explained that she is frustrated with her day program staff for being bossy and changing the rules often, which resulted in her—at the age of 29—being yelled at for using a plastic knife, which was newly forbidden at her day program. Regarding health, one of Ana's answers was a loud and clear rejection of the medicalization of her life: "less doctor appointment more work [sic]."

If I had discounted Ana's way of engaging with the photovoice project, her rejection of paternalism and medicalization would have been lost in the shuffle. In later conversations, Ana expanded on her answers and shared that she was frustrated with her sister, who tells Ana she needs to lose weight even though she is a pack-a-day smoker. As Ana put it, "is it better to eat and live or smoke and die?" And to readers worried that methodological flexibility robs a research project of comparable data: I write this passage a few days after helping Ana pack for a move from her group home to her own apartment. Sweaty and bent over a box of art supplies, I looked up when Ana called my name. Holding her disposable camera, she insisted that we take a selfie to mark this new and exciting period of her life. Ana assured me when I asked if she had taken other photos that I should "be patient." The photographic data, it seems, will soon be available.[1]

## Hiring a research assistant with Down syndrome

I met my research assistant, Ben, through his position in one of the local health clinics serving individuals with Down syndrome. After working closely together at the clinic for 3 months I approached him about being a research assistant. After working with my institutional review board to do adapted ethics training, we began to work together. I needed someone to ensure that my research materials were written in plain language, and that the kinds of questions I asked would resonate with both adolescents and adults with Down syndrome. Ben and I have spent a lot of time together going over questionnaires and thinking through the mechanics of the interview process. He also acted as

[1] This type of close relationship between researcher and participant is not uncommon in experience-near anthropological research. Although there is limited space to reflect here, the blurring of such boundaries when working with participants with cognitive differences is likely another important topic for debate.

a key informant, sharing his perspective on health care, romantic relationships, and other topics helpful for better understanding all my informants.

Researchers of intellectual disability ought to view the research process itself as a political and ethical project, especially given the long history of abuse and mistreatment of those with intellectual disability to which able-bodied medical and social science researchers have contributed (Carlson, 2013). In hiring Ben, I hoped to signal to my participants and the academic community that "assuming competence" is a broader project than treating our research participants as engaged interlocutors. It also involves including stakeholders with intellectual disabilities as *researchers* with valuable insight. More than once, I relied on Ben's data analysis to either confirm or reject my instincts about particular participants. In one case, I believed that a 15-year-old girl with Down syndrome had a particularly close, and positive, relationship with her sister. Ben pointed out that her strong relationship with her sister might mean she didn't have any other close friends. Given that many adolescents with intellectual disabilities struggle with forming peer relationships as a result of social stigma, Ben's analysis provided a new direction for understanding family relationships in a broader social context.

To prepare Ben for his role as a research assistant, we undertook several weeks of training. Having Ben write the research objectives down in his own words was also beneficial and helped him to take ownership of the project and his role as a research assistant. In one of our earliest meetings, shown in Figure 17.4, Ben came up with his own succinct framing of the research: "People with Down syndrome are experts and know more than parents and [doctors]." He carried this framing with him throughout the project, and it served as my reminder to be flexible regarding methods and to be a better listener even when I struggled to understand certain opinions.

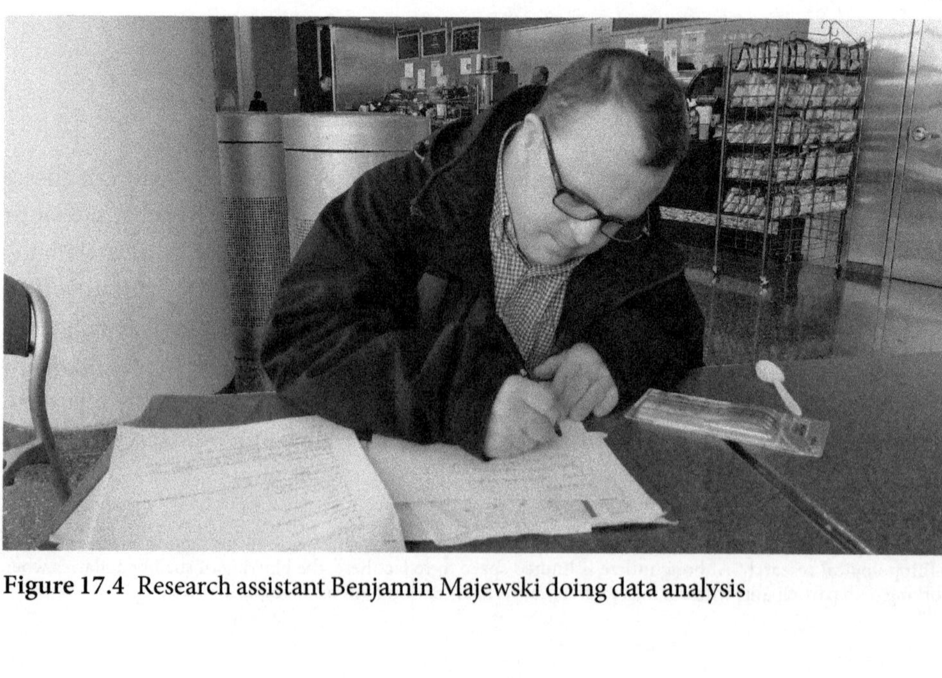

**Figure 17.4** Research assistant Benjamin Majewski doing data analysis

## Beyond Down syndrome: Ethnography and intellectual disability

The aim of the present project was to understand how adolescents and adults with Down syndrome navigated healthcare decision-making and relations of care within the context of social inequity. As demonstrated in the previous sections, adopting a position of maximum methodological flexibility provided valuable insights into how individuals with Down syndrome navigated their own physical and mental health. Doing so also shed light on how different social networks and familial contexts influence healthcare access. Although such findings stand alone as useful insights into the lifeworlds of those with intellectual disabilities, they also illustrate how re-thinking our assumptions regarding what constitutes "research participation" can be useful for building on existing social science theory and intervening in broader conversations with clinical and policy audiences on the topic of intellectual disability. As Vincanne Adams (2016) notes in her edited volume *Metrics: What Counts in Global Health*, health research communities are often fixated on scalable quantitative data that are only loosely based on, or entirely disconnected from, on-the-ground realities. Quantitative data become an end in themselves and do not necessarily need to address actual health and social disparities, and only need to be presented in such a way that improvement is documented and more funding is provided. Adams and other contributors to her volume are not rejecting quantitative data collection entirely, merely suggesting that the ethnographic stories we leverage as "affective evidence" are well positioned to "not just serve metrics, but actually discredit or force them to be reconsidered," and to "create space for rethinking what we mean by evidence and by metrics or how to undo them" (Adams, 2016, p. 49). By adapting research methods for use with participants with intellectual disabilities, the "affective evidence" is more attuned to on-the-ground realities, and therefore can be used creatively to challenge and critique the ways in which intellectual disability is framed and understood in health disparities research. Such data are not only powerful as a refutation of certain health policies, but also as a resource for re-imagining how qualitative data become evidence for quantitative health assessments.

## Conclusion

The work of Donna Haraway is helpful in drawing this chapter to a close. Although not a scholar of intellectual disability, her critique of the Anthropocene, defined by her as a patriarchal and human-centered vision of an unlivable future, is helpful for grounding a theoretically robust accounting of the methods we choose to use for interlocutors with intellectual disability. While offering her accounting of research in which the focus is on relational and embodied forms of surviving and thriving in inequitable environments, she states: "It matters what thoughts think thoughts. It matters what knowledges know knowledge. It matters what relations relate relations. It matters what worlds world worlds. It matters what stories tell stories" (Haraway, 2016, p. 35). In other words, the frameworks that researchers use to create knowledge ought to be as carefully constructed as our research findings. By urging us to think deeply about the theoretical positions that we bring to the table as we embark upon ways of knowing and researching, Haraway offers a profound bit of advice for those engaged with interlocutors with intellectual disabilities: beyond the typical urge for reflexivity in ethnographic work (Song, 2006), she is calling on us to question the roots of long-accepted ways of understanding the world around us—including, I argue, the deep histories and assumptions about competency, personhood, and subjecthood upon which our methods are built.

## References

Adams, V. (ed.) (2016). *Metrics: What Counts in Global Health.* Durham, NC: Duke University Press.

Baynton, D. C. (2013). "Disability and the Justification of Inequality in American History," in Davis, L. J. (ed.) *The Disability Studies Reader*. New York: Routledge.

Caldwell, K. (2014). "Dyadic Interviewing: A Technique Valuing Interdependence in Interviews with Individuals with Intellectual Disabilities." *Qualitative Research*, 14/4: 488–507.

Carlson, L. (2009). *The Faces of Intellectual Disability: Philosophical Reflections*. Bloomington, IN: Indiana University Press.

Carlson, L. (2013). "Research Ethics and Intellectual Disability: Broadening the Debate." *Yale Journal of Biology and Medicine*, 86/3: 303–314.

Cohen, A. (2017). *Imbeciles: The Supreme Court, American Eugenics, and the Sterilization of Carrie Buck*. New York: Penguin Books.

Ervin, D. and Merrick, J. (2014). "Intellectual Disability and Developmental Disability: Healthcare Financing." *Frontiers in Public Health*, 2/160: 1–3.

Closser, S. and Finley, E. P. (2016). "A New Reflexivity: Why Anthropology Matters in Contemporary Health Research and Practice, and How to Make It Matter More." *American Anthropologist*, 188/2: 385–390.

Haraway, D. (2016). *Staying with the Trouble: Making Kin in the Cthulucene*. Durham, NC: Duke University Press Books.

Jackson, M. (2012). *Lifeworlds: Essays in Existential Phenomenology*. Chicago, IL: University of Chicago Press.

Kafer, A. (2013). *Feminist, Queer, Crip*. Bloomington, IN: Indiana University Press.

Kittay, E. F. (2011). "The Ethics of Care, Dependence, and Disability." *Ratio Juris*, 24/1: 49–58.

Kittay, E. F. (2005). "At the Margins of Moral Personhood." *Ethics*, 116/1: 100–131.

Kleinman, A. (1989). *The Illness Narratives: Suffering, Healing, and the Human Condition*. New York: Basic Books.

Newman, S. D. (2010). "Evidence-Based Advocacy: Using Photovoice to Identify Barriers and Facilitators to Community Participation After Spinal Cord Injury." *Rehabilitation Nursing*, 35/2: 47–59.

Poveea, K., Bishop, B. J., and Robertsa, L. D. (2014). "The Use of Photovoice with People with Intellectual Disabilities: Reflections, Challenges, and Opportunities." *Disability and Society*, 29/6: 893–907.

Simplican, S. C. (2015). *The Capacity Contract: Intellectual Disability and the Question of Citizenship*. Minneapolis, MN: University of Minnesota Press.

Song, H. (2006). "Seeing Oneself Seeing Oneself: White Nihilism in Ethnography and Theory." *Ethnos: Journal of Anthropology*, 71/4: 470–488.

Wang, C. and Burris, M. A. (1997). "Photovoice: Concept, Methodology, and Use for Participatory Needs Assessment." *Health Education and Behavior*, 24/3: 369–387.

SECTION 4

# COMMENTARIES

# 18

# Are Patients with Psychiatric Disorders "Uniquely" Vulnerable in the Context of DBS Research?

## Commentary on Klein (Chapter 13)

*Laura B. Dunn and Paul E. Holtzheimer*

Brain–computer interfaces are here, and the field of psychiatry—and neuroscience more broadly—will need to grapple with the ethical challenges they bring. To take one example, closed-loop deep brain stimulation (DBS) for psychiatric illnesses (e.g., depression or obsessive–compulsive disorder) entails feedback from implanted electrodes; this feedback, in turn, influences, in a patient-tailored way, the treatment of the psychiatric illness by the implanted stimulation device. As investigators look toward these "next-generation" DBS approaches (Widge, et al., 2018), renewed enthusiasm is emerging for DBS for psychiatric disorders, even after disappointing results from controlled trials of DBS for treatment-resistant depression (Holtzheimer et al., 2017; Dougherty, 2018).

In Chapter 13, "Informed Consent for Next-Generation Deep Brain Stimulation Psychiatric Research: Engaging End Users to Understand Risks and Improve Practice," Eran Klein outlines six specific challenges related to informed consent for next-generation DBS for psychiatric disorders, and illustrates these ethical challenges using qualitative data from DBS research participants. Further, Klein argues that these challenges can be addressed, in part, through intentional engagement around ethical issues with those who are using (end users), or might use (potential end users), such devices.

There are several noteworthy and intriguing aspects of this chapter. First, as Klein notes, several ethical challenges related to DBS have been previously described (Lipsman et al., 2012). These challenges can be classified as stemming from (1) characteristics of the population being studied (i.e., potentially vulnerable populations; decision-making capacity in psychiatric illness) and (2) characteristics of the intervention being studied (i.e., scientific uncertainty in psychiatric DBS).

Along with others, our team discussed the potential vulnerability of patients with treatment-resistant depression in the research context—whether due to desperation, lack of alternatives, impaired decision-making capacity, or other influences (Christopher et al., 2012). In our own work, we found that, among adults who were considering enrollment in DBS research for their treatment-resistant depression, there were a number of considerations that affected their decision-making. These included "perceived lack of other treatment options, desire to take initiative, beliefs about DBS as a novel treatment, possibility of DBS efficacy, hoped-for improvements, potential risks and disadvantages of DBS or clinical trial participation, and altruism" (Christopher et al., 2012). However, we did not find any evidence of impaired decision-making capacity or reduced voluntariness (Fisher et al., 2012). Similar to Klein, we argued that, "the emerging research area of DBS can be advanced in an ethically sound manner, provided that safeguards and processes for discussing trials with participants are carefully and proactively enacted" (Christopher et al., 2012).

The discussion by Klein of different types of vulnerability merits further attention. While some of the qualitative data that Klein presents appear consistent with the forms of vulnerability, one has to ask whether these patients are uniquely vulnerable—are they vulnerable in ways that patients with other illnesses are not? This has not been adequately studied, in our opinion, and deserves more empirical attention. In our own study, one potential source of vulnerability emerged in relation to participants' appreciation of the scientific uncertainty of the experimental treatment. Among the chronically severely depressed patients we interviewed, several seemed to overestimate the level of scientific certainty regarding benefits of the experimental DBS protocol. For example, when asked, "How likely do you think it is that you personally will benefit from being in this study?," one participant replied, "I've been told that they have had good results so far so I have reason to believe I will benefit as well" (Fisher et al., 2012). Other participants, however, were more pessimistic, for example, "I am skeptical about positive impact because of [my] poor responses to other treatments," while many were neutral, making comments such as, "There does not exist enough data to make any meaningful estimation of the benefits I may experience" (Fisher et al., 2012). Whether such findings are unique to patients with treatment-resistant depression or other psychiatric disorders considering a brain-based intervention such as DBS is unknown, however. Of note, patients with cancer enrolling in early-phase clinical trials express similar sentiments (Sulmasy et al., 2010)—and may be even more optimistic than the patients we interviewed—raising the distinct possibility that so-called "vulnerability" has less to do with specific diagnoses, and more to do with a sense of "desperation" for effective treatment that some participants (or their families) may experience, combined with optimism about the scientific potential of the experimental treatment.

However, all of the participants scored very well on the MacArthur Competence Assessment Tool for Clinical Research (MacCAT-CR), which assessed understanding, appreciation, reasoning, and choice (the four component abilities of decision-making capacity) in relation to the DBS research protocol. Every participant could correctly respond—when directly asked—to a question that asked whether it was possible that they might not personally benefit from the study. We summarized some of our findings as follows:

> It might be most useful to compare TRD [treatment-resistant depression] subjects with those with other serious illnesses considering early phase or invasive research in an effort to identify which, if any, of the phenomena we explored are specific to DBS for TRD research. This is particularly important at a time when multiple brain-based interventions—for example, gene therapy trials that include sham surgery—are being mounted for a variety of neurological and neurodegenerative disorders (Fisher et al., 2012)

Klein goes on to argue that next-generation DBS brings with it additional ethical issues that need to be described and ultimately addressed—namely, "effects on agency, authenticity, and family relationships." For instance, their qualitative research found that some people who were being treated with DBS questioned whether changes in their emotions or behavior were due to the DBS itself, or whether they, in fact, had control over these emotions and behaviors. In terms of family relationships, they found that implantation of the device may have led to some unexpected effects on family interactions, including some that, despite improvements in the patient's mood, were negative. The strength of the data they present is that they interviewed patients who had undergone the intervention and were living every day with its effects. This example of ethics research that engages directly with end-users of brain-based devices is important, as it points toward aspects of the intervention that may need to be openly discussed in an informed consent discussion. However, as we have argued, it will also be important to compare brain-based intervention research with other forms of research; we do not want to end up engaging in ethics "exceptionalism" as a result of failure to conduct rigorous studies on ethics-related questions.

## References

Christopher, P. P., Leykin, Y., Appelbaum, P. S., Holtzheimer, P. E., 3rd, Mayberg, H. S., and Dunn, L. B. (2012). "Enrolling in Deep Brain Stimulation Research for Depression: Influences on Potential Subjects' Decision Making." *Depression and Anxiety*, 29: 139–146.

Dougherty, D. D. (2018). "Deep Brain Stimulation: Clinical Applications." *Psychiatric Clinics of North America*, 41/3: 385–394.

Fisher, C. E., Dunn, L. B., Christopher, P. P., Holtzheimer, P. E., Leykin, Y., Mayberg, H. S., Lisanby, S. H., and Appelbaum, P. S. (2012). "The Ethics of Research on Deep Brain Stimulation for Depression: Decisional Capacity and Therapeutic Misconception." *Annals of the New York Academy of Sciences*, 1265: 69–79.

Holtzheimer, P. E., Husain, M. M., Lisanby, S. H., Taylor, S. F., Whitworth, L. A., McClintock, S., Slavin, K. V., Berman, J., McKhann, G. M., Patil, P. G., Rittberg, B. R., Abosch, A., Pandurangi, A. K., Holloway, K. L., Lam, R. W., Honey, C. R., Neimat, J. S., Henderson, J. M., DeBattista, C., Rothschild, A. J., Pilitsis, J. G., Espinoza, R. T., Petrides, G., Mogilner, A. Y., Matthews, K., Peichel, D., Gross, R. E., Hamani, C., Lozano, A. M., and Mayberg H. S. (2017). "Subcallosal Cingulate Deep Brain Stimulation for Treatment-Resistant Depression: A Multisite, Randomised, Sham-Controlled Trial." *Lancet Psychiatry*, 4/11: 839–849.

Lipsman, N., Giacobbe, P., Bernstein, M., and Lozano, A. M. (2012). "Informed Consent for Clinical Trials of Deep Brain Stimulation in Psychiatric Disease: Challenges and Implications for Trial Design." *Journal of Medical Ethics*, 38: 107–111.

Sulmasy, D. P., Astrow, A. B., He, M. K., Seils, D. M., Meropol, N. J., Micco, E., and Weinfurt K. P. (2010). "The Culture of Faith and Hope: Patients' Justifications for Their High Estimations of Expected Therapeutic Benefit When Enrolling in Early Phase Oncology Trials." *Cancer*, 116/15: 3702–3711.

Widge, A. S., Malone, Jr., D. A., and Dougherty, D. D. (2018). "Closing the Loop on Deep Brain Stimulation for Treatment-Resistant Depression." *Frontiers in Neuroscience*, 12: 175.

# 19

# Ongoing Consent for the Inverse Problematic to Loss of Capacity

## Commentary on Sankary and Ford (Chapter 1)

*Caitlin Courchesne and Judy Illes*

In Chapter 1, Lauren Sankary and Paul Ford provide a timely perspective on strategies to obtain ongoing consent for individuals whose capacity may diminish over time. They address the importance of accommodating research protocols for individuals belonging to groups historically eschewed from research participation on account of heightened vulnerability, building upon a body of bioethics inquiry that recognizes a need to reconceptualize what it means to be vulnerable as a research participant (Luna, 2009; Luna and Vanderpoel, 2013; Bell et al., 2014). The authors suggest an enhanced consent protocol to protect the rights and autonomy of research participants with neurodegenerative disease while enrolled in experimental trials of neuromodulatory devices. Here, we apply Sankary and Ford's concept of ongoing consent to a patient population with an inverse cognitive trajectory: children and adolescents who gradually gain capacity to consent over time.

Research into diseases of childhood and conditions to which children are particularly susceptible is essential in order to improve their treatment options. Nevertheless, the developmental immaturity of children and adolescents undermines their ability to advocate for their own interests during the course of clinical research. As articulated by the Council for International Organizations of Medical Science and the World Health Organization, "research involving children or adolescents spans a wide range of individuals, from infants through to those just short of legal maturity, with very different physical, cognitive and emotional capacities" (World Health Organization, 2017, p. 66). In keeping with the theme of implanted neural devices, we apply Sankary and Ford's concept of ongoing consent for children and adolescents with treatment-refractory epilepsy, a condition for which neural devices present viable yet relatively understudied modalities of seizure management.

Since the mid-2000s, children and adolescents with treatment-refractory epilepsy have been recruited to clinical trials of implantable neural devices—also known as brain–computer interfaces (BCIs)—such as vagal nerve stimulation, responsive neurostimulation, and deep brain stimulation. Globally, clinical trials of BCIs for treatment-refractory epilepsy have, remarkably, recruited children as young as infants, while upper eligibility age limits extend into late adolescence (Table 19.1). Children who lack communicative abilities surely will not benefit from attempts to obtain assent: total parent proxy consent is the only appropriate strategy when children are too

**Table 19.1** Clinical trials registered on ClinicalTrials.gov (2005–2018) involving invasive brain procedures and children (NCT IDs: NCT03446664, NCT03062514, NCT02632149, NCT02602899, NCT02378792, NCT02089243, NCT02004340, NCT01846741, NCT01378611, NCT01118455, NCT00782249, NCT00522418, NCT00215215)

| Trial title | Condition(s) | Intervention(s) | Study design | Trial site(s) | Recruitment age | Phase | Funded by | Study start date–study completion date | Intervention length (months) |
|---|---|---|---|---|---|---|---|---|---|
| Microburst Vagus Nerve Stimulator (VNS) Therapy Feasibility Study | Epilepsies, partial epilepsy tonic–clonic epilepsy | Microburst stimulation device | Single group assignment, unmasked | United States | 12 years and older (child, adult, older adult) | Phase 1 | Industry | February 2018–June 2021* | 12 |
| Trial to Evaluate the Safety and Effectiveness of Vgus Nerve Stimulation for Children with Refractory Epilepsy | Refractory epilepsy | Vagus nerve stimulation | Randomized, parallel assignment, double-masked | China | 3–6 years (child) | NA | Industry | October 2017–December 2019* | 24 |
| Trial to Assess Vagus Nerve Stimulation Therapy in Children with Lennox–Gastaut Syndrome | Lennox–Gastaut syndrome | Vagus nerve stimulation | Single group assignment, unmasked | China | 3–14 years (child) | Early phase 1 | Industry, other | Oct0ber 2016–October 2017 | 6 |
| Deep Brain Stimulation of the Anterior Nucleus of the Thalamus in Refractory Epilepsy | Refractory epilepsy | Deep brain stimulation | Single group assignment, unmasked | China | 12–60 years (child, Adult) | NA | Industry, other | April 2015–December 2017 | 12 |
| Clinical Trial of Vagus Nerve Stimulation for Treatment of Refractory Epilepsy | Refractory epilepsy | Vagus nerve stimulation | Randomized, parallel assignment, double-masked | China | 6–60 years (child, adult) | Early phase 1 | Industry, other | August 2014–December 2017 | 24 |

| | | | | | | | | | |
|---|---|---|---|---|---|---|---|---|---|
| Controlled Randomized Vagus Nerve Stimulation (VNS) Therapy Versus Resection (CoRaVNStiR) | Epilepsy | Vagus nerve stimulation; resective surgery | Randomized, parallel assignment, single-masked | China | 12–60 years (child, adult) | NA | Other | June 2014–July 2017 | 12 |
| Transcutaneous Auricular Vagus Nerve Stimulation for Pediatric Epilepsy | Epilepsy | Ear vagus nerve stimulation | Randomized, parallel assignment, quadruple-masked | China | 2–18 years (child, adult) | NA | Other | November 2013–December 2016 | 6 |
| VNS Therapy Automatic Magnet Mode Outcomes Study in Epilepsy Patients Exhibiting Ictal Tachycardia (E-37) | Epilepsy | Vagus nerve stimulation | Single group assignment, unmasked | United States | 12 years and older (child, adult, older adult) | NA | Industry | July 2013–August 2015 | 18 |
| Does VNS Interact with the Serotonergic and Immune System in Children With Intractable Epilepsy? | Refractory epilepsy in children | Vagus nerve stimulation | Randomized, parallel assignment, triple-masked | The Netherlands | 4–18 years (child, adult) | Phase 2, phase 3 | Industry, other | March 2006–March 2013 | 6 |
| Trial to Assess Vagus Nerve Stimulation Therapy vs. Anti-Epileptic Drug (AED) Treatment in Children With Refractory Seizures | Epilepsy | Vagus nerve stimulation; anti-epileptic drug (AED) | Randomized, parallel assignment, unmasked | Austria, Belgium, Germany, Sweden, United Kingdom | Up to 17 years (child) | Phase 4 | Industry | October 2004–January 2010 | 12 |
| Trial Comparing Different Stimulation Paradigms in Patients Treated With Vagus Nerve Stimulation for Refractory Epilepsy | Epilepsy | Vagus nerve stimulation | Randomized, parallel assignment, unmasked | Belgium, United States | 16 years and older (child, adult, older adult) | NA | Other | October 2005–December 2015 | 12 |

(*continued*)

**Table 19.1** Continued

| Trial title | Condition(s) | Intervention(s) | Study design | Trial site(s) | Recruitment age | Phase | Funded by | Study start date–study completion date | Intervention length (months) |
|---|---|---|---|---|---|---|---|---|---|
| Study Comparing Best Medical Practice With or Without VNS Therapy in Pharmacoresistant Partial Epilepsy Patients | Epilepsy/partial epilepsy | Vagal nerve simulation; best medical practice AED | Randomized, parallel assignment, unmasked | Belgium, Canada, France, Germany, Italy, The Netherlands, Norway, Spain, Sweden, United Kingdom | 16 years and older (child, adult, order adult) | Phase 4 | Industry | February 2006–July 2008 | 24 |
| Effectiveness Study Comparing Treatment With Drug(s) or Adjunctive VNS Therapy for Pharmacoresistant Partial Seizures | Epilepsies, partial | Vagus nerve stimulation | Randomized, parallel assignment, unmasked | United States | 12 years and older (child, adult, older adult) | Phase 4 | Industry | February 2005–November 2007 | 12 |

*Estimated completion date. NA, not available.

young to understand the nature of their illness or communicate their preferences. Still, ethics committees have a responsibility to assess not only the procedural risks that device trials may pose to young research participants, but also the comprehensiveness, rigor, and reflexivity of proposed parent consent procedures.

In the case of intractable epilepsy, parent-proxies themselves fall under Kipnis' (2001) definition of medical vulnerability, a state of desperation resulting from their child's lack of response to previous courses of conventional anti-epileptic drugs. Parents of young children recruited into neural device trials therefore require clear explanations of the perceived risk–benefit ratio of the trial, the potential benefits that the research poses, and discussions of study end points—including early withdrawal procedures—prior to the onset of the trial. Ethics consultation may additionally benefit parents who must make medical decisions for children incapable of providing assent.

Of the BCI trials listed in Table 19.1, 12 years is the most recurrent minimum age for trial eligibility. Recent psychometric assessment of children eligible for clinical trial enrolment suggests that at and above 12 years of age, most minors are likely to be competent to make informed medical decisions based on the following four domains of capacity: (1) expressing a choice about participation; (2) understanding the disclosed information about the nature and procedures of the research; (3) reasoning in the process of deciding about participation, with the ability to compare alternatives in the light of consequences; and (4) appreciating the impact of decisions made at one point in time on future states and contexts (Hein et al., 2014). These four domains require the acquisition of appropriate skills that each mature at different time points along the course of development. On one hand, expressing a choice, whether verbal or non-verbal, requires the ability to communicate, a skill that begins to develop in early childhood and refines throughout adolescence. On the other hand, appreciation of the consequences of a decision requires abstract thinking, a network-level skill that refines with age and experience (Grootens-Wiegers et al., 2017).

Decision-making in older children involved in BCI trials need not be entirely independent from their caregivers. Apart from instances of coercion, sharing the decision-making process with caregivers honors the biological maturity and rights to physical autonomy of adolescents, yet also preserves the values shared across family units. In this context, physical autonomy extends to the rights of adolescents to have control over how their body looks, moves, or feels. In cases that involve invasive experimental interventions such as BCIs, clinicians and researchers must build trusting relationships with adolescent participants and anticipate that their preferences may vary considerably from those previously reported or those of their parents over the course of a clinical trial. This has been explored in the past for the case of incidental findings in neuroimaging research (Di Pietro and Illes, 2013). Research involving implantable neural devices merits special attention to signs of dissent from the child, as adults receiving BCIs for epilepsy management have postoperatively reported losses of control, confidence, and feelings of self-estrangement (Gilbert et al., 2017). At the crossroads of developing a sense of self, adolescents should be encouraged to report confidentially poor adjustment or changes in self-perception to trusted members of their research team over the course of a BCI trial. In turn, these disclosures should be met with increased social and psychological support or explant procedures if deemed appropriate and non-life threatening.

As neurodegeneration poses the threat of loss of capacity, neurodevelopment embraces a certain level of capacity and decision-making evolution and achievement. Neither case represents fully predictable phenomena, abilities, or end points, but what they share is the significant potential for benefit from advancements in neurotechnology. They also share the fundamental ethics considerations of autonomy, respect, and access, and new ethics challenges that accompany technologies that may profoundly alter persons and preferences over time.

## Acknowledgements

CC is a graduate student in the Faculty of Medicine at the University of British Columbia. She is supported by the Canadian Institutes of Health Research (Canadian Graduate Scholarship-Master's). JI is Canada Research Chair in Neuroethics. This work was supported in part by the National Institutes of Health Research Project Grant #1RF1MH117805-01, Informing Choice for Neurotechnological Innovation in Pediatric Epilepsy Surgery (JI).

## References

Bell, E., Racine, E., Chiasson, P., Dufourcq-Brana, M., Dunn, L.B., Fins, J.J., Ford, P.J., Glannon, W., Lipsman, N., Macdonald, M.E., and Mathews, D.J. (2014). "Beyond Consent in Research: Revisiting Vulnerability in Deep Brain Stimulation for Psychiatric Disorders." *Cambridge Quarterly of Healthcare Ethics*, 23/3: 361–368.

Di Pietro, N.C. and Illes, J. (2013). "Disclosing Incidental Findings in Brain Research: The Rights of Minors in Decision-Making." *Journal of Magnetic Resonance Imaging*, 38/5: 1009–1013.

Gilbert, F., Cook, M., O'Brien, T., and Illes, J. (2017). "Embodiment and Estrangement: Results From a First-in-Human 'Intelligent BCI' Trial." *Science and Engineering Ethics*, https://doi.org/10.1007/s11948-017-0001-5.

Grootens-Wiegers, P., Hein, I. M., van den Broek, J. M., and de Vries, M. C. (2017). "Medical Decision-Making in Children and Adolescents: Developmental and Neuroscientific Aspects." *BMC Pediatrics*, 17/1: 120.

Hein, I.M., Troost, P. W., Lindeboom, R., Benninga, M. A., Zwaan, C. M., Goudoever, J. B., and van Lindauer, R. J. L. (2014). "Accuracy of the MacArthur Competence Assessment Tool for Clinical Research for Measuring Children's Competence to Consent to Clinical Research." *JAMA Pediatrics*, 168/12: 1147–1153.

Kipnis, K. (2001). *Vulnerability in Research Subjects: A Bioethics Taxonomy, in National Bioethics Advisory Commission (NBAC), Ethical and Policy Issues in Research Involving Human Participants. Volume II: Commissioned Papers.* Rockville, MD: NBAC.

Luna, F. (2009). "Elucidating the Concept of Vulnerability: Layers Not Labels." *International Journal of Feminist Approaches to Bioethics*, 2/1: 121–139.

Luna, F. and Vanderpoel, S. (2013). "Not the Usual Suspects: Addressing Layers of Vulnerability." *Bioethics*, 27/6: 325–332.

World Health Organization, Council for International Organizations of Medical Sciences (CIOMS) (2017). *International Ethical Guidelines for Health-Related Research Involving Humans.* Geneva: CIOMS.

# 20

# Differing Understandings of Informed Consent

## Commentary on Howell and Shogren (Chapter 3)

*Jack Trammell*

The history of disability in the West is largely a 2000-year-old or longer dialogue intimately connected to consent. Owing to the chronic power imbalance between people with disabilities and the ablest majority, the conversation has most often been one-sided. In Chapter 3, Britteny Howell and Karrie Shogren implicitly suggest that the only way to change that overarching ablest ontology, which still influences the development of research methodology and consent, is to consider different understandings of what informed consent is (and thus also how we obtain it). They maintain that ethical research cannot be conducted without developing those understandings and methodologies more overtly, completely, and richly.

In Shakespearean terms, twenty-first-century researchers are often "hoist by their own petard" when they design studies that rely on informed consents, but can only achieve them through means that are not always consensual. Many studies are, as the authors point out, designed to reduce the very disparities that contribute to the suppression of the disabled voice, yet also struggle methodologically to pass the first hurdle of true informed consent. They also are forced to coexist in a scholarly environment where disability is often ignored. In cases with guardians, proxies, or other representative counsel, the problem is particularly exacerbated. The variation of understandings of consent within universities, disciplines, and even amongst individual researchers and doctors complicates the task.

The authors identify one of the key tensions to be debated but perhaps never fully resolved, which is how to define acceptable levels of risk. All human research is inherently risky, and, in particular, in the social sciences where studies often focus on marginalized or stigmatized populations. In some cases, proxies or guardians must examine the risk for their family member or ward, and they also are subject to the variation in interpretation that is inherent in accessing human risk. Howell and Shogren make it clear that effective communication is key, but that consent is also predicated on accurate assessment and a shared agreement about meanings, definitions, and terms. Beyond communication, the authors call for "capacity building" (allowing a bigger bandwidth for consent) and "adapted consent" (targeting specialized populations with specialized consents).

A key principle in all conversations about consent is also the concept of right to participation. The Disability Rights Movement has adopted from its origins the idea that full participation in all meaningful, and "everyday" activities (the language of the Americans with Disabilities Act) is the ultimate goal to be achieved. The right to participate in research may seem somewhat removed from the right to public transportation, or the right to a free and public education. In reality, the progress in disability accommodation and awareness that has been made in the past several decades, particularly in the West, simply raises the bar higher, and tantalizingly closer to a fuller inclusion. That includes the right to participate in research. The authors of this chapter locate that higher bar, and argue that we are obligated to reach it, and then push it higher. The subject/participants voice must be heard as part of that process.

The degree of paternalism still identifiable in research ethics is an impediment to moving the bar, and a residue from centuries of second-class status of people with disabilities. Whether considering people with intellectual disabilities, or individuals with other disabilities such as mental health concerns, the default mindset carried forward to this point still often fails to address what the authors refer to as the critical "socio-ecological" variables, and this design flaw persists into present studies and current research programs.

Some professionals, such as medical doctors, might argue that the socio-ecological variables are much harder to measure, and oversimplify a process that should involve more concrete knowledge from well-known medical and psychological domains. Howell and Shogren show research, however, that documents how potential subjects who are blocked from participating due to guardianship, proxy, or capability concerns about self-determination often rate their exclusion as more harmful than do other parties involved. Clearly, their voice is not always heard, or the determining authority in the choice that is made.

The authors find many of these realities in the current research paradigm "troubling," as indeed we all should. The checkered history of eugenics, progressivism, and large-scale wellness initiatives is filled with mistakes, discrimination, and outright abuse. It's not just that we should hold ourselves to a higher standard (as Institutional Review Boards (IRBs) justifiably intend), it's that we need to make the standard as complex as the subjects it applies to. We need to hold ourselves accountable in the academy for our difficulty in understanding intellectual disabilities, mental health concerns, and other disabilities.

There should be no unnecessary limitations placed on people with disabilities in their participation that are there due to a lack of awareness, sophistication, or care in design by the parties actually conducting the research. This is a potential form of passive harm and/or discrimination, completely unintended, seldom identified by IRBs, and which the authors maintain is much more common than we think. In erring on the side of what we think is caution, there are many cases where we actually initiate a kind of injury (not recognizing in an ecological and social way a subject's own complex agency and their right to express it).

This may at first seem somewhat contradictory and quixotic. But if one accepts the basic premise that we need to develop more sophisticated understandings and mechanisms to measure consent, then the only way to avoid the petard-hoisting is to engage in much closer examination of the ethical and methodological assumptions that undergird all current understandings of what consent is, and not be afraid to question them, modify them, and validate them. We owe this to all peoples who legally have the right to participate in any major life activities.

# 21

# The Mindset of Surrogates and Inclusivity Research

## Commentary on Howell and Shogren (Chapter 3)

*Deborah R. Barnbaum*

### Surveying the strengths

There are myriad strengths in Britteny Howell and Karrie Shogren's well-researched and thoughtful essay. They do an excellent job mustering empirical evidence that the systematic under-representation of persons with intellectual disability (ID) results from a variety of factors, including a lack of understanding on the part of Institutional Review Boards (IRBs) and proxy decision-makers about the capacities and strengths of persons with ID. Rather than rely on surrogate decision-makers, Howell and Shogren endorse supported decision-making as means of helping persons with ID retain greater agency. They appear to endorse teach-back methods to foster greater understanding of informed consent documents, but rightly point out that some assessments to test capacity to consent create greater burdens for, and a heightened level of paternalism towards, persons with ID. Participant models that involve persons with ID in all aspects of the research process—creating research methodologies, serving on IRBs, conferring with researchers during the research process—will go great lengths towards more equitable participation. Throughout, Howell and Shogren endorse models that focus on strengths and capacities, rather than on deficits.

### Three bases of surrogate consent, and what they tells us about surrogates' paternalism

One challenge to equitable enrollment cited by Howell and Shogren is that 50% of persons with ID have legal guardians charged with making proxy decisions on their behalf. Even when persons with ID are legally authorized to make decisions for themselves, some consent documents are not written to be accessible to persons with ID, and, again, a guardian is charged with offering consent. Howell and Shogren observe that these surrogate decision-makers are often reluctant to enroll persons with ID.

While Howell and Shogren point out that, ideally, surrogates are not used, and persons with ID are permitted to enroll in research on their own, this is not always possible.

Using Howell and Shogren's terminology, I will refer to the person with ID who is unable to consent as a "ward," and the surrogate decision-maker as a "guardian." There are three philosophical justifications for surrogate consent. Recognizing these three standards may contribute to more equitable participation of persons with ID in research.

The first is to make a decision based on a *substituted judgment*. In this case, the guardian makes a choice based on the ward's individual beliefs, preferences, and desires (Beauchamp and Childress, 2013, p. 227). Responsible decision-making using the substituted judgment standard requires the guardian to articulate not what the guardian wants, but what the ward would say that the ward wants, were the ward in a position to articulate a choice. Hence, the guardian is substituting the ward's beliefs, preferences, and desires for their own. In relying on the individual beliefs, preferences, and desires of the ward, the substituted judgment standard privileges the principle of autonomy.

The second is to make a decision based on a *best interest standard*. In this case, the guardian makes a choice based on what is in the ward's best interest (Beauchamp and Childress, 2013, p. 228). According to the best-interest standard the principle of beneficence is paramount.

The third is to make a decision in virtue of the ward being a member of a given community, and, in particular, a *community of illness*, and what the ward would want in virtue of that community membership (Brown, 2006). It is not ward's individual values that determine the correct surrogate decision, as in the substituted judgment standard. Rather, it is the conjecture that as a member of a community of illness, the ward would want what would be in *the best interest of that community of illness*. The assumption is that the ward has an affinity with others in the ward's community, and would want to help fellow community members. While the community-of-illness standard attempts to replicate what the ward would want, similar to the substituted judgment standard, this standard relies on communitarian values rather than on individualistic values embraced by the principle of autonomy, *per* the substituted judgment standard.

While there is discussion as to which of these three standards should have preference in any given situation, my purpose here is not to argue for the superiority of one of these standards over the others, merely articulating the distinction among the three.

Given this mapping of ways in which guardians can make decisions on the part of wards, how do surrogates who make decisions on the part of persons with ID fare? Not well, unfortunately. Howell and Shogren cite Swaine et al. (2011), to demonstrate that legal guardians of persons with ID are considerably less likely to agree to research participation on the part of persons with ID than are persons with ID. They observe that this points to a troubling failure of legal guardians to share the same values and preferences as their wards. This failure may account for the inability of legal guardians to make genuine substituted judgments on behalf of persons with ID.

Howell and Shogren cite the findings of McDonald et al. (2015) that guardians consistently overestimate the risks of harm in research participation. Surrogate decision-makers who are unable estimate risks and harms to accurately will be unable to employ the best-interest standard.

Finally, Howell and Shogren cite McDonald et al. (2013), who observe that persons with ID recognize research participation as a way of helping others, as well as a way to contribute to knowledge about persons with ID. Community inclusion is a value shared by many persons with ID, according to Dean et al. (2016), as cited by Howell and Shogren. Were surrogate decision-makers aware of these facts, they would be in a position to employ the community-of-illness standard. The fact that surrogates are not endorsing research participation at the rates that persons with ID would prefer raises the possibility that the community-of-illness justification may be similarly under-utilized.

## Using the three bases of surrogate consent to promote inclusion

I agree with Howell and Shogren that involving persons with ID in the consenting process, without surrogate decision-makers, is the best way to contribute to autonomy for persons with ID. But in lieu of consent from persons with ID, it may be helpful to communicate with surrogates prior to their determination about research participation by their wards, about three possible justifications for their decisions, so the surrogates can clarify the basis for their decision. Imagine a situation in which a legally authorized guardian denies their ward's participation in research, even though the ward expresses a preference to participate. Was the guardian's decision based on a *substituted judgment*, and, if so, *can the surrogate articulate the values of the person with ID that would preclude research participation*? Was this decision based on the *best-interest standard*, and, if so, *is the surrogate's assessment of the benefits and harms of research participation accurate, or exaggerated*? Was the decision based on the *community-of-illness standard*, and, if so, *does the surrogate have a good sense of the person with ID's identification with, valuing of, and desire to help a community of other individuals with ID*? As Howell and Shogren point out, half of persons with ID have legal guardians who are charged with making decisions on their behalf. Giving guardians a conceptual framework that allows them to articulate the basis for their decision may help them better represent those for whom they speak.

## References

Beauchamp, T. L. and Childress, J. F. (2013). *The Principles of Biomedical Ethics*. New York: Oxford University Press.

Brown, B. F. (2006). "Proxy Consent for Research on the Incompetent Elderly," in Mapps, T. A. and DeGrazia, D. (eds.) *Biomedical Ethics*, 6th ed. New York: McGraw Hill, pp. 240–247.

Dean, E. E., Fisher, K. W., Shogren, K. A., and Wehmeyer, M. L. (2016). "Participation and Intellectual Disability: A Review of the Literature." *Intellectual and Developmental Disabilities*, 54/6: 427–439.

McDonald, K. E., Kidney, C. A., and Patka, M. (2013). "'You Need to Let Your Voice be Heard': Research Participants' Views on Research." *Journal of Intellectual Disability Research*, 57/3: 216–225.

McDonald, K. E., Schwartz, N. M., Gibbons, C. M., and Olick, R. S. (2015). "'You Can't be Cold and Scientific:' Community Views on Ethical Issues in Intellectual Disability Research." *Journal of Empirical Research on Human Research Ethics*, 10/2: 196–208.

Swaine, J., Parish, S. L., Luken, K., and Atkins, L. (2011). "Recruitment and Consent of Women With Intellectual Disabilities in a Randomised Control Trial of a Health Promotion Intervention." *Journal of Intellectual Disability Research*, 55/5: 474–483.

# 22

# Drawing Distinctions Among Different Types of Research on Persons with Autism

## Commentary on Richman (Chapter 5)

*Deborah R. Barnbaum*

### Several strengths

Professor Richman does us a service by laying out a philosophical analysis of "autonomy" and its limitations as a basis for informed consent. Richman does an impressive job examining the elements of informed consent, and the ways in which capacities of persons with autism ("autists," per his terminology) may challenge traditional notions of informed consent. His discussion of voluntariness and its limitations among autists when consenting to research is particularly compelling, as well as his concerns that guardians should be wary of subtle coercion.

Richman's observation about possible mismatch between the goals of the autist who participates in research, and the goals of parents/guardians or researchers, is instructive. Quoting Jonas, Richman argues that authentic consent requires the goals of the *research participant* and the goals of the *researcher* align. A mismatch can occur when the ultimate goal of research into autism spectrum disorder (ASD) is a cure or elimination of autism. Per Richman, "A great many autists find their autism to be a neutral or positive part of who they are." As such, research geared toward fundamentally changing who an autist is may be viewed differently from the perspective of the research participant and the researcher.

Since the focus of Richman's chapter is on autonomy considerations his concerns regarding the "mismatch" focus on the way in which research goals might not reflect the authentic preferences of research participants. However, there is another way of making sense of this mismatch—it may be that the mismatch occurs when there is a gulf between what researchers believe is beneficial to research participants and their cohorts, and what participants see as beneficial to themselves or fellow autists. Later I expand on this possibility by examining a distinction among different types of research on autists.

## A distinction worth making

Richman raises the concern that some research on autists—research that aims at a cure, or that eliminates some behaviors considered soothing by autists—is research to which many participants may object. A distinction among types of research on autists would further elaborate on the ways in which some research may be objectionable, but some may be unobjectionable, and, in fact, welcome to the autist community. Like Richman, I will restrict my discussion to autists participating in research on autism itself. Additionally, my distinction is among types of interventional research, and not epidemiological research that does not directly engage autists. Let us draw the following distinction:

(1) Research on comorbidities associated with ASD, such as testing a new probiotic to treat gastrointestinal (GI) problems commonly associated with ASD.
(2) Research on programs that allow autists to better navigate the neurotypical world, such as testing a 3-month "work skills" program that teaches autists how to navigate shared break rooms, team meetings, and supervisor evaluations.
(3) Research on interventions designed to treat core deficits in autism, such as medications designed to augment executive function or theory of mind.

The first category of research is designed to benefit directly persons with ASD. While it may be up for debate whether ASD is harmful for autists, in light of many autism advocates' view that ASD is not, in fact, a disability, it is widely understood that the comorbidities associated with autism (GI problems, seizure disorders) *are* harmful for autists. Thus, this first category of research may directly help some of the persons in the study, as well as help future cohorts of those participants. Insofar as there is little debate as to the benefit of this research, either from the point of view of autists or the neurotypical community, this first type of research is not controversial.

The second category of research is more complex. On one hand, it may directly benefit participants and their future cohorts. On the other hand, this research is premised on the belief that the burden of conforming to the world of neurotypicals should be borne by persons who are neurodiverse—"oppressive socialization," using Sisti and Stramondo's terminology (2015). This may be true in some cases (there probably cannot be two sets of rules for driving cars, one each for members of the neurodiverse and the neurotypical communities), but not in others (the burden to communicate appropriately employee evaluations to otherwise excellent employees should be on the supervisor, not the neurodiverse employee). As such, this second category of research may be of direct benefit to autists who participate, and to future cohorts of persons with autism, but it may not be. This type of research needs to be assessed on a case-by-case basis, as it may prove to not align with the interests of autist participants.

The third category of research—the one that Richman spends the most time on—is the most complex because it is not at all clear that such research will be of benefit to autists, and may, in fact, be harmful. Research meant to "cure" persons of autism is predicated on the view that ASD is always harmful for autists, a view Richman observes to be "profoundly offensive" to some autism advocates. Beyond research that aims to cure autism, other research that might fall into this category could include research to reduce "stimming" behaviors, potentially annoying to neurotypicals, but which may serve a valuable calming purpose to some autists. Restricting hand flapping may soothe neurotypical sensibilities at the dinner table, but for some autists, hampering stimming may do more harm than good. This is an example of changing an autist's behavior being more disabling than autism itself, a point that Richman attributes to Milton and Moon (2012). Richman's claim that participants should "identify" with the goals of the researchers becomes salient at this juncture. If an autist holds that being "cured" of autism, or stimming behaviors, would do them harm, that view must be respected. A further complication arises when a given participant believes their life would be better without the core deficits that contribute to autism, or without stimming behaviors, a view not universally shared among autists. Thus, this third type of research is the most ethically challenging.

The point in drawing this three-fold distinction should be clear: The ethics of each of these types of research is different, precisely because of the differences amongst the possibility of benefit, and possibility of harm, associated with each.

Richman's essay was focused primarily on ways autonomy may be compromised in ASD, and autonomy's implications for research that may ultimately lead to a cure for autism. A discussion of different *types* of research that autists might participate in, and the ethical implications of each, based on a conception of who benefits from each type of research, would have been a welcome addition to this impressive chapter.

## References

Milton, D. and Moon, L. (2012). "The Normalisation Agenda and the Psycho-Emotional Disablement of Autistic People." *Autonomy, the Critical Journal of Interdisciplinary Autism Studies*, 1.

Sisti, D. and Stramondo, J. (2015). "Competence, Voluntariness, and Oppressive Socialization: A Feminist Critique of the Threshold Elements of Informed Consent." *International Journal of Feminist Approaches to Bioethics*, 8/1: 67–85.

# 23

# A Critical Lens on Disability and Consent

## Commentary on Patterson and Block (Chapter 6) and on Mehmood (Chapter 14)

*Allison Bloom*

In their two chapters, Stephanie Patterson and Pamela Block (Chapter 6) and Saira A. Mehmood (Chapter 14) draw from their scholarly experiences to reflect on debates about disability and research participation. As Patterson and Block note, an exploitative history of biomedical research has necessitated institutional and federal standards to prohibit unethical research on unwilling and uninformed participants. However, all three authors question the notion of "vulnerability" as a measure for determining the capacity for consent among people considered part of the "disability community." Across this varied—and often fluid—community of people who might consider themselves (or be otherwise categorized as) disabled, they ask what it means to "be vulnerable" or to "consent." Moreover, both chapters offer practical suggestions that aim to take this assessment of disability, vulnerability, and consent into critical consideration with respect to policy and research design. Drawing on these insights, I suggest additional areas for further reflection and the need for a more critical lens on the meaning and experience of disability within protocols for consent.

Patterson and Block foreground the issue of how generalizations are made about people with disabilities. They urge researchers to look at an individual's "daily sociocultural framework" as a means for gauging concerns about a person's ethical participation in a particular research setting. This point is especially relevant when we consider the important distinction in disability theory between "debility" and "disability." Through this framework, "debility"—which Julie Livingston (2005) uses to include impairments alongside chronic illness and aging—refers to how some people may be less capable of certain activities than others, while "disability" acknowledges how societies are built around an assumption of what all people can do; consequently, people with debilities are rendered disabled by these social structures (Livingston, 2005; Shakespeare, 2006). Therefore, not only do we need to consider a person's "daily sociocultural framework" to understand their potential relationship to a research study, but we also need this consideration to understand what circumstances may render them disabled, and how research itself can be further disabling when this critical lens is neglected.

We can see this complex triangulation between disability, debility, and consent through a telling example from Block's own research. Block and her research coordinator faced significant resistance to a project by an Institutional Review Board member who did not believe anyone with a traumatic brain injury (TBI) could ever consent to participate in research. Yet for this same project, Block's research coordinator had a TBI, after which she went on to obtain her master's degree. This example embodies the socially constructed nature of "disability" and the cross-disciplinary need for a more critical lens on variations in disability experiences.

Patterson and Block further suggest that focusing on "the capacity to consent and the power to resist manipulation" in general—rather than disability status—are more accurate benchmarks for research design. The point is not that people with disabilities should be treated the same as those without, but that everyone comes into a research environment with their own advantages and disadvantages. Thus, as they succinctly describe, "There is nothing inherently vulnerable in the state of being physically disabled or even cognitively disabled that would render an individual incapable of autonomous decision-making—these decisions must be made on a case-by-case basis."

This discussion highlights how structural inequalities are important dimensions to consider when developing protocols around consent. Disabled individuals with access to resources and prestige may not fit with the definition of "vulnerable" in the way that someone with far less privilege would, disabled or not. Based on my own professional and research experiences with immigrant survivors of domestic violence—women who were often undocumented, impoverished, and with few social supports—many extremely vulnerable people may suffer physically, cognitively, or emotionally with debilities that go unidentified and unaccommodated for much of their lives. Therefore, receiving a diagnosis for a debilitating injury, cognitive impairment, or chronic illness and being recognized by clinicians, social workers, and researchers as "disabled" is already a marker of access to resources. Disability is just one dimension within a much larger web of considerations around inequality and consent.

Through this "case-by-case" approach, the researcher will also encounter vastly different cultural conceptions of disability. These conceptualizations must also be taken into account when gauging someone's disability experience. The way someone's family understands and responds to a debility, for example, or the way an individual conceptualizes their debility, have a profound effect on that person's cognitive and physical relationship to the world. Furthermore, not only is disability a culturally contingent experience, but as Mehmood also observed, it can be a fluid one—particularly as people age, most will find themselves at some point disabled. Thus, with respect to disability, rather than a singular burden on the part of the researcher, determining capacity to consent must also be approached as a dialectical exchange. That person's own perception of their debilities in relation to the world around them must be taken into account.

While working on a "case-by-case basis" is important, this still leaves questions around design and implementation. Mehmood provides helpful insights on these practical dimensions. During her study at a center serving people with chronic mental illness in New Orleans, like Patterson and Block, she came to question the vagueness of vulnerability and consent. As a medical anthropologist, she emphasizes how ethnographic methods are useful for assessing participants not only on a "case-by-case" basis, but for also assessing how capacity to consent may shift over time.

Mehmood's methods ought to serve as a reminder to researchers of a key tenet for long-term research: that consent should be an ongoing process throughout the duration of the study. Among her research participants, their everyday lives were ever-shifting and complex, so that the instruments required by her protocol were insufficient. Instead, ethnographic methods gave much-needed depth to her consent protocols. Working with a population living with chronic mental illness, many participants would go in and out of psychosis and experience different levels of impaired cognition. Her solution was to break the research up into phases, each with a new conversation around consent. While applying ethnographic methods to consent protocols is time consuming, the benefits are worthwhile. Mehmood was able to get to know what members were like in and out of psychosis, and better understand when they were too sick or vulnerable to consent. As such, her methods highlight the ever-shifting nature of a human-research setting. Building on her findings, I underscore for researchers how, in order for consent to be ethical, it should not just be a singular step in a protocol. Approaching consent in a processual way not only reveals shifts in cognition or abilities that can inform a research protocol, but also reveals deeper information around how someone's disability is constructed by their surroundings, and how that person's own relationship to their disability shifts over time. Along with Patterson and Block, Mehmood's findings emphasize how researchers must reflexively assess their processes for determining consent in the context of disability.

These insights, along with the suggestions I have made here, point to the usefulness of a more critical lens on disability when developing these research protocols. Accounting for a participant's particular experience and understanding of disability both enhances the ethicality of that research and provides an avenue for knowledge production within the study itself. This reflexive and critical lens thereby offers a fruitful and more nuanced approach to addressing vulnerability, disability, and consent.

## References

Livingston, J. (2005). *Debility and the Moral Imagination in Botswana*. Bloomington, IN: Indiana University Press.

Shakespeare, T. (2006). *Disability Rights and Wrongs*. New York: Routledge.

# 24

# Repurposing Ethnography to Assess Consent Capacity

## Commentary on Mehmood (Chapter 14)

*Megan S. Wright*

### Introduction

Saira Mehmood illustrates how participant observation, an ethnographic method, can be applied to assess research consent capacity for persons with chronic mental illness who use mental health services at a non-profit organization. Through observation of and interaction with prospective participants and organization staff members, Mehmood was able to get a sense of a mental health service user's decisional capacity and vulnerability. While this is a novel and beneficial approach to assessing consent capacity, questions remain about its application, appropriateness, and usefulness in other contexts.

### Benefits of Multi-Method Assessments of Consent Capacity

The Institutional Review Board (IRB) that provided oversight of Mehmood's qualitative research required her to use decision tree and quiz instruments to assess prospective research participants' consent capacity during the process of obtaining voluntary, informed consent prior to conducting interviews. Mehmood notes problems in using such tools, however, which include causing prospective participants to feel anxious if the instruments are in the form of a quiz and the IRB's implicit assumption that persons without chronic mental illness would answer the questions correctly.[1] Thus, she opted only to use the instruments when "there was a gray area"; that is, when a prospective participant had experienced psychosis but at a later point expressed that they wanted to participate in the research.

Instead, Mehmood relied upon multiple other methods to assess capacity to consent to participate in research. First, she used the mental health staff's judgment of whether

[1] It is unclear whether the tools described in Chapter 14 to evaluate decisional capacity are validated, either for the general population or for persons with chronic mental illness. It would seem highly problematic for IRBs to require use of tools that are not evidence-based.

a prospective participant's demeanor, which could seem to a lay person to indicate decisional impairment, was actually normal for that person (i.e., the person's baseline). Interestingly, however, Mehmood simultaneously critiques relying on staff for information about mental health clients because the staff may make unfounded assumptions about them. Mehmood does not reconcile these contrary views of the helpfulness of staff assessments about service users.

Second, during the participant observation that preceded other parts of data collection, Mehmood also played games such as Monopoly and Rummikub with prospective research participants. Playing games with prospective participants helped Mehmood get a sense of their literacy level, as well as change in their cognitive status over time. Low literary can indicate a need to change the process of conveying information about the research study. Poorer play compared with a previous game may indicate increased cognitive impairment, which has implications for consent capacity.

There were several benefits to using participant observation, which included interaction both with prospective research participants and mental health staff who provided informal capacity assessments of the participants, prior to conducting the interviews. First, consent capacity can be assessed over a period of time rather than at one point in time, which may permit more people to participate in the research even if they sometimes experience psychosis. Second, seeing the participant in a variety of settings may indicate a vulnerability that may not be as apparent in a one-on-one informed consent conversation immediately preceding a qualitative interview. Evaluating behavior in a broader context can thus function as a safeguard to ensure voluntary, informed consent is obtained.

## Appropriate application of ethnographic method to assess consent capacity

Mehmood notes that a period of participant observation long enough to assess capacity is "time-consuming and work[s] best in non-clinical research projects." While time constraints are an obvious limitation on this method of assessing consent capacity, it is not as clear why clinical research projects as a category may not benefit from this approach. There are other limitations to using participant observation to identify decisional impairments and assess consent capacity, however.

First, to be able to use participant observation, consent from prospective participants or waiver of informed consent requirements from an IRB is necessary.[2] In the former case, using participant observation to assess consent capacity is impossible because one would already need consent to be doing the ethnography (i.e., consent would be required to assess consent capacity, which is illogical). In the latter case, permission

[2] This requirement may differ depending upon jurisdiction, however. In Canada, for example, research ethics boards may not require informed consent for exploratory research that includes observation of the type Mehmood describes.

to conduct participant observation without the consent of research participants who are being observed and interacted with would be dependent upon the IRB and the organization being studied. It is not guaranteed that an investigator would be granted this permission.

Second, to be able to use ethnographic methods, one must have received training in ethnography. Researchers whose training has not included ethnographic methods, even if they have been trained in conducting interviews, thus may not be able to use this consent assessment tool appropriately. The potential scope of use may thus be limited to a very small subset of investigators.

Third, it is unclear how participant observation would be useful in assessing consent capacity for potentially vulnerable or decisionally impaired persons when they are not in an institutional or organizational setting. For example, researchers may wish to interview persons who have dementia, a condition that may impair decisional capacity, who reside at their homes, and recruit such participants through a treating physician. There would be no opportunity to spend months observing and interacting with prospective research participants in this instance and many others.

Finally, the ability to use participant observation to assess decisional impairments may be dependent upon the risk–benefit profile of the research question. If the research design contains greater risk to participants than asking them questions about their lives (e.g., clinical trial of a drug or device), then perhaps an IRB should require a more formal capacity assessment as a safeguard.

## Remaining questions and concerns

Just as investigators using ethnography should be trained in the method, it seems reasonable to expect that investigators assessing the consent capacity of a person who may have decisional impairments should be trained in conducting such assessments. Put differently, for certain populations of research subjects, is it appropriate for a qualitative researcher with no expertise in assessing decisional capacity to perform such an assessment? Are there other safeguards that should be considered?

Perhaps an independent professional trained in evaluating decisional capacity should assess capacity during the informed consent process. Independent capacity assessors would bring their expertise to the question of capacity to participate in research, which provides an additional safeguard for the welfare of the prospective research participant. They would also presumably be free of conflicts of interest that exist in the investigator–participant relationship wherein the investigator may be biased toward finding the subject capable of consenting to research so that the investigator is able to collect data and complete their research. Adding another party to the consenting process brings up questions of practicability and resource constraints, however.

# 25

# Using Ethnographic Methods

## Commentary on Mehmood (Chapter 14)

*Jack Trammell*

Universal design principles began in architecture, but are now becoming more widely adopted in areas like higher education, or even in corporate settings. The philosophy behind universal design is that the design process itself can anticipate many diverse human needs in advance of or instead of spending resources on new construction and later retrofit. Likewise, in education, universal design principles suggest that re-conceptualizing consent may alleviate some of the chronic challenges related to conducting research with subjects with intellectual disabilities or other stigmatized populations. Saira Mehmood, in her chapter "Using Ethnographic Methods to Determine Capacity to Consent in Individuals Diagnosed With Chronic Mental Illnesses" (Chapter 14), proposes that the use of ethnographic methods to determine consent can help redefine and classify what participant consent is, most specifically in populations with chronic mental illness.

In the three-phase ethnographic project the author conducted, participant observation played a key role. Many previous efforts at inclusion, including participation in major research projects, have been based intentionally or mostly unintentionally on the assumptions of the deficit model, which seeks to change, cure, or "treat" individuals, rather than to understand fully their behavior and intelligence in complete and ethical context. Such problematic assumptions result in obvious challenges to obtaining true consent in at-risk populations owing to the possibilities that participants may not understand more traditional measures, questions, or formats; even if participants understand the consent formats intellectually, they may not completely connect with them on a practical level, where, arguably, the most meaningful spectrum of consent takes place.

The author spent many hours with the study subjects, participating in the same activities as they did, observing and noting various individual behaviors and conversations as a supplement to the information coming from stigma scales and more structured interviews. There was a concerted effort to understand the subjects before trying to understand the consent. This highlights a wider need that the author clearly identifies, which is the need for new methodologies and techniques that specifically target intellectual disability (ID) and other stigmatized populations for more sophisticated, flexible, and inclusive forms of consent.

Of course, if such changes were simple many of them would have already been implemented. The complexity of consent, coupled with the lack of detailed guidance in earlier research or in earlier agency policies, clearly places the onus for such changes on researchers with careers and agendas that take them into researching ID, or stigmatized subjects. This onus is appropriate from a historical perspective; it is problematic if it is stagnant, inflexible, or routinized to bureaucracy. The author highlights a decision tree that was used to help determine a subject's capability to give consent in this study; there is clearly an imperative for researchers in this area to be more proactive in defining and accommodating for true consent, even if it means more methodological and overall work in preparing a study.

It will, perhaps, make some stakeholders nervous to re-conceptualize consent, in part as more of a judgment or a more subjective evaluation by the researcher, or "expert." Many advocates for people with ID, or other stigmatized populations, have a justifiable skepticism about doctors, psychologists, or counselors whose expertise might override the patient's voice, agency, and true needs. In fact, there is a history of this happening that is widely recognized in the literature. In using diary excerpts later in the project, the researcher in this study was able to see the results of her initial evaluations and later consents, and this post hoc examination is often missing in the broader consent problems mentioned earlier.

The author also stresses the importance of creative thinking. Using simple board games and card games as a "warm up," the author was able to watch "decisional capacity" before starting more formal consent procedures. This is not, in fact, the typical way consents are implemented, but it demonstrates the need to re-conceptualize, and to rethink, how previous understandings of consent may have been biased by notions about intelligence and ability that inadvertently colored (and still do) research designs and implementation that might otherwise seem very sound, and pass muster with Institutional Review Boards (IRBs) and other panels.

My conclusion from Mehmood's work is that we need to pause, and allow ourselves to recognize that some of what we have considered best practice in the past may not work "best" now for special populations, particularly those with stigmatized identities. Consent is a basic human right (or should be), and is the part of all human subject research that transcends other variables in ethical importance (in my opinion), and where, unfortunately, the track record of the sciences and social sciences is a tainted history that does not inspire confidence if examined by twenty-first-century standards. We have learned as we have stumbled, of course, and the existence of IRBs is a reaction to those challenges.

But the IRB process and related initiatives are subject to their own subjectivities, time, and place, and the author of this study believes that, ultimately, rethinking consent will save time and be more beneficial for all parties involved. This suggests an overarching need for a "universal design" in research methodology that is sorely lacking at this time.

# 26

# Joining Voices

## Commentary on Kohler (Chapter 17)

*Anne Kohler and Benjamin Majewski*

In Chapter 17 "Assuming Capacity," one section details the process of recruiting, hiring, and training a research assistant with an intellectual disability to provide other researchers with a blueprint for doing the same. The chapter is necessarily written from Anne Kohler's perspective as principal investigator. This commentary brings in Benjamin Majewski's perspective as a researcher with Down syndrome. When the researchers started thinking about how to write a commentary together on Ben's experience working as a research assistant, Anne felt it was important to ensure that Ben would be able to share his experiences without being constrained by the very academic conventions that this volume critically examines. How to demonstrate his careful engagement with the process of research? They decided upon a loosely guided conversation in which Ben would be given the chance to reflect on his role as a research assistant. In what follows they discuss the role of research for people with Down syndrome, consent, research methodology, and the challenging and rewarding dimensions of social science research. Anne's questions are in bold, and Ben's responses in unbolded text.[1]

---

**So, what's it been like being a research assistant?**

It's been a lot of fun.

**Yeah?**

It's been a lot of fun. I've learned a lot of different things that I haven't really done before.

**Like what?**

Data analysis, highlighting and coding, doing a lot of interviews. Yeah, and doing our research, and it's something that I really enjoy doing, really. And I will look back and reflect on how much of an impact it's been for me. Now I know what it's like to see people

[1] The transcript has been lightly edited for clarity and conciseness.

with Down syndrome, to know that with my help and the research that we're doing? To see people with Down syndrome—wow, what a difference. And from my work as a research assistant, it makes me feel sad now that you're leaving [ . . . ] And it's a good time to look back on what our work means for people with Down syndrome, and how our work can make a big impact on them.

**So, what do you think our work does mean for people with Down syndrome? In your view?**

It helps me to learn more, and to learn to see that there is a lot of work that needs to be done.

**Definitely. So, what would you say to someone who didn't think that you should involve someone with Down syndrome as a research assistant?**

I would say that you should hire more researchers [and] self-advocates to be research assistants. There is so much that they can do.

[ . . . ]

**So, what has been something that's been difficult or challenging about being part of the research, or being a research assistant?**

The work that we do can be challenging. Doing coding, and all that stuff. I really haven't done that before, and now I kind of know that I can do it, that I can actually do something with pen and paper.

**Yeah, and you were great at it too. Yeah, so it was challenging but to me it was rewarding to work together, and to figure it out. So, why do you think research is important?**

Because I think it's everywhere, and you definitely see it. It informs. We see it in hospitals, we see it in science labs, we see it in the world, the world today. [ . . . ] So, just going back home tonight, get into bed, I will be thinking to myself "wow, I get it, I made a difference today."

[ . . . ]

**So, what would you say to someone—maybe if someone says "it's not important to do research on Down syndrome"?**

That is not true. It's false. There's a lot of work to do. There's so much. There's research, everywhere, and there's so much to do to make a difference.

**What would you hope to see come out of research on Down syndrome? What do you think the goal for you would be of research on Down syndrome?**

That's a tough one. I really haven't had a goal before, but I know what a goal is. A goal for me would be—I'm not really sure yet.

**That's okay! So, we know research solves a problem, right? And answers a question—so, what problems, are there any problems you would want to see solved or questions you would want answered about Down syndrome?**

Well, there's a lot, there's a lot of problems. Being out in the world—there's going to be issues along the way. And we have to deal with them, and try to move on, try to solve one problem so it won't escalate even further. So, what I try to do is not let that happen, and just stay at it. Stay positive.

**Yeah. So, we're going to write a book chapter—so, it's very short, maybe a couple of pages, and a lot of our conversation will be part of the book chapter. But is there anything you want the world to know about you, or about being a research assistant, or about having Down syndrome that you want to share in the book chapter?**

I am someone who has Down syndrome, is a research assistant and resource specialist at a Down syndrome clinic. It's a lot of fun, but there are a lot of challenges that you are going to face. [ ... ] So, I think it's important for me but also for people with Down syndrome that there's so many jobs you can do. Research assistant, resource specialist, a bus boy. Bus boys, researchers, research assistants, anthropologist—there are so many jobs for people with Down syndrome, so many jobs. They can do anything.

**They can do anything, you're right. Do you think inclusion is important?**

Inclusion is very important. We want to be included, to be on the team. And to think outside of the box, you know? Two outs, bases loaded, and—go Red Sox! [ ... ] Again, I think what is important is that we benefit others. Benefit from being and working in a hospital, in a hospital setting, a restaurant, or [a grocery store], or a pizza place. There [are] so many jobs for a lot of people.

**Do you think being included in research is important?**

Oh, of course! Research is everywhere.

**Yeah. So, tell me about this presentation that you're now going to be giving in clinic.**

So, I'm going to do this a lot more in clinic. I will use my PowerPoint.

**And what are you trying to teach other adults with Down syndrome?**

I'm trying to teach that there is research out there for people with Down syndrome, and they can say "oh, I want to be a research assistant, I want to do that." And then I will tell them about it. You have to fill out an application. There's a lot more to do!

**Definitely. And you're going to—so, one of the most important things is that it's peoples choice [to participate], right? Why is it so important that people can chose whether or not to participate in research?**

Well, consenting, getting permission.

**You know that maybe 50 or 60 years ago people didn't use to ask permission from people with Down syndrome to participate?**

Maybe that was the case then!

**But not now?**

Not now!

# 27

# What Stories Tell? In Praise of Anthropology

## Commentary on Kohler (Chapter 17)

*Leonardo Carbonieri Campoy*

When it comes to disability, it is usually understood that anthropology, the discipline in which Anne Kohler and I both work, offers the knowledge that disabled people have more potential and capability than often others have imagined. Going deep into the "native's point of view" (Geertz, 1983) and presenting the particular contexts under scrutiny without presuppositions or impulsive judgments, anthropologists seek to make the reader question the idea that disability could be understood by the "missing," as a "monstrosity" or a condition of being "less human" than that which is usually taken as normal or typical.

Chapter 17 makes us think about how this kind of knowledge can be produced. Kohler argues that the possibility of knowing the lives of people with intellectual disabilities without reproducing values and conceptions of normality depends heavily on the way we do our research. Here is where the trick, or the magic, of anthropology happens. It is not on its theories or even on its methods, but on a constant quest for a perspective by which our interlocutors are not interpreted through stereotypes or preconceptions socially impinged on them. We are persistently trying to understand the people we work with by their own terms.

Reading Chapter 17 and considering my own research experiences, I reaffirmed an assumption that I already held, one which states that it takes a lot of effort to build this kind of understanding. After all, Kohler reminds us, we anthropologists were mainly raised in a social setting built on exclusionary conceptions of normality. If we do not watch ourselves, we can project these conceptions on our studies. Kohler rightly points to where the danger of this projection lies: on the notions of personhood.

Perhaps unconsciously, anthropologists may expect people with intellectual disabilities to speak about their lives and perspectives in the same way as they would themselves, practicing intellectual skills and abilities as they themselves would do it. In the discrepancy between what the research participants present and what anthropologists expect of them, the exclusionary classification may emerge, as if sentences were not being well said, words were not being correctly used, memory was not working well—in short as if narratives were not being properly deployed. Anthropologists might wonder whether the narratives of people with intellectual disabilities can be taken as "good data."

Instead of expecting specific ways of talking, thinking, and memorizing from our interlocutors, that is to say, of enacting their personhood, can we anthropologists rethink our own ways of doing research with people with intellectual disabilities? Instead of asking if their narratives are "good or bad data," can we question if the methods we use to collect them are "good or bad methods?"

That is the question that orients Chapter 17, to which Kohler offers interesting answers. If Bourdieu et al. (1991) propose an epistemological vigilance for research in social science, Kohler advances this project by proposing, for intellectual disabilities, not only a methodological, but especially an ontological vigilance on the part of anthropologists. If, as Bachelard (1986) asserts, the method of research is already a determinant of theory, then the ways in which we investigate intellectual disability are decisive for how we conceive the being in the world of certain people. As Kohler points out:

> [...] in adapting or creating new methods, I believe it is worth rooting such changes in a thorough accounting of how we, as researchers, theorize the personhood of people with intellectual disabilities.

In this sense, the three methodological adaptations that Kohler has crafted in her own research experiences with people with Down syndrome seek to approach the unique ways in which people with intellectual disabilities communicate their narratives and live their lives. Assisted interviewing, adapted photovoice, and hiring a person with intellectual disability as a research assistant are the tools Kohler has conceived to let her perception be driven by the ways her interlocutors understand themselves.

The third is especially notable, since it highlights the political and ethical aspects of doing research with people with intellectual disabilities. Wanting to be sure that her research approach would make sense to her interlocutors—the language of the questionnaires, interview process, and so on—Kohler hired Ben, a young man with Down syndrome, to work with her.

Hiring a research assistant with Down syndrome highlights the political and ethical aspects that are articulated in the whole project of adapting methods to study with people with intellectual disabilities. After all, anthropology, just as any other academic discipline, is not completely neutral or objective (Latour, 1993). We do know that the representations we elaborate on are embedded in political and ethical positions. The point is to have a clear view of these positions and to make sure that we commit ourselves with them on the research process and on its final products. I understand that Kohler and I share the same position: we want to tell stories of the personhoods of people with intellectual disabilities together with them. We want their participation, the most we can get, in the elaboration of narratives about them. To put it simply, we understand that it is the right way of doing anthropology.

For me, here resides the power of anthropology: telling peoples' stories, refusing encasement and its confines, including the values, systems, experts, institutions, and, we may say, consecrated theories and methods. By that refusal, the legitimation of our work does not come from some elite knowledge-maker, self-appointed to speak on behalf of benighted populations. It comes from the participation of this population on the production of our work. With that, we put ourselves in the position to be able to criticize these same elite knowledge-makers.

Kohler concludes by reflecting on how ethnographic data produced by methodological adaptations can be translated to policy audiences. She argues that such adaptations, by bringing the anthropological view closer to people with intellectual disabilities, can refute certain health policies, as well as serve as a source for re-imagining quantitative claims about the health conditions of people with intellectual disabilities.

I agree. In suggesting an anthropological therapy for autistic children (see Chapter 8), I understand that I share Kohler's views: criticizing the mainstream institutions that diagnose, treat, and produce quantitative data about intellectual disabilities by proposing practical alternatives, ones that we believe can be more attentive to the identities and conditions of people with ID. While I underpin my proposal with stories of consultations of autistic children, Kohler constructs her argument with a focus on the narratives of people with Down syndrome. These stories and narratives are what anthropology can promote. Faced with medical categories, quantitative data, and health policies that seem to speak about disabled people from a distant and static point of view, our efforts are to take a closer look at these people's lives. Stories and narratives are the way to go to anthropology achieve this look. A look that resonates with those being looked at.

## References

Bachelard, G. (1986). *The New Scientific Spirit*. Boston, MA: Beacon Press.
Bourdieu, P., Passeron, J.-C., Chamboredon, J.-C. (1991). *The Craft of Sociology*. Berlin: De Gruyter.
Geertz, C. (1983). "From the Native's Point of View": On the Nature of Anthropological Understanding. In: Geertz, C. (ed.) Local Knowledge. New York: Basic Books, pp. 55–71.
Latour, B. (1993). *We Have Never Been Modern*. Boston, MA: Harvard University Press.

## References

# 28

# "Caught Between the Suffering and the Good"

## Commentary on Campoy (Chapter 8)

*Melissa Park and Donald Fogelberg*

### Caught between suffering and the good

Chapter 8 by Leonardo Campoy does not address the ethical pragmatics of research, such as ensuring informed consent and/or using participatory action methods to engage individuals with cognitive differences as co-researchers. Instead, he takes a different tack, asking us consider what we, as researchers, *do* with our findings beyond the dissemination of its results. Specifically, he poses the question: "Why can't an anthropology of health services go beyond words and writings to suggest actions … ," which echoes Behar's (1996) reflections about the ethical call to action of the situations in which ethnographers find themselves. Often framed within rhetorics of social accountability or responsibility, the proliferation of applied humanities programs aligns with a recent shift in anthropology's focus from the *suffering subject*—archetypal figures depicted as "living in pain, in poverty, or under conditions of violence or oppression"—to attend to the good—"well-being, imagination, empathy, care … " (Robbins, 2013, p. 448). Campoy's suggestion is, however, more radical, as he proposes that anthropology could constitute a therapeutic intervention. This arc raises a larger concern: What happens when *responsive* ethnographic research gets "caught" between a concerted focus on the social structures which debilitate human experience and the *care,* itself, that researchers should extend (or not) to research participants through action.

### Terministic screens

Campoy argues that the methods and positioning of the *participant observer* endow anthropologists with (1) a unique positioning within healthcare contexts; (2) a positioning from which they can understand and translate between professionals, children with autism, and their parents—a translational process he suggests could be a "communicational therapy." However, as Burke (1966) noted, a system of terms can act as a screen that favors specific interpretations (and actions) over others. The power of positivist–scientific terms (e.g., "therapy") is not just rhetorical, but linked to the legal, professional, and financial systems which regulate healthcare practices and, ultimately, overshadow the types of experience that one might think anthropology is actually about (Park, 2008). Positivist–scientific terms—already privileged within clinical settings—obligate a set of related actions, such as defining measureable objectives and providing evidence that they have been met. Such an end goal could detract from an anthropological appreciation of the very human experience of illness and/or disability and, specifically, as Kleinman (2006) so well articulated, the very *experiences that really matter*.

## Excavating translational practices

Arguably, anthropological methods allow for extended time in the field that can shift attention to how suffering is not purely individual but social; created and sustained through discursive practices and the "ordinary" (Das, 2006). Yet, Campoy provides a solution without a thick-enough description to support his argument that a failure of translation was at the heart of the suffering he sought to alleviate. The data he draws from are thin, based on four participant observations that never extend beyond the clinic. In contrast, a series of ethnographies following African American children with disabilities and their families in the community before, during, and after healthcare encounters documented the translational practices *already* being done by families and clinicians alike (Mattingly, 2018). Based on over 15 years of participant observations, interviews, and collective narratives, the "Boundary Crossing" studies illustrate how parents of children with disabilities use the terms of biomedicine to engage clinicians in collaborative care, and revealed the equally diligent work of clinicians to translate biomedical procedures into narrative form in attempts to partner up. These translational practices are not reflected in *chart talk* (Mattingly, 1998), because they exist outside the logic of health services and are therefore considered illegitimate (Mattingly and Lawlor, 2001). Perhaps in order to answer Campoy's question of how anthropology, specifically, and research, more broadly, might go beyond words and writings to actions, we might first reflect on how research findings can inform everyday ethical actions.

## Enacting care

Understanding why the particular persons with whom we conduct our research are moved to do what they do from an experiential perspective not only deepens our understanding of the structural constraints in and of health services, but also illuminates how persons create the type of experiences to transform them (Mattingly, 2017). Such experience-near, thick descriptions of what persons with disabilities and families are already doing could be infused into healthcare curricula earlier, potentially re-shaping, even re-purposing health systems to support rather than constrain creative action. Anthropologist and autist Dawn Prince (2010) contrasts her experience of becoming an academic anthropologist with that of being born one. As an academic anthropologist she learned how to segment experience. Conversely, her experience as a "born anthropologist" underscores the *responsiveness of bodily sensing* itself to the situations in which we find ourselves. She first describes the fluidity by which she experiences the world around her, how the smells, sights, and sounds flood into her own self in ways also echoed by other autist advocates (Baggs, 2007; DJ in Rooy, 2017):

> These experiences profoundly inform the ways that I look at anthropology and, over time, redefined anthropology as part of my living body, my desire to create a cohesive world for future generations, to be a *good* anthropologist (Prince, 2010, p. 61).

She then writes about how her son, who has a diagnosis of autism, begins to rock, tantrum, and self-injure when he enters school, becoming "contextually autistic." We take her statement to both explicitly (and implicitly) raise a question—one that carries significant ethical implications: Listening to the wisdom of one's own bodily sensing as being already inherently connected to others (human and otherwise) asks us to reconsider definitions of impairment grounded solely within individual bodies or definitions of inclusion that assume divisions, directionalities, or hierarchies (Park, 2015). More than just proposing participatory methodologies or creating yet another practice profession, this would create a scale of inclusion in which it becomes increasingly difficult to maintain any categories at all, where the best "good" that anthropology might offer is not in any act of translation or communication therapy, but the ways we, ourselves, can listen.

## References


Baggs, A. (2007). "In My Language," https://www.youtube.com/watch?v=JnylM1hI2jc (accessed March 11, 2019).

Behar, R. (1996). *The Vulnerable Observer: Anthropology That Breaks Your Heart*. Boston, MA: Beacon.

Burke, K. (1966). "Terministic Screens," in Burke, K. (ed.) *Language as Symbolic Action: Essays on Life, Literature, and Method*. Los Angeles, CA: University of California Press, pp. 42–62.

Das, V. (2006). *Life and Words: Violence and the Descent Into the Ordinary*. Los Angeles, CA: University of California Press.

Kleinman, A. (2006). What Really Matters: Living a Moral Life Amidst Uncertainty and Danger. Oxford: Oxford University Press.

Mattingly, C. (1998). "In Search of the Good: Narrative Reasoning in Clinical Practice." *Medical Anthropology Quarterly*, 12: 273–297.

Mattingly, C. (2017). "Autism and The Ethics of Care: A Phenomenological Investigation Into the Contagion of Nothing." *Ethos*, 45/2: 250–270.

Mattingly, C. (2018). "The Art of Medicine: Health Care as a Cultural Borderland." *The Lancet*, 391: 198–199.

Mattingly, C. and Lawlor, M. (2001). "The Fragility of Healing." *American Anthropologist*, 29/1: 30–57.

Park, M. (2008). "Making Scenes: Imaginative Practices for a Child With Autism in an Occupational Therapy Session." *Medical Anthropology Quarterly*, 22/3: 234–256.

Park, M. (2015). "Autism Spectrum Disorder and the Manifold Ethnomethodologies of Engagement [Panel]: What moves us: the manifold practices of connectedness between children with autism, their family and therapists in the community and clinic." *American Anthropological Association Conference*, Denver, CO.

Prince, D. E. (2010). "An Exceptional Path: An Ethnographic Narrative Reflecting on Autistic Parenthood from Evolutionary, Cultural, and Spiritual Perspectives." *Ethos*, 38/1: 56–68.
Robbins, J. (2013). "Beyond the Suffering Subject: Toward an Anthropology of the Good." *Journal of the Royal Anthropological Institute*, 19: 447–462.
Rooy, R. (2017). *Deej*. Rooy, R. (director). Rooy Media LL.

# 29

# Toward a Research Ethics Culture of Inclusion and Participation

## Commentary on All Chapters

*Eric Racine*

As a co-editor of this volume, I have learned much from the different contributions about the inclusion and participation of individuals with cognitive differences and impairments which sometimes result in diminished decision-making capacity (or perceptions thereof). Here, I will take for granted the value of research concerning people with cognitive differences and impairments, which is well illustrated in many chapters. I will present and discuss how the culture of research and research ethics poses fundamental challenges to the promotion of inclusive and participatory research. Many of the contributions speak to these issues in different ways, and I here step back and speculate about how we could potentially make progress in tackling these challenges.

### Problematic culture of research and research ethics

A first is to recognize the existence of a problem and many contributions illustrate how the culture of research and research ethics presents challenges to the inclusion and participation of people with cognitive impairments as genuine agents. Some of these include underestimation of the capacity of individuals with cognitive impairments to give consent (Chapters 2 and 14); complexities (some legitimate, some less) in multi-site research, as understandings of cognitive impairment vary (Chapters 3 and 16); and struggles with the notion of vulnerable populations and the concept of vulnerability as a tool intended to protect research participants from abuse (Chapters 1, 6, 7, and 13) but which has unintended implications of over-protectionism (Chapters 10 and 17). All of these challenges (and others) seem to share an underlying cause: the emergence of a research ethics culture which has stressed protection as a fundamental driving value over others, such as inclusion and participation (Emanuel and Grady, 2007; Friesen et al., 2017; Mathews et al., 2018). Historically, protection has been a legitimate response to abuses, including some involving individuals with cognitive impairments. However, I believe that it is now serving as an unscrutinized goal for research ethics guidelines and practices, and that the strict focus on protective measures hinders reflection upon what ethics in research *should be*. Moreover, this protectionist understanding of ethics has been fueled by the legal-minded concerns of academic institutions triggered by worries about litigation and risk exposure, notably in research where sensitive issues and marginalized populations are at stake (Trudel and Jean, 2010; van den Hoonaard and Hamilton, 2016). This has led to a culture of regulatory research ethics (the paradigm of "regulatory protectionism" (Emanuel and Grady, 2007)), which has institutionalized ethics as soft law with bureaucratic and administrative overtones.

The development of regulatory ethics has had the dramatic consequence of taking away a significant portion of ethics from research ethics. Ethics can be properly considered a discipline which openly and critically questions values guiding problematic attitudes and human behaviors, and which uses evidence to support the development of responses that promote the greater well-being of those concerned (Gouinlock, 2002). By this definition, research ethics is only "half-baked" ethics. It does respond to a number of problem situations, and it does promote important goals. However, the field of research ethics has limited its understanding of problem situations to the experiences of only certain stakeholders; it often excludes research participants themselves (Dresser, 2006), as well as researchers who are enculturated to defer their judgments to committees (van den Hoonaard and Hamilton, 2016). It has thus failed to really examine what research participants need and want out of research ethics and how research might fit into their processes of realizing their own agency (Dresser, 2006). The same could be said to some extent about researchers themselves (McDonald et al., 2014; Deslauriers et al., 2010). As many chapters illustrate (Chapters 3, 10, and 16), research ethics has remained overly narrow in focus, with limited investigations into the broader interactions between research and other social systems. The stiffening of research ethics has the unfortunate drawback of making more flexible and personalized approaches—which are often needed to foster the agency of research participants with cognitive impairments and differences—difficult.

Unfortunately, reforms to research ethics policies are often not at all guided by any kind of evidence about the effectiveness of various approaches (Trudel and Jean, 2010; McDonald et al., 2014; Beagan and McDonald, 2005; Deslauriers et al., 2010). Given this, it might be most promising to develop alternative practices for discussion and further reflection on foundational issues. This is where I think the innovations shared in this volume (Chapters 12–17) are remarkably promising and encouraging. They present a path to a renewed research ethics, one that starts from the experiences of researchers and research participants and opens discussion about what research is considered to be and what it implicitly or explicitly values and promotes. Whether this deeper ethics will replace the mainstream regulatory paradigm is an open question. I doubt it would in the short term, owing to the vested stakes in the status quo favoring regulatory ethics. However, although current research ethics may be suboptimal, it should not offset the responsibility, and to some extent, the opportunity, of researchers to own their ethics and develop thoughts and practices that reflect more profoundly the deeper tradition of ethics.

## Supporting a change of culture and practices

The call for a deeper research ethics seen in many chapters of this book (e.g., Chapters 10, 12 15, 16, and 17) should be viewed as an ally by those wanting to reflect on and restate the importance of the commitment of research to human knowledge. Indeed, the failure to develop a more intrinsically motivated research ethics culture (despite having research ethics guidelines) is caused by the same forces that prevent research from being driven by the quest for knowledge. Professions (e.g., medicine, nursing, law, engineering) and some disciplines (e.g., anthropology, sociology) have developed their own statements about their values, while, in comparison, researchers have seen research ethics developed externally, mostly by funding agencies and state departments, potentially explainable by the fact that research is not considered a profession (in the narrow sense of the term). Empowering researchers to develop their own ethics beyond the regulatory would not solve everything, but could perhaps allow for the development of a deeper, more intrinsic motivation to have ethics flourish and reflect what researchers want to project and commit to. This ethics could be developed in greater collaboration with research participants and funding agencies but would have the merit of emphasizing where responsibilities lie—since researchers need to take ownership of their actions and their implications—and of possibly giving greater credence to the genuinely open-ended and reflexive aspect of ethics while avoiding reduction to guidelines, a codes, or the like. Many contributions in this book point to this more quotidian and reflexive ethical life for research and researchers (Chapters 8, 9, 14, and 15). They also reflect promising ways of engaging with mid-level ethics in research in the interstice between high-level guidance provided by research ethics guidelines and actual experienced situations.

I recognize the somewhat sweeping nature of the claims I have made in this commentary but hope they can instill reflection upon problematic foundational aspects of research ethics, so markedly apparent in the context of research with people with cognitive impairments. In my opinion, research ethics should critically reflect on whether research promotes a *quality* of human development within in its own activities and interactions with research participants.

## Acknowledgments

The writing of this chapter was supported by a career award from the Fonds de recherche du Québec—Santé (FRQ-S). Thanks to Wren Boehlen for helpful feedback on a previous version of this manuscript, and to Ariel Cascio for the same reason and for her leadership in the development of this volume.

## References


Beagan, B. and McDonald, M. (2005). "Evidence-Based Practice of Research Ethics Review?" *Health Law Review*, 13/2–3: 62–68.

Deslauriers, C., Bell, E., Palmour, N., Pike, B., Doyon, J., and Racine, E. (2010). "Perspectives of Canadian Researchers on Ethics Review of Neuroimaging Research." *Journal of Empirical Research on Human Research Ethics*, 5/1: 49–66.

Dresser, R. (2006). *Silent Partners: Human Subjects and Research Ethics*. New York: Oxford University Press.

Emanuel, E. J. and Grady, C. (2007). "Four Paradigms of Clinical Research and Research Oversight." *Cambridge Quarterly of Healthcare Ethics*, 16/1: 82–96.

Friesen, P., Kearns, L., Redman, B., and Caplan, A. L. (2017). "Rethinking the Belmont Report?" *American Journal of Bioethics*, 17/7: 15–21.

Gouinlock, J. (ed.) (2002). *The Moral Writings of John Dewey*. Amherst: Prometheus Books.

Mathews, D. J. H., Fins, J. J., and Racine, E. (2018). "The Therapeutic 'Mis'conception: An Examination of Its Normative Assumptions and a Call for Its Revision." *Cambridge Quarterly of Healthcare Ethics*, 27/1: 154–162.

McDonald, M., Cox, S., and Townsend, A. (2014). "Toward Human Research Protection That is Evidence Based and Participant Centered," in Cohen, I. G. and Fernandez Lynch, H. (eds.) *Human Subjects Research Regulation: Perspectives on the Future*. Cambridge, MA: MIT Press, pp. 113–126.

Trudel, P. and Jean, M. S. (2010). *La malréglementation: une éthique de la recherche est-elle possible et à quelles conditions?* Montréal: Les Presses de l'Université de Montréal.

van den Hoonaard, W. C. and Hamilton, A. (eds.) (2016). *The Ethics Rupture: Exploring Alternatives to Formal Research-Ethics Review*. Toronto: University of Toronto Press.

# 30

# Vulnerability, Empowerment, and Dissent

## The Importance of Saying No: Commentary on All Chapters

*M. Ariel Cascio*

The chapters in this volume showcase important theories in ethics and important empirical research that addresses the issue of research participation for persons who might be considered vulnerable (by researchers, research ethics committees, or gatekeepers) by virtue of something to do with cognition—be it intellectual disability, mild cognitive impairment, autism, mental illness, or otherwise. For the purposes of this commentary, I consider vulnerability in a relational and contextual framework (Mackenzie and Stoljar, 2000; Racine et al., 2017). Everyone is potentially vulnerable, but that vulnerability has meaning only within relationships and context; people are vulnerable *to* something, *by virtue of* something, and/or *with respect to* someone else. Vulnerability is closely linked to empowerment and dissent. One of the central concerns of research ethics is that people might be vulnerable to "coercion or undue influence" (Department of Health and Human Services, 2009) making them more likely to agree to participate in research they do not want to do. Saying yes more easily than no is also a particular concern for some participants with cognitive differences and disabilities, especially those who have been institutionalized (Harris, 2003). As I will explain, empowering people to participate in research is an important concern and motivator for this volume. My point in this commentary is to highlight the implicit complement to this point—empowering people to refuse to participate in research is an important part of managing vulnerability in research.

The participants described in these chapters have often been labelled vulnerable for a number of reasons linked to the mind, brain, or nervous system. As many contributors have noted, often researchers or research ethics boards conclude that people with cognitive disabilities, mental illness, or other forms of neurodivergence should be protected by being excluded from research. Sometimes this conclusion comes from rather vague presumptions about competence, as ethics boards presume participants with autism (Chapter 7) or traumatic brain injury (Chapter 6) may not be capable of consenting. Sometimes it comes from specific concerns, for example those about state of mind, attention, comprehension, and risk appreciation (Chapter 13) participants; theory of mind, executive function, and communication (Chapter 5); or significant communication differences between participants and researchers (Chapters 8 and 12). Both theoretical and empirical work in this volume reveals problems with these assumptions.

Many authors also address broader societal concerns about research inclusion and justice, arguing that excluding people with cognitive disabilities, mental illness, or other forms of neurodivergence from research can reproduce other forms of social exclusion and perpetuate marginalization. Excluding people from research might exclude them from benefitting directly from research, and excluding certain types of people from research might exclude their communities from benefitting indirectly from the findings. Participating in research is also a way in which people represent their needs and interests, and so exclusion from research can mean exclusion from representation, also understood as an important component of justice (Fraser and Honneth, 2003).

Despite the many values of research participation, it is not the right choice for all people all the time. Potential participants should be empowered to say yes or no to a study. Participation may be a bad choice owing to lack of competence to consent and absence of a proxy (Chapter 2); lack of diligence by guardians giving proxy consent (Chapter 2); experiencing an acute symptom of psychosis (Chapter 14); and conflicts between researchers and participants (Chapter 5). The latter takes on a particular tone in the context of autism research, my own area of expertise. Many adults on the autism spectrum have had bad experiences with research, such as not having been afforded much opportunity to assent or dissent as children (Chapter 7). Many researchers aim towards curing, preventing, or eliminating autism, whereas many autistic people do not share these goals (Chapter 5). Potential participants may refuse to participate for these reasons. Furthermore, people may simply not be interested, itself a sufficient and important reason to decline.

Respecting dissent is an ethical obligation, but researchers may see refusal as a challenge or a sign of unsuccessful recruitment. Researchers encounter much pressure to recruit, some from research design and some from institutional pressures to graduate, secure jobs, and obtain funding. Much ink has been spilled (perhaps ironically) about publish or perish. Despite these pressures, others have suggested that perfect or high success rates in recruitment might be suspect. Cameron and Murphy (2007) explain, "For consent to be working there must be evidence that potential participants choose not to take part. [ . . . ] In a field where research participants are recognized as a vulnerable group, documenting nonparticipant rates is vital. Recording nonparticipation rates is one way of checking whether compliance is occurring through the power relationship which inevitably exists in a research project." In this way, a potential participants' refusal can be read as a success—evidence that the consent process works—and a publishable one at that. It is noteworthy that in this volume, many detailed refusals to participate are in success chapters (Chapters 12 and 15). These chapters also not only address the disappointment, stress, and worry researchers (Chapter 15) or family members (Chapter 12) may experience as a result of such refusal, acknowledging these reactions, but also the necessity to move past them.

While research ethics literature tells researchers to be mindful of participants' vulnerability and exhorts researchers to act with care, it provides few concrete details about everyday interactions. How do you tell if someone does not want to participate, especially if they communicate differently than you do? What tone and language can you use to be persuasive and supportive, but not coercive, in the face of potential participant discomfort or disinterest? How do you talk to a parent who is disappointed their child cannot participate? In short, how do you create a space to say no? The authors in this volume have given future researchers something concrete to draw from, be it adapted ethics training (Chapter 17), accessible recruitment and other materials (Chapter 16), ethnographic attention to capacity (Chapter 14), the use of alternative and augmentative communication (Chapter 12), and so on.

In short, including people with cognitive differences in research (especially research which interests them and affects their daily lives) is an important goal for which researchers studying cognitive disability, mental illness, and neurodiversity should strive. However, researchers should also not see a refusal to participate as inherently a failure of inclusion. Ethical, inclusive research also empowers potential participants to decline and creating a space for saying no should also be seen as a success.

## References

Cameron, L. and Murphy, J. (2007). "Obtaining Consent to Participate in Research: The Issues Involved in Including People With a Range of Learning and Communication Disabilities." *British Journal of Learning Disabilities*, 35/2: 113–120.

Department of Health and Human Services (2009). "Protection of Human Subjects Title 45 Code of Federal Regulations Part 46," https://www.hhs.gov/ohrp/regulations-and-policy/regulations/45-cfr-46/index.html (accessed March 11, 2019).

Fraser, N. and Honneth, A. (2003). *Redistribution Or Recognition?: A Political–Philosophical Exchange*. London: Verso.

Harris, J. (2003). "Time to Make up Your Mind: Why Choosing is Difficult." *British Journal of Learning Disabilities*, 31/1: 3–8.

Mackenzie, C. and Stoljar, N. (2000). *Relational Autonomy: Feminist Perspectives on Automony, Agency, and the Social Self*. Oxford: Oxford University Press.

Racine, E., Aspler, J., Forlini, C., and Chandler, J. A. (2017). "Contextualized Autonomy and Liberalism: Broadening the Lenses on Complementary and Alternative Medicines in Preclinical Alzheimer's Disease." *Kennedy Institute of Ethics Journal*, 27/1: 1–41.

# Index

*For the benefit of digital users, indexed terms that span two pages (e.g., 52–53) may, on occasion, appear on only one of those pages.*

Notes
Abbreviations used

| | |
|---|---|
| ASD | autism spectrum disorder |
| FASD | fetal alcohol spectrum disorder |
| IDD | intellectual and developmental disabilities |
| ID | intellectual disability |
| MCI | mild cognitive impairment |
| MID | mild intellectual disability |